Psychiatry

for Primary Care

Physicians

Second Edition

Edited by
Larry S. Goldman, MD
University of Chicago

Thomas N. Wise, MD
Inova Health Systems, Fairfax, Virginia
Georgetown University School of Medicine
Johns Hopkins School of Medicine

David S. Brody, MD
Drexel University College of Medicine

AMA *press*

AMA Press

Vice President, Business Products: Anthony J. Frankos
Publisher: Michael Desposito
Senior Acquisitions Editor: Barry Bowlus
Director, Production & Manufacturing: Jean Roberts
Director, Marketing: J. D. Kinney
Marketing Manager: Reg Schmidt
Director, Sales: Amy Roberts
Developmental Editor: Jane Piro
Copyeditor: Mary Kay Kozyra
Senior Production Coordinator: Boon Ai Tan
Senior Print Coordinator: Ronnie Summers

Internet address: www.ama-assn.org

Additional copies of this publication may be ordered by calling 800 621-8335. Mention product number OP100203.

ISBN 1-57947-410-1

Library of Congress Cataloging-in-Publication Data

Psychiatry for primary care physicians / edited by Larry S. Goldman,
Thomas N. Wise, David S. Brody. — 2nd ed.
    p. ; cm.
Includes bibliographical references and index.
  ISBN 1-57947-410-1
  1. Psychiatry 2. Primary care (Medicine). 3. Mental
illness — Diagnosis. 4. Mental illness — Treatment.
  [DNLM: 1. Mental Disorders — diagnosis. 1. Mental Disorders — therapy
3. Primary Health Care.   . WM 141 P9745 2004]   I. Goldman, Larry S. II.
Wise, Thomas N. III. Brody, David S., 1947-
  RC454.4.P7912 2004
  616.89—dc22

                                                    2003017178

The authors, editors, and publisher of this work have checked with sources believed to be reliable in their efforts to confirm the accuracy and completeness of the information presented herein and that the information is in accordance with the standard practices accepted at the time of publication. However, neither the authors, editors, and publisher, nor any party involved in the creation and publication of this work, warrant that the information is in every respect accurate and complete, and they are not responsible for any errors or omissions or for any consequences from application of the information in this book.

In light of ongoing research and changes in clinical experience and in government regulations, readers are encouraged to confirm the information contained herein with additional sources, in particular as it pertains to drug dosage and usage. Readers are urged to check the package insert for each drug they plan to administer for any change in indications and dosage and for additional warnings and precautions, especially for new or infrequently used drugs.

BP70:03-P-081:11/03

CONTENTS

INTRODUCTION

Primary care physicians play a key role in the identification and management of mental health disorders. More patients with mental health disorders will seek help from their primary care physicians than from a mental health specialist. As a result, almost 40% of patients seen in the primary care setting will experience a significant mental health problem. It is therefore critically important that primary care physicians be able to recognize and diagnose common mental health disorders and activate patients to seek and adhere to treatment for these problems. As the literature continues to document the impact of mental health problems on the development and outcomes of a variety of medical diseases, such as coronary artery disease, diabetes mellitus, and asthma, medical subspecialists will also need to develop and apply these skills.

In recent years, primary care physicians have become increasingly involved in the management of mental health disorders. Both the number of primary care visits for mental health disorders and the number of psychotropic prescriptions written by primary care physicians have increased dramatically over the past 10 years. Currently, primary care physicians write more than 70% of the selective serotonin reuptake inhibitor prescriptions in the United States. These trends inspired us to develop the first edition of this book 5 years ago and, if anything, they are more prominent today.

There is still tremendous pressure on primary care physicians to assess and manage psychiatric disorders themselves rather than to refer to specialists. Some of the pressure comes from patients, who want help from someone they know and trust; at times, they may also wish to avoid the stigmatization they associate with receiving psychiatric care. Other pressures come from the health care system itself, which may place logistical or financial barriers in the way of psychiatric care. Timely, competent psychiatric consultations and treatment services are far from uniformly available for many primary care physicians' use. Although managed care organizations in some parts of the country have reduced disincentives to make specialty referrals, the psychiatric care may itself still be tightly managed; the patient may have mental health benefits that are limited in scope, duration, or monetary total; or the care may be "carved out" to a mental health entity unconnected to the patient's primary health care system.

Despite the continuing pressures, the ease by which primary care physicians can acquire appropriate skills and current information to effectively render such care themselves remains far too low. Primary care training programs and medical organizations have increased their offerings of psychiatric information, but with infrequent exceptions these are inadequate for the quantity and scope of psychiatric problems seen in primary care settings. In the meantime, much of the research in psychiatry that was moving apace 5 years ago has continued to generate new psychopathological information and therapeutic advances. For these reasons, we felt that a second edition of this book was worthwhile.

ABOUT THIS EDITION

We have made a few important changes in this edition. First, we have included two chapters on some of the "basic science" of psychiatry, namely, development and psychological frameworks for understanding behavior. We feel these chapters will allow physicians to have a greater depth of understanding of many clinical phenomena they see daily, and they may also play an important role for medical student readers who are trying to master this material in their preclinical years. We have also added a chapter on childhood psychiatric disorders for those primary care physicians who see children and adolescents, and we have expanded what was only a section of one chapter in the first edition into a separate chapter in this edition to better highlight the handling of office-based psychiatric emergencies. The increased appreciation of the special mental health needs of women and of the elderly—and new findings in these areas—have led us to turn both of these topics into separate chapters for each group. Finally, we have included a chapter summarizing a variety of resources that can help busy primary care practitioners enhance the psychiatric care that they provide.

We have retained the heart of the book, namely the chapters covering evaluation and management of various psychiatric disorders. As before, many of these have been written jointly by a primary care physician and a psychiatrist. These chapters reflect updates in nomenclature, assessment, outcomes, pathophysiology, comorbidity, and therapeutics since the first edition. Finally, we have retained the two chapters on somatic and psychological treatments, and there is much new information in both of these.

As before, we have striven to make the information in this book not only timely but also practical and easy to access. We have again asked the authors to make liberal use of bullets, tables, diagrams, and clinical vignettes to make the material understandable and useful. We have supplied additional reading suggestions for each chapter for those readers who wish to learn more about particular topics, and we have continued to omit footnotes and in-text citations to improve the ease of reading. We have tried to cover the most important psychiatric material that comes up in the practices of family physicians, internists, and obstetrician-gynecologists, and we also believe this book can also play an important role in undergraduate and graduate medical education.

We hope that these goals have been met successfully.

Larry S. Goldman, MD
Chicago, Illinois

Thomas N. Wise, MD
Falls Church, Virginia

David S. Brody, MD
Philadelphia, Pennsylvania

ABOUT THE EDITORS

Larry S. Goldman, MD

Dr Goldman graduated from the University of Illinois School of Medicine in 1978. His residency in general psychiatry and a fellowship in consultation-liaison psychiatry at the University of Chicago Hospitals followed. He taught full-time at the University of Illinois from 1985 to 1988 and at the University of Chicago from 1988 to 1994. From 1995 to 1999, Dr Goldman served as the Director of the Department of Mental Health for the American Medical Association. He is currently Professor of Psychiatry and Director of Adult Psychiatry at the University of Chicago. He is a diplomate of the American Board of Psychiatry and Neurology and a fellow of the American Psychiatric Association.

Thomas N. Wise, MD

Dr Wise is Medical Director of Behavioral Services at the Inova Health Systems in Fairfax, Virginia. He is also Professor and Vice Chair of the Department of Psychiatry at Georgetown University School of Medicine as well as Associate Professor of Psychiatry at The Johns Hopkins School of Medicine. Dr Wise is editor in chief of *Psychosomatics, The Journal of Consultation and Liaison Psychiatry*. A native of Reno, Nevada, Dr Wise graduated from Dartmouth College and Duke University School of Medicine.

David S. Brody, MD

Dr David Brody is a graduate of Temple University School of Medicine. He completed an Internal Medicine residency program at University Hospitals in Cleveland and was a Robert Wood Johnson Foundation Clinical Scholar at Case Western Reserve University School of Medicine. He has served as the Director of the Division of General Internal Medicine at Temple University School of Medicine and the MCP Hahnemann School of Medicine. He has also been the Chairman of Medicine at the Mercy Catholic Medical Center. Currently Dr Brody is a Professor of Medicine and Director of Quality Improvement at the Drexel University School of Medicine. He is a diplomate of the American Board of Internal Medicine.

CONTRIBUTORS

Michael Ankrom, MD
Assistant Professor of Geriatrics and
    Gerontology
The Johns Hopkins Hospital
Baltimore, MD

Jeffrey I. Bennett, MD
Assistant Professor of Psychiatry
Southern Illinois University
Springfield, IL

George R. Bergus, MD
Associate Professor and Co-Director
Department of Family Practice/
    Psychiatry Residency
University of Iowa
Iowa City, IA

David S. Brody, MD
Professor of Medicine
Director, Quality Improvement
Drexel University School of Medicine
Philadelphia, PA

Ravi T. Chandran, MD
Pulmonary Critical Care and Sleep Associates
Seneca, SC

K.N. Roy Chengappa, MD
Associate Professor of Psychiatry
University of Pittsburgh School of Medicine
Pittsburgh, PA

Greg Clary, MD
Assistant Clinical Professor
Director of Clinical Services
Duke University
Durham, NC

Steven Cole, MD
Professor of Psychiatry
Head, Division of Medical and Geriatric
    Psychiatry
Stony Brook Health Sciences Center
Stony Brook, NY

Edwin Cook, MD
Professor of Psychiatry
University of Chicago
Chicago, IL

Bezalel Dantz, MD
Assistant Professor of Internal Medicine
    and Psychiatry
University of Chicago
Chicago, IL

Stuart J. Eisendrath, MD
Professor of Clinical Psychiatry
Director of Clinical Services
Langley Porter Psychiatric Hospital and Clinics
University of California, San Francisco
San Francisco, CA

Brenda Erickson, MD
Durango, CO

Mitchell D. Feldman, MD, MPhil
Associate Professor of Medicine
Director, Faculty Development Program
Division of General Internal Medicine
University of California, San Francisco
San Francisco, CA

Sanford Finkel, MD
Clinical Professor of Psychiatry
University of Chicago
Chicago, IL
Medical Director
Council for the Jewish Elderly
Chicago, IL

Charles V. Ford, MD
Professor of Psychiatry
Neuropsychiatry Clinic
University of Alabama at Birmingham
Birmingham, AL

Jackie Gollan, PhD
Assistant Professor of Psychiatry
University of Chicago
Chicago, IL

Larry S. Goldman, MD
Professor of Psychiatry
Director of Adult Psychiatry
University of Chicago
Chicago, IL

Marjorie Greenfield, MD
Associate Professor of Obstetrics and
    Gynecology
Case Western Reserve University School of
    Medicine
Cleveland, OH

Steven R. Hahn, MD
Professor of Clinical Medicine and
    Instructor in Psychiatry
Albert Einstein College of Medicine
Director, Primary Care Internal Medicine
    Residency Program
Albert Einstein College of Medicine at Jacobi
    Medical Center
Bronx, NY

Bharat Jain, MD
Director
Westmoreland Sleep Disorders Center
Greensburg, PA
Director
Frick Hospital Sleep Disorders Center
Mt Pleasant, PA

Roger G. Kathol, MD
Adjunct Professor, Departments of Internal
    Medicine and Psychiatry
University of Minnesota
Minneapolis, MN

K. Ranga Krishnan, MD
Professor and Chairman,
Department of Psychiatry and Behavioral
    Sciences
Duke University
Durham, NC

Kurt Kroenke, MD
Professor of Medicine
School of Medicine
Indiana University
Indianapolis, IN
Senior Research Scientist and Director of
    Fellowship Training
Regenstrief Institute for Health Care
Indianapolis, IN

Hochang Benjamin Lee, MD
Assistant Professor
Neuropsychiatry and Memory Group
The Johns Hopkins Hospital
Baltimore, MD

Bennett Leventhal, MD
Professor of Psychiatry
Chief, Child Psychiatry
University of Chicago
Chicago, IL

David C. Lewis, MD
Professor of Medicine and Community
    Health
Donald G. Millar Professor of Alcohol and
    Addiction Studies
Brown University
Providence, RI

Mack Lipkin Jr, MD
Professor of Clinical Medicine
Director, Primary Care Internal Medicine
    Residency Program
New York University Medical Center/
    Bellevue Hospital
New York, NY

Constantine G. Lyketsos, MD, MHS
Academic Director
The Copper Ridge Institute
Professor of Psychiatry and Behavioral
    Sciences
*The Johns Hopkins University School of
    Medicine*
Director, Inpatient Neuropsychiatry and
    The Johns Hopkins Hospital
The Johns Hopkins Hospital
Baltimore, MD

Prakash S. Masand, MD
Clinical Professor of Psychiatry
Director, Program for Continuing Medical
    Education
Director, Psychopharmacology
    Consultation Program
Duke University
Durham, NC

Clifton K. Meador, MD
Executive Director
Meharry-Vanderbilt Alliance
Chief Medical Officer
St Thomas Hospital
Nashville, TN

Norman S. Miller, MD
Professor of Psychiatry
Director of Addiction Medicine
Michigan State University
East Lansing, MI

Kenneth N. Panitch, MD
Department of Family Medicine
Jefferson Medical Care
Cherry Hill, NJ

Alan Ravitz, MD
Associate Professor of Psychiatry
Director, Inpatient Child Psychiatry
University of Chicago
Chicago, IL

Phillip R. Reeves, MD
Psychiatry Resident
Department of Psychiatry and Human
    Behavior
Jefferson Medical College and Hospital
Philadelphia, PA

Miriam B. Rosenthal, MD
Associate Professor Emerita of Psychiatry
    and Obstetrics and Gynecology
*Case Western Reserve University School of
    Medicine*
University Hospitals of Cleveland
Cleveland, OH

Michael J. Roy, MD, MPH
LTC, MC, US Army
Director, Division of Military Internal
    Medicine
Associate Professor of Medicine
*Uniformed Services University of the Health
    Sciences*
Bethesda, MD

R. Taylor Segraves, MD, PhD
Chairman, Department of Psychiatry
The Metro Health Medical Center
Professor of Psychiatry
Case Western Reserve University
Cleveland, OH

Robert M. Swift, MD, PhD
Associate Chief of Staff,
    Research and Education
VA Medical Center
Providence, RI

Troy L. Thompson II, MD
Professor of Psychiatry and Human
    Behavior
Jefferson Medical College and Hospital
Philadelphia, PA

Thomas M. Wise, MD
Medical Director of Behavioral Sciences
Inova Health Systems
Fairfax, VA
Vice Chair, Department of Psychiatry
Georgetown University School of Medicine
Associate Professor of Psychiatry
The Johns Hopkins School of Medicine
Washington, DC

Joel Yager, MD
Professor, Vice Chair for Education
Department of Psychiatry
University of New Mexico
Albuquerque, NM

William R. Yates, MD
Professor and Chair, Department of
  Psychiatry
University of Oklahoma College of Medicine
Tulsa, OK

Chapter 1

Psychological Frameworks in Health and Illness

Jackie Gollan, PhD
Larry S. Goldman, MD

WHAT IS PSYCHIATRY?

Psychiatry is a confusing discipline for medical students, residents, and primary care physicians. There are two main reasons for this confusion. First, there is the implicit problem of mind vs body. These two terms—*mind* and *body*—denote the contrast between a subjective experience of thought and feeling (mind) in opposition to the brain, an objective organ of the body. For the physician the most salient difference between mind and body is the method of investigation. Investigation of mindful activities includes observations and questions that elucidate what the individual is thinking and how that individual feels. The brain and nervous system are studied by physical examination and laboratory and imaging studies.

The second major factor complicating psychiatry is the existence of many factions that appear to argue with one another about what the ultimate "truth" (ie, cause of mental phenomena) is and how to approach a patient with pathologic feeling states, thoughts, or behaviors. Thus, is psychiatry more of a biological specialty or a derivative of psychology and its various theories of the mind? The obvious answer is that both approaches are necessary and complement each other. This chapter provides a review of several major psychological theories that help structure the psychosocial problems that affect patients. These theories allow the physician—via empathic listening—to understand the patient. Thus, the psychodynamic approach relies on a theory that focuses on an individual's life story: in the context of conscious and unconscious themes and conflicts, symptoms arise. The cognitive-behavioral approach is based on learning theory and elucidates how individuals develop automatic, often counterproductive, thoughts and attitudes that lead to pervasive depression or anxiety or to dysfunctional behaviors. The final approach expands the focus from the individual patient to a broader social system, with particular emphasis on the family and how norms, boundaries, and communications occur.

Few would argue that every aspect of human behavior, including feelings and thoughts, is ultimately a product of chemical processes in the brain. In the future, it will likely be possible to pinpoint the exact localization and set of neurochemical events that are involved when an individual thinks about the chicken crossing the road. Although this will be scientifically gratifying (whether it will be of clinical utility or emotionally satisfying is another matter, of course), it is simply impossible at this time to understand most complex behavioral phenomena in such terms. As a result, several other conceptual frameworks have been proposed.

The models in common use today have been retained not because they represent a set of scientifically validated truths but because they have proved helpful in "explaining" and working with many day-to-day psychological experiences, both normal and pathological. Complex phenomena such as human feelings, thoughts, and behavior can often be understood by any of a number of theoretical frameworks. The most common paradigms also form the theoretical basis for several of the most important types of psychotherapy used in clinical practice. Although the frameworks themselves are heuristically useful, the specific therapies that have emerged from them have in many cases been empirically validated as efficacious treatments for specific psychiatric disorders.

The psychodynamic model is the framework that has been used for the longest time in psychiatry, and even in general clinical medicine. This model is derived from more than 100 years of psychoanalytic theory and practice. Its former hegemony in medicine was eliminated by the development of behavioral and cognitive approaches to understanding human behavior. This represents a shift from the emphasis on unconscious mental states found in psychodynamic frameworks to emphases on overt behavior and conscious thought processes. The main advantage of this paradigmatic shift from the abstract to the concrete has proved to decrease the focus on inferential (and possibly less reliable) processes to observable and reliable phenomena. A third framework, the systems approach, relies on theoretical concepts from both of the other frameworks, with emphasis on examining individual behavior as representative of the history, values, beliefs, and expectations of a particular social group. However, the systems approach is distinct, because it focuses on how these behaviors play out within groups of individuals (a couple, a family, a hospital ward, etc) rather than within a single individual. The systems approach also emphasizes communication and transactional aspects among those individuals in the system.

This chapter provides a broad overview of each of these three frameworks. The primary concepts and terms are explained and their translation into clinical operations is made explicit. These translations are illustrated using clinical examples of these concepts being used in each framework. The differences between these models in clinical care are also compared.

PSYCHODYNAMIC THEORY AND PRACTICE

Sigmund Freud is generally considered to be the father of psychoanalysis, which was the progenitor framework for psychodynamic thought. Freud's ideas borrowed heavily from Charcot, Janet, and others, but he built extensively on their earlier concepts. These men were in large part struggling to understand patients with neurological symptoms who proved not to have organic neurological disease. At the end of the 19th century, Freud and Joseph Breuer developed a psychological explanation for some of these phenomena. Freud then began to generalize his ideas to other parts of everyday life and to neurotic (internal conflict) symptom formation. He made it clear that severe mental illnesses such as schizophrenia were organic in etiology. Unfortunately, the irrational exuberance of some of Freud's disciples led to attempts to understand and treat almost any mental illness (and even some physical ones) with psychoanalysis.

Freud and the early analysts were largely concerned with impulses and internal mental processes at the oedipal level of development (see below). However, subsequent theorists emphasized mental states earlier in development (Melanie Klein, Donald Winnicott, and others); the internal attempts to harness and channel impulses (ego psychologists such as Anna Freud); and the real-world, external interpersonal results of these internal processes (Harry Stack Sullivan, Karen Horney, and others). A more recent development (originated by Heinz Kohut and others) is self-psychology, which focuses on the effects of deficient parental empathy in development.

Psychodynamic thinking rests on two models of the mind, the topographic and the structural. The former emphasizes the role of unconscious processes in thoughts, feelings, and behaviors. The latter posits the existence of specific mental structures whose interactions determine an individual's thinking, feeling, and actions.

Topographic Model

The *topographic model* of the mind (Figure 1-1) postulates that certain mental events occur out of conscious awareness and that even these events can have important influences on conscious, volitional behavior. Desires and feelings originating in the unconscious (primary process thinking) can intrude on our putatively rational ways of analyzing and responding to the world (secondary process thinking). For example, we are far more likely to "forget" an appointment with a dentist than a date with someone to whom we are attracted. The implication of this model is that much of what we do is not as logical as we like to think. The therapeutic implication is that helping patients gain access to the unconscious motivations and feelings of which they are unaware may ameliorate some of their problems.

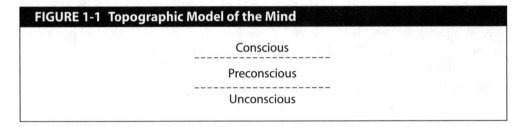

FIGURE 1-1 Topographic Model of the Mind

Structural Model

The *structural model* (Figure 1-2) postulates a dynamic interplay among three components of the mind. It is the repository of drives, instincts, and impulses, both conscious and unconscious. The id is the childlike part of each person that insists on doing what it wants when it wants regardless of the consequences. The *superego* is the conscience or moral engine that incorporates parental and societal values about proper behavior; it also includes the ideal mental model of what we aspire to be. Inadequate development of the superego leads to antisocial behavior and lack of guilt for transgressions. Some patients seem to have overdeveloped superegos and lead constricted lives devoid of pleasure because they see any enjoyment as wrong or sinful. The *ego* is the adjudicating part of the mind that acts to balance the demands of reality, the wishes of the id, and the restrictions imposed by the superego. An important part of the ego is the so-called ego ideal, which embodies the hoped-for appearance, values, and aspirations of a person. A neurosis

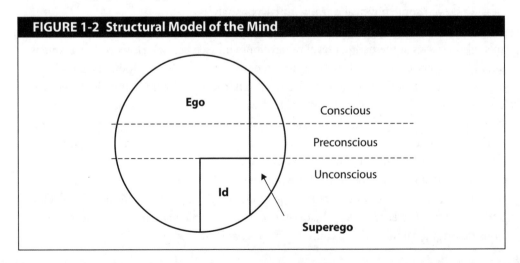

FIGURE 1-2 Structural Model of the Mind

results from an imbalance among these elements or from a maladaptive way of resolving a conflict among them.

Just as there is a sequence of developmental steps in childhood affecting motor skills, language, and cognitive processing, psychodynamic theory postulates a separate line of development involving these mental structures. A newborn is seen as little more than an unregulated id. Over the first 6 years or so of life there is gradual development of the ego to help the child conform to the demands of the environment and parental expectations. A large part of superego development is thought to be the incorporation of parental attitudes and values. Certain key steps in this process that correspond to various environmental demands and the child's ways of dealing with them have been described. It is thought that people who find it difficult to master these steps may be especially prone to struggle with unresolved issues associated with these steps later in life. A return to using tools from an earlier stage of development in the face of stress is referred to as *regression*. These developmental issues are covered in greater detail in Chapter 2.

The *oral* stage of development corresponds to early infant issues of the taking of things into the mouth: the breast, food, and other objects. Because it is a time of relative dependency and passivity, those who fail to master it are thought to be inclined to excessive reliance on other people or even inanimate objects (such as food or drugs) for emotional succor later in life. The *anal* stage corresponds to the period of toilet training, when issues of cleanliness, order, control, and submission may come to the fore. People who have troubles during this time are thought to be prone to develop personalities characterized by emotional and financial miserliness as well as excessive preoccupation with rules, order, and morality. The *oedipal* stage of development is concerned with romantic and erotic feelings toward one's parents and the handling of feelings of jealousy by virtue of the parents' positive feelings toward each other that are competing with the child's feelings. Unresolved issues during this stage of development are proposed to interfere with the achievement of successful intimate, romantic relationships later in life.

Another key tenet of psychodynamic thinking is that people who are particularly unhappy in their current lives are especially prone to seek out people who resemble key figures from earlier in their lives, often parental figures. This may be an attempt to "replay" a particularly gratifying relationship, or it may be an attempt to recreate a problematic one in order to master the traumatic elements of it. At times, the appraisal of a person in one's life may be colored by these past relationships, and the person may be treated as if he or she were the figure from the past. This tendency to bring past figures into the present is referred to as *transference*. This may be seen in medical settings when certain patients selectively focus on aspects of their doctor and regard him or her as more of a caregiver or nurturer, stern authority figure, sadistic harm-inflictor, or potential romantic partner than is realistic or appropriate. The physician is, of course, not exempt from such feelings and may develop distorted appraisals about particular patients; this is referred to as *countertransference*.

Psychoanalysis and Psychodynamic Psychotherapy

A psychodynamic model is the basis for psychoanalysis and psychodynamic psychotherapy (also called insight-oriented psychotherapy). All of these treatments seek to help the patient understand that the basis of his or her problems stems from unconscious conflicts and unresolved issues from earlier in life. The treatment acts by highlighting the patient's maladaptive patterns, identifying the unconscious aspects, and consciously setting about doing things differently (sometimes by also reconstructing and working through the origins of these issues from earlier in life). The patient-therapist relationship is considered a critical element in the patient's progress, and the nature of this relationship is often an important focus of the therapy. *Interpersonal psychotherapy* is a time-limited, focused psychotherapy that draws on psychodynamic theory but tends to focus largely on current interpersonal relationships. It has been found empirically to be therapeutic for some types of depression and certain other conditions. *Brief focal psychotherapy* is another time-limited form of psychotherapy based on psychodynamic principles whereby acute symptom formation is felt to be due to an internal psychic conflict. Examples of possible indications include conversion disorder, certain posttraumatic states, pathological bereavement, or acute inhibitions (eg, writer's block).

In terms of treatment strategies, psychodynamic psychotherapy focuses on the unconscious processes underlying behaviors and conscious thoughts, rather than on the thoughts themselves. The length of treatment varies according to the clinical problems, but most treatment requires intensive participation spanning years. Techniques range from free-association about early childhood experiences, interpretation of defenses, focus on understanding transference reactions, and brief interventions targeted at specific issues. In general, these approaches require a high level of understanding on the part of the patient, high ego strength, and a willingness to experience intense emotions.

Defense Mechanisms

Defense mechanisms are mental operations that are generally carried out automatically (ie, unconsciously) to help people deal with unpleasant thoughts or feelings. Many defense mechanisms have been described, and they are used frequently, even by people without psychopathology. Each person uses his or her own characteristic or typical set of defense mechanisms, although at times other mechanisms may be employed. Defense mechanisms often fall into one of the four categories listed in Table 1-1; these groupings often reflect overall levels of psychological well-being or functioning. Some empirical evidence supports the idea that patients who tend to use several defense mechanisms from a particular cluster generally function at around that level. These levels are not fixed; patients may employ higher-level defenses as they recover from an acute illness, mature with aging, or undergo changes in psychotherapy.

It is beyond the scope of this chapter to describe and illustrate all of the defense mechanisms in detail. However, the following examples highlight common mechanisms and how they may be expressed in medical situations.

Case Vignettes

Splitting.   A patient is admitted to the hospital for treatment of subacute bacterial endocarditis. She is cooperative for a few days but soon begins to be very demanding and belittling of the nursing staff. At the same time, she remains very cordial and cooperative with the physician caring for her. The nurses angrily tell the doctor to set limits on the patient and consider discharging her, even though she is not stable. The doctor, failing to understand why the nurses are so displeased with this patient, complains to the nursing supervisor about their lack of helpfulness on the case.   *(continued on page 8)*

Table 1-1 Defense Mechanisms

Mechanism	Description
Psychotic	
Delusions	Fixed beliefs contrary to reality not shared by others
Hallucinations	Sensory experiences without external stimulus provoking them
Schizoid fantasy	Excessive preoccupation with inner fantasy world instead of reality
Immature	
Projection	Attributing one's feelings or beliefs to someone else
Projective identification	Projection along with acting in a manner to induce behavior in the other person that confirms the projection
Introjection	Taking on attributes of another that are highly dissonant with oneself
Idealization	Seeing another in an unrealistically positive way
Splitting	Seeing others unrealistically as either with no flaws ("all good") or far more flaws than they actually possess ("all bad")
Denial	Thinking and acting as if something true is not; if belief is strong enough and reality sufficiently contradictory, denial may be psychotic in nature
Acting out	Dealing with unwanted feelings by maladaptive behaviors
Neurotic	
Intellectualization	Dealing with unwanted feelings by excessive focus on the intellectual or rational aspects of a situation
Reaction formation	Acting and feeling in a manner opposite to one's actual feelings
Rationalization	Offering a plausible, superficial explanation that hides a deeper, more meaningful one
Displacement	Transferring one's feelings about someone or something to another person or situation
Identification	Adopting the characteristics of another person as one's own
Avoidance	Actively taking steps to evade thoughts or exposure to an unwanted situation or feeling
Repression	Unintentionally keeping information or feelings out of awareness
Dissociation	A splitting of consciousness to keep ideas, feelings separated
Magical thinking	Connecting events in a childlike, preabstract way
Conversion	Translating a psychic conflict into physical symptoms
Mature	
Suppression	Deliberately keeping information or feelings out of awareness, usually in a time-limited fashion (eg, deferring thinking about something)
Sublimation	Transforming unwanted feelings, wishes into more acceptable ones
Humor	Looking for comic aspect of an otherwise conflictual situation, feeling
Altruism	Subordinating one's feelings or needs to those of another person

Note: This list of defense mechanisms reflects some the more commonly described ones in the literature but is not meant to be exhaustive.

Projection. A very driven young businessman is on a fast track to a lucrative partnership in his firm. His physician treats the businessman's entire family, and it is clear that the man's family relationships are being seriously neglected. The patient is found to have an irregular heartbeat and a murmur. The physician outlines the potential causes, some quite serious, and suggests the patient undergo a series of investigations. The patient angrily rails against the doctor's suggestion, complaining that the doctor does not really care about him and asserting that the tests are being recommended only to increase the doctor's income.

Denial. A medically sophisticated middle-aged man with a strong family history of colon cancer begins to develop hematochezia. He reassures himself for several months that the bleeding is nothing more than hemorrhoids. Eventually, his partner convinces him to have the bleeding investigated.

Magical thinking. A family medicine resident wears a particular shirt on one of his first nights on-call in his second year. The call is uncharacteristically undemanding, and he gets to sleep much of the night. He then takes all of his subsequent calls wearing the same shirt, convinced it will bring him a quiet call night.

Reaction formation. A young man has to undergo multiple painful reconstructive procedures for a congenital deformity. After each operation and hospitalization, he gives his surgeon generous gifts that he can ill afford.

Intellectualization. A middle-aged woman is diagnosed with an unusual malignancy with a very poor prognosis for survival. She shows little emotional reaction to the news or to her subsequent tumultuous course. Nonetheless, she spends hours each day doing research in medical libraries and on the Internet, trying to learn more about all forms of cancer and basic principles of cancer biology.

Conversion. A woman with several children undergoes a tubal-ligation procedure. Her marriage dissolves soon afterward; she then marries another man who is childless and very eager to have children of his own. Her obstetrician confirms that it is all but impossible for her to become pregnant again. Over the next few weeks, she begins to develop nausea every morning, her abdomen becomes distended, and she experiences a "kicking" sensation in her abdomen from time to time.

Sublimation. In her early childhood, a physician watched her father experience a cardiac arrest and die while she stood by helplessly. She becomes an emergency medicine physician and an expert on the use of defibrillators in public places.

COGNITIVE AND BEHAVIORAL THEORIES AND THERAPIES

Over the past 30 years, there has been a significant growth in the acceptance of cognitive and behavioral (CB) theories and therapies. Historically, CB approaches were developed as alternative models to the prevailing psychodynamic approaches of the 1960s. These approaches underwent intense empirical scrutiny and are now considered to be the more popular psychological theories of the day. Moreover, application of CB models has produced a variety of effective psychosocial treatments (eg, psychological therapies with demonstrated efficacy in comparison to pill placebos or active medications). Such empirically validated approaches to child and adult-based psychotherapy are exemplified in cutting-edge therapies for depression; anxiety, eating, personality, and substance use disorders; sexual dysfunctions; insomnias; and relationship distress.

Numerous influences explain the paradigmatic shift from psychodynamic theories to behavioral and cognitive theories during the 1960s and 1970s. During this time, the focus shifted from studying unobservable and inferred psychological mechanisms to measuring visible behaviors and recording cognitive processes. The impetus for developing behavioral and cognitive approaches stemmed from the following:

- The introduction of social learning theory, which proposed that cognitive processes were crucial in the acquisition and regulation of behavior (an idea developed by Albert Bandura)
- Growing dissatisfaction with the lack of operational definitions and empirical support for psychoanalytic theories and treatments
- The introduction of research supporting the roles of social and physical environment, cognitive information processing variables, and neurophysiological factors

Finally, in terms of transporting psychological theories into the clinical setting, even as late as the mid-1980s, there were few long-term follow-up studies measuring the effectiveness of psychoanalytic therapies. Moreover, controversy regarding the length, expense, and lack of demonstrated efficacy of psychodynamic treatment prompted the development of CB treatments. Only within the past 15 years has considerable progress in the development of specific and time-limited psychotherapy protocols using cognitive-behavioral treatment (CBT) models been made. Moreover, the clinical use of these models has become standard in official treatment guidelines, such as those outlined in the American Psychiatric Association's practice guidelines for the treatment of psychiatric disorders.

CB models propose that an individual's health and illness are derived from learning via interaction with the social and physical environment. Learning, which is conceptualized as a process that alters the risks of vulnerability and resilience to illness, is considered to be essential for physical survival and psychological well-being. Compared to other models of health and illness, eg, the psychoanalytic viewpoint, CB models aim to explain how behavior is acquired and maintained (learned), rather than develop explanations of why the behavior exists. In the following sections, the basic principles of behavioral and cognitive theories and how they translate into clinical practice are described.

Behavioral Model

The behavioral model is based on the premise that new capacities are acquired through exposure to new stimuli. In some ways, this model is akin to the developmental model of the immune system: learning (eg, immunity) is obtained via exposure to new stimuli (eg, pathogens). Behavioral models propose that exposure to new environmental stimuli produces a learning history and that this learning history is continually updated via new experiences and environmental feedback. From the behavioral point of view, external reinforcement is necessary for learning to occur.

Three definitions elucidate the key factors that facilitate the process of learning:

- *Stimulus* refers to events that happen in the environment. Characteristics of the stimulus (eg, positive or negative qualities) and the significance of the stimulus for the individual influence the potential for the potency of the stimulus.
- *Response* refers to any behavior that occurs in reaction to the stimuli. Responses can be defined by motoric, emotional, cognitive, and visceral characteristics.
- *Learning/conditioning* is any change in behavior resulting from experience. Changes can include the timing, frequency, intensity, and coordination of a specific behavior. In the

context of behavioral models, learning refers to increased understanding about self, others, and the world. Learning might include forming an association that occurs automatically. The concept of learning extends beyond the process of acquiring information in academic forums (eg, training as a physician). Illustrations of generalized learning from the medical field include seeing a patient who acquires anticipatory anxiety and nausea before radiation therapy or observing a patient increase his or her compliance with complex medical regimens when encouragement and support are received.

Specific models of learning explain the method of acquiring and regulating learning. *Nonassociative learning* occurs through general experience in the absence of paired events. Examples include *habituation* (response decreases with repeated exposure to stimulus; eg, getting accustomed to painful fertility shots); *sensitization* (response increases with repeated exposure; eg, responding more quickly to emergencies after repeated exposure to previous emergencies); and *observational learning* or *modeling* (learning by observing someone else demonstrate behavior and seeing the consequences; medical training often incorporates observational learning in medical procedures, eg, a resident adopting an attending's interviewing technique that he observed because patients responded so well to it).

Classical conditioning model. Without question, the classical (respondent) conditioning model is one of the most influential theories of learning. This explanatory paradigm was developed from Pavlov's research on digestion processes among dogs. Pavlov noted that his experimental dogs salivated in response to the taste, sight, and smell of meat powder and also when meat powder was not present. After a series of paired presentations of food in the experimental room, his dogs salivated as soon as they entered the experimental room and saw the experimenter. Pavlov defined this phenomenon as "a conditioned reflex." He found that when an unconditioned stimulus (sound of a bell) was repeatedly paired with a conditioned stimulus (food) an unconditioned response (salivation) was naturally elicited. Ultimately, after a series of paired presentations of the bell and food, the unconditioned stimulus (bell) also independently produced the salivation response (now referred to as a conditioned response) (Figure 1-3). When a conditioned response consistently occurs in response to a conditioned stimulus, associative learning has occurred. It is worth noting, however, that classical or respondent conditioning does not involve the acquisition of new responses, rather the pairing of an existing response to a new stimulus. Classical conditioning explains the acquisition of involuntary reflexes (eg, increased heart rate at the sight of favorite foods) and more complex responses in humans (eg, increased heart rate when driving or speaking in public). Classical conditioning also explains the acquisition of substance addictions, specific preferences and aversions, and phobias.

Instrumental learning theory. Another essential behavioral model includes the theory of instrumental learning, also known as the operant conditioning theory of learning. Originally developed by Edward L. Thorndike, cats were placed in puzzle boxes that required them to pull on string to escape from the box and to obtain food. As the number of trials increased, the cats elicited correct responses more quickly. Thorndike, B.F. Skinner, and other researchers who became interested in the trial-and-error nature of learning suggested that connections develop between responses and stimuli as a

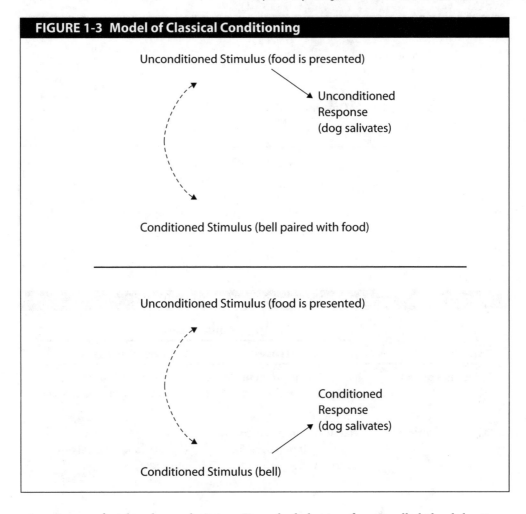

FIGURE 1-3 Model of Classical Conditioning

Unconditioned Stimulus (food is presented)

Unconditioned
Response
(dog salivates)

Conditioned Stimulus (bell paired with food)

Unconditioned Stimulus (food is presented)

Conditioned
Response
(dog salivates)

Conditioned Stimulus (bell)

consequence of trial-and-error learning. Since the behaviors functionally helped the cats obtain a goal, the phenomenon is now referred to as instrumental learning. Most behaviorists agree that behaviors are complex and emitted based on the consequences that follow. Skinner offered the following concepts to explain the acquisition and maintenance of behavior (see Figure 1-4).

- *Reinforcement* is defined as an increase of behavior (see Table 1-2).
- *Positive reinforcement* refers to an increase of behavior when something valued, positive, or necessary is presented at the same time or shortly after the occurrence of a specific behavior. Providing positive reinforcement is an effective strategy for increasing medication compliance and session attendance.
- *Punishment* refers to a reduction or suppression of a behavior by delivering an unpleasant stimulus at the same time or shortly after the behavior occurs. Punishment is the least likely to effectively eliminate behavior because punishment suppresses responses rather than actually eliminating the origin of the response. Moreover, punitive responses often generate secondary problems that may distract from learning (spanking a child is a punitive measure that often generates resentment that interferes with clear conveyance of the parent's expectation for appropriate behavior). A simple example of punishment includes a verbal reprimand from a teacher or parent.

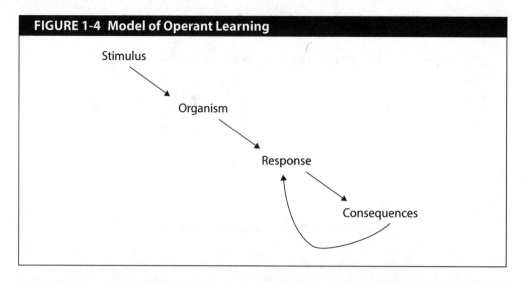

FIGURE 1-4 Model of Operant Learning

Table 1-2 Behavioral Reinforcement Procedures

Procedure	Consequence	
	Behavior Increases	**Behavior Decreases**
Stimulus Applied	Positive reinforcement (eg, good grades)	Positive punishment (eg, getting grounded for bad behavior)
Stimulus Removed	Negative reinforcement (eg, using lotion to reduce sunburn)	Negative punishment (eg, time out, removal of privileges)

- *Negative reinforcement* refers to removing an unpleasant stimulus whenever a response occurs, which strengthens the response. A simple example is turning off an alarm clock or using a pain cream to relieve sunburned skin. Avoiding performance situations that evoke anxiety is another prime example.
- *Extinction* occurs when the removal of an expected positive reinforcer results in a reduction of unwanted behavior. A simple example is ignoring an adolescent's tantrum about using the car. A medical example is psychiatric seclusion, or time out, for an individual who is behaving inappropriately and who values interactions with the staff. Disadvantages include extinction burst (the behavior temporarily increases) and that this process occurs slowly.

Behavioral psychotherapy focuses on changing behavior by helping individuals "unlearn" previously acquired associations that linked stimuli and maladaptive behaviors. There is little consideration for the thought processes, either conscious or unconscious, that underlie the psychological condition. This type of therapy is especially indicated for treating anxiety disorders. Methods include systematic desensitization, where there is systematic pairing of relaxation with increasingly anxiety-evoking situations (eg, the patient is gradually exposed to increasing numbers of spiders), implosion (eg, lots of imagined spiders all at once), and flooding (eg, introducing lots of real spiders all at once). Behavioral therapy is also used to modify behaviors by conditioning patients with negative or positive feedback. The targeted application of negative feedback is illustrated in aversive therapy, which pairs alcohol with an aversive stimulus (eg, disulfiram [Antabuse], an emetic medication that induces strong nausea in response to the taste of alcohol). This approach is effective for treating addictive and self-injurious behaviors. Additional treatments that use principles of operant conditioning involve increasing a desirable behavior through positive reinforcement and decreasing an undesirable one with punishment or extinction. Exemplar techniques include modifying behavior with contingency contracts (eg, a formal written agreement between two or more people that clearly defines the behaviors that are to be modified and the rewards and punishments that will result if these behaviors are not modified); token economies in which desirable behaviors are increased by issuing tokens that can be exchanged for desired items; and social skills training (SST), which is classified as a type of behavioral modification that incorporates techniques of operant and classical conditioning and social learning.

Cognitive Models

Cognitive models propose that individuals acquire new information by forming and using conceptual representations of themselves and others in the world. Cognitive models of learning emphasize internal thought processes that occur during learning and give less attention to the idea that external reinforcement is a necessary condition for learning to occur. Cognitive models propose that learning can occur without performance (latent learning), through observation, and via an "aha experience" (insight). The cognitive model also proposes that individuals behave in ways that are consistent with their beliefs and assumptions. In this way, individuals respond to cognitive representations of events rather than to the actual events and, further, that learning is cognitively mediated. These core beliefs, which develop early in life as a result of biological, developmental, and environmental factors, influence how individuals classify and categorize their experiences. When under stress, maladaptive cognitive processing may occur.

Cognitive psychotherapy therefore focuses on conscious thought processes. It is primarily based on two principles: (1) cognitive processes are a primary determinant of behavior and (2) cognitive restructuring (modifying assumptions and beliefs) may achieve behavioral and emotional change and alleviate illness. The cognitive model views psychiatric symptoms as being produced by inappropriate patterns of thought or cognitive distortions. For example, most depressed people automatically interpret situations in negative ways (see Table 1-3 for examples). If individuals can be trained to recognize and change these illogical thought patterns, their symptoms will improve. Cognitive psychotherapy is indicated for moderately depressed patients without psychosis. However, it is time limited and generally occurs weekly over 15 to 25 weeks (longer for individuals who present with personality disorders or more chronic issues).

Cognitive-Behavioral Treatments

Integration of the CB models has produced a set of effective CBTs. The CBT therapies propose that cognitive processing mediates emotional and behavioral dysfunction and that certain types of cognitions can be monitored. In this way, dysfunctional emotional and behavioral processes may change when cognitions are modified. In addition, attention is given to classical conditioning and operant principles of learning. Examples of CBT therapies include rational emotive therapy (RET) and CBT for depression. In

Table 1-3 Cognitive Errors

Distortion	Description
All-or-nothing thinking	Seeing things in black and white categories. If performance or situation is less than expected, then it is perceived as a total failure, unacceptable, etc.
Overgeneralization	Seeing a single negative event, no matter how minor, as part of a never-ending pattern of defeat.
Mental filter	Exclusively focusing on one negative to the exclusion of others so that one's vision of reality becomes exclusively focused on this one issue.
Disqualifying the positive	Rejecting positive experiences by insisting that they do not count for some reason or another. One can then maintain a consistent negative self-bias even though everyday experiences contradict that perception.
Jumping to conclusions	Making a negative interpretation even though there are no definite facts that convincingly support the conclusion.
Mind reading	Creating arbitrary conclusions that people, situations, and things are reacting to one negatively.
The fortune-telling error	Anticipating that situations will not turn out well and that one will feel convinced that one's prediction is already an established fact.
Magnification	Exaggerating the importance or relevance of things (including failure, incompletion, someone else's achievements).
Catastrophizing	Amplifying the consequences of ambiguous or negative events or situations.
Minimization	Inappropriately reducing personal skills (or someone else's) and strengths until they are negligible factors.
Emotional reasoning	Issuing greater importance to the negative feelings than is realistic: "I feel bad, therefore it must be true."
"Should" statements	Making statements about self and others that reflect expectations of behavior or situations ("I *should* be more competent. I *need* to be happy all the time."). "Should" or "must" statements directed at the self usually produce feelings of guilt. Similar statements directed at others often generate feelings of anger and resentment.
Labeling and mislabeling	An extreme form of overgeneralization. Rather than describing the situation, assigning labels to the person or self ("I am a terrible person not worthy of love from another."). Typically, this includes using colorful language to express strong emotions.
Personalization	Viewing self as the origin or cause of a problem. Assuming someone's opinion is more valuable or more correct than one's own.

general, the appeal of CBTs is that they employ clear, simple, and testable theories. They also use reliable measures for evaluating pretreatment status and response to treatment. Finally, CB models are useful in understanding the acquisition of learning and regulation of behavior with diverse populations across different age groups (eg, children, adolescents, and adults).

SYSTEMS FRAMEWORK

The systems framework of examining behavior regards individuals as operating in a social context that is, to a large extent, shaped by the history, values, beliefs, and expectations of a particular social group. Each individual occupies a niche within the group, acts on the basis of group influences, and in turn influences the group. In the clinical setting, the unit of study is the group itself, rather than the individual members of the group as separate actors. This framework is most commonly applied to families or at times subgroups of families, such as a couple in a close relationship. Less commonly, a health care unit such as a hospital ward or clinic can be examined to understand the effects the system has on a particular individual, usually the patient. This systems approach forms the basis for many types of therapy for couples and families and may occasionally be used by a consultant to examine patient or staff behavior in the health care setting, sometimes with therapeutic ends. The focus here is on families because this is the unit most often examined in medical situations.

A family can be thought of as an open system in which individual members have reciprocal effects on one another and, as a unit, is influenced by and influences the environment beyond the family. A clinician interested in understanding a patient within a family context would assess the key aspects discussed in the following paragraphs.

Structure

Family structure is a function of the family *constellation* and how the family is organized. With regard to the constellation, families can spread out horizontally within a single generation and vertically across multiple generations. In addition, family may include members who are related by neither blood nor marriage (eg, same-sex couples, adopted children, godparents, "play cousins," etc). The critical factor in assessing membership is to determine who within the broadest umbrella of family (around an identified patient) provides meaningful influence on the patient or on others who can in turn affect the patient. At times, this might include deceased relatives, neighbors, and others. Usually, there are core family members with daily influences, but more peripheral figures can at times step in to play a key role (eg, an estranged "black sheep" who is recruited back to the family to donate an organ in order to make amends). In times of illness, others who are not normally part of the family, such as health care team members or assisting community members, may become part of the family structure.

Family organization refers to the within-family rules concerning hierarchy, power, and roles. These rules may be drawn from the prevailing culture or subculture or they may be idiosyncratic to a particular family. Cohesion, another key element of family organization, reflects the balance between connectedness and separation within the family. Cohesion is a strong predictor of how well a family will cope with an illness.

Function

Key aspects of family function include boundaries, communication, and adaptability. *Boundaries* refer to the family's internal rules concerning differentiation and autonomy between family members on one hand and between the family and the rest of the community on the other. Families are disengaged when the interpersonal distance between members is too great: The individual members tend to feel isolated, and the family may have trouble rallying when there is a crisis, such as an illness. In families in which the interpersonal distances are too small (said to be enmeshed), differences among family members are minimized and expected to be subordinated to the greater family good. In enmeshed families, privacy and autonomy are regarded as threatening and there is little appreciation for each individual's uniqueness or particular needs. Included in the assessment of boundaries are generational boundaries, ie, the family rules that differentiate parental and child roles.

Communication is clearly critical for families to operate under normal circumstances and when faced with demands such as illness. Communication among family members always includes both a content aspect (which is typically explicit) and a relational aspect (which is often implicit), which operate to define or modify the relationship(s) among those communicating. Communication can be verbal or nonverbal and may vary in clarity and directness. A parental statement to a child such as "drink your milk" is a direct verbal message that includes only a request (or demand), but it implicitly transmits the message that the parent has more power or authority and can compel the child to comply. An angry shaking of the head by the child in return is a nonverbal response that also questions whether the parent has the power to enforce the desired outcome (drinking the milk).

Adaptability is a function that balances the family's ability to adapt to new life circumstances, including developmental tasks, with the family's need for enduring rules and values. Families are often described on a continuum from rigid to chaotic in terms of their adaptability. Overly rigid families lack the flexibility to deal effectively with new demands created by an illness. Chaotic families also do poorly because they may not be able to create the organization needed to execute orderly responses required for effective adaptation, making adherence to a medical regimen problematic.

Situation Within the Family's Life Cycle

Just as an individual undergoes a series of developmental steps throughout his or her lifetime, so families have a succession of phases. Table 1-4 illustrates this succession by

Table 1-4 Example of a Family Life Cycle

- Two young people separately leave their homes
- The two commit to a long-term relationship as a couple
- Family with younger children
- Family with adolescents
- Children leave the family
- Couple and family in later life

presenting the onset of a family—here the joining of two young adults in a committed relationship. As is the case with individual development, families move through developmental steps at varying rates and not necessarily in the order shown, depending on life events. Steps may be skipped or revisited, too. The family's experience of and adaptation to illness will be colored by the event's position in the family life cycle. For example, a life-threatening illness of a member of a young adult couple with young children, financial strains, and parental care responsibilities will produce quite different effects from a life-threatening illness that affects an older couple with adult children, financial stability, and already-deceased parents of both partners.

Belief Systems

Although families and the individuals within them have many different belief systems (faith, customs, morality, etc), the belief systems about health and illness become paramount when someone in the family develops symptoms. Beliefs shape whether the symptoms are genuine, serious, and deserving of health care or sympathy. Once the family enters the health care system, its beliefs about the meaning and causes of an illness influence its acceptance of the condition and health care recommendations. Differences in beliefs among family members—or between the family and health care providers—may lead to family (or patient-doctor) schisms in reacting to the illness, especially if the differences are unrecognized or especially strong. For example, if one family member regards another's illness as largely psychosomatic, there may be little encouragement for seeking medical care and there may be a lack of sympathy or even overt hostility. Similarly, a family that believes an illness can be treated with dietary manipulations or prayer alone will be unlikely to follow recommendations regarding medications or surgery.

The elements described here could be part of a family assessment as it applies to a particular patient's medical situation. This approach should be the norm when dealing with children and adolescents and is applied routinely by family physicians, pediatricians, and child psychiatrists. Such an approach may also be valuable when an adult patient is sufficiently involved with his or her family system and when additional individual frameworks for understanding the situation do not clarify matters. If the assessment seems unduly complex, a specialist in families may be brought in as a consultant. Such a specialist will also be helpful if an assessment suggests that a family-based intervention is indicated.

Finally, the same type of approach (with some modifications) can be applied when considering small health care units. Just as with families, medical team members have their own rules about organization, their own ways of functioning, their own life cycles, and their own belief systems. System-oriented consultants can be very valuable to the administrator of a health care team when team problems are identified. Similarly, problems between an individual patient and a health care team may best be analyzed and resolved using this type of systems approach.

SUMMARY

Psychodynamic, cognitive, and behavioral psychotherapies differ in their primary indications, focus, and techniques. However, each approach offers useful frameworks for evaluating and understanding the acquisition and maintenance of behavior and, more broadly, how health and illness develop. With these theoretical approaches, students and professionals can understand how behavior is motivated; how early development influences adult functioning; the principles that explain development, personality, and behavior; and the psychological mechanisms that are key components of psychotherapy.

ADDITIONAL READING

American Psychiatric Association. *Practice Guidelines for the Treatment of Psychiatric Disorders: Compendium 2000*. Washington, DC: American Psychiatric Association.

Barlow DH. *Clinical Handbook of Psychological Disorders: A Step-by-Step Treatment Manual*. New York, NY: Guilford Press; 2001.

Beck AT, Rush AJ, Shaw BF, Emery G. *Cognitive Therapy of Depression*. New York, NY: Guilford Press; 1979.

Brenner C. *Elementary Textbook of Psychoanalysis*. Rev ed. New York, NY: Anchor; 1974.

Carter E, McGoldrick M, eds. *Individual, Family, and Social Perspectives*. 3rd ed. Boston, Mass: Allyn & Bacon; 1998.

Clark D, Beck A, Alford B. *Scientific Foundations of Cognitive Theory and Therapy of Depression*. New York, NY: John Wiley & Sons, Inc; 1999.

Crouch M, Roberts L. *The Family in Medical Practice: A Family Systems Primer*. New York, NY: Springer-Verlag; 1985.

Ellis A, Dryden W. *The Practice of Rational Emotive Therapy*. New York, NY: Springer Publishing Co; 1987.

Freud A. *The Ego and the Mechanisms of Defense*. Rev ed. New York, NY: International Universities Press; 1966.

Freud S. *New Introductory Lectures on Psychoanalysis*. New York, NY: W W Norton & Co; 1965.

Gurman AS, Jacobson NS. *Clinical Handbook of Couple Therapy*. New York, NY: Guilford Press; 2001.

MacKinnon RA, Michels E. *The Psychiatric Interview in Clinical Practice*. Philadelphia, Pa; WB Saunders Co; 1971.

McHugh PR, Slavney PR. *The Perspectives of Psychiatry*. 2nd ed. Baltimore, Md: The Johns Hopkins University Press; 2002:1–330.

Rolland JS. *Families Illness & Disability: An Integrative Treatment Model*. New York, NY: Basic Books; 1994.

Tasman K, Lieberman JA, eds. Cognitive and behavioral therapies. In: *Psychiatry*. Philadelphia, Pa: WB Saunders Co; 1997.

Wilson GT, Pike KM. Eating disorders. In: Barlow DH, ed. *Clinical Handbook of Psychological Disorders: A Step-by-Step Treatment Manual*. 3rd ed. New York, NY: Guilford Press; 2001.

Wolpe J. *The Practice of Behavior Therapy*. 3rd ed. New York, NY: Pergamon Press; 1985.

Chapter 2

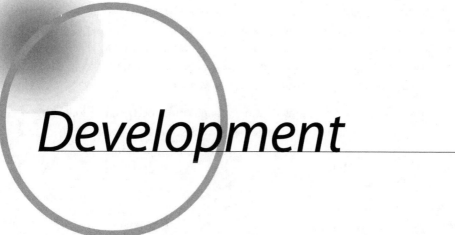

Development

Alan Ravitz, MD
Edwin Cook, MD
Bennett Leventhal, MD

The following basic concepts and principles underlie most thinking about human development:

- The term *life cycle* describes an order of the life course that occurs within the context of a basic sequence or unfolding of steps. Many of the steps are common to everyone, but the nature of the unfolding is unique to each individual. This basic sequence recurs for each succeeding generation over time. A life cycle can be thought of as applying to individuals, families, and even illnesses. It is a basic tenet that development occurs throughout life, from prenatal development until death.
- *Life structure* is the underlying pattern of a person's life at any given point in the life cycle. Its primary components include occupation, intimate relationships, and family and other social roles. It encompasses a person's relationships with significant others in the broader social system (group, institution, culture, nation, etc). The life structure evolves over the life cycle, and the relative importance of different components (eg, intimate relationships vs occupation) changes over time.

This chapter examines development using a longitudinal perspective, following successive age periods and discussing the different developmental components during each phase of life. These components include motor skills, communications, and cognitive development. Table 2-1 gives an overview of some of these components and their timelines. Theories that have influenced the thinking about these stages will be included at each appropriate point in the discussion.

When reading material about development, be critical in assessing the developmental theories as opposed to things that have been empirically examined, such as milestones. This discussion provides the primary care physician with a roadmap to identify normal development, behavior, and cognitive capacity. Problems that present can then be defined along this developmental path and further investigated.

TABLE 2-1 Key Developmental Milestone Overview

Gross Motor		Fine Motor	
Sit unassisted	6 months	Pincer grasp	12 months
Walking	12 months	Scribble	18 months
Stairs (1 ft/step)	36 months	Circle	36 months
Bicycle	6 years	Square	48–54 months
Language		**Cognitive**	
One word	12 months	Identify colors	36 months
Two-word phrases	24 months	Orientation	6–8 years
Sentences (three words)	36 months	Alphabet	5 years
		Primer reading	6 years
		Add single digits	7 years

TEMPERAMENT

Temperament is defined as a persistent behavioral style that consists of a group of related traits, including behavioral tendencies and response predispositions, that are stable over time. Research on temperament began with Stella Chess and Alexander Thomas, two psychiatrists who identified certain essential behavioral traits. These traits included mood quality and quantity, activity level, rhythmicity, approach or withdrawal, adaptability to change, threshold of responsiveness, intensity of reaction, degree of distractibility, and persistence in the face of obstacles. By examining these traits in children, Chess and Thomas identified three temperamental types. Children with difficult temperaments manifested negative responses to new stimuli, difficulty adapting to change, intense responsivity, low rhythmicity, and troubled mood. Children with easy temperaments manifested the opposite characteristics. A third group of children, identified as slow-to-warm-up, manifested characteristics of a difficult temperament on introduction to new situations but eventually became more comfortable once they warmed up. More recent work in this field has begun to identify some of the biochemical and genetic underpinnings of these elements of temperament.

Chess and Thomas found that individual temperamental type is less predictive of future psychological health than the goodness of fit between a child's capacities and temperament and the environmental expectations to which that child is exposed. This formulation offers an explanation for why some children do better in certain families and other children do worse. Chess and Thomas also found that both children and parents can change over time if caretaking circumstances are modified. Parenting traits that are likely to enhance goodness of fit include parental self-confidence, recognition of individual differences in children, flexibility, a willingness to experiment and seek advice, a willingness to offer loving care, avoidance of feeling personally victimized by children, and a willingness to accept children as they are.

PRENATAL DEVELOPMENT

Several issues are important to the development of the child before conception. Examples include chromosomal abnormalities or pregnant women taking known or suspected teratogens. More common adverse outcomes during pregnancy are due to poor nutrition (especially in areas of starvation) and behaviors that are unhealthy for the mother and also affect the developing fetus. Although cocaine and other illicit drugs are not helpful for development and all drugs, illicit or licit, are to be avoided during pregnancy, the two most common teratogenic substances of abuse are licit ones, namely alcohol and nicotine. Heavy alcohol ingestion may lead to fetal alcohol syndrome (FAS) with midfacial hypoplasia, mental retardation, and hyperactivity. It is less clear whether minimal ingestion of alcohol leads to adverse consequences, known as fetal alcohol effects (FAE), in which the consequences are behavioral teratogenicity. A recent finding is that maternal nicotine use increases the risk for problems with aggression in offspring, when other factors such as maternal responsiveness to the infant are controlled.

An important element of prenatal development is the psychological preparation process by the parents, siblings, and extended family. Obviously, there are a variety of reactions to the anticipated arrival, ranging from eager expectation with positive fantasies about the child who will be born to a sense that the child is not only unplanned but unwanted. Obviously, the birth of the child may occur within the context of a loving relationship between a couple, a conflictual relationship between a couple, or to a single mother. In all cases, support from extended family members is important, and the presence of a supportive maternal grandmother has been shown to be a protective factor for single mothers.

INFANCY (BIRTH TO AGE 3)

Much emphasis has been placed on bonding between babies and their parents during the first days of life. Previously, it was extrapolated from studies of imprinting in some non-human vertebrate species that there was a critical period for bonding between human infants and their caregivers. However, there has not been shown to be an ethologically critical period but rather a sensitive period in humans. It appears more important that a consistent and warm caregiver is present throughout infancy.

An interesting aspect of the first 2 months of life is the relative lack of concern the child has for social interaction. This abruptly ends at week 6 to week 8 with a social smile. Shortly thereafter, sleep becomes more organized, much to the relief of parents.

The first 12 to 18 months of life are referred to as the *oral period*, partly because the tendency to put something in one's mouth is one of the most common behaviors of a child. One of the most important tasks for parents during this period is to become sensitive to the child's various communicative signals. For example, a distressed 3-month-old is likely to be either hungry, too full, or wet. Parents learn to interpret the specific manifestation of distress so as to address the appropriate problem in an effective manner.

Eric Erikson developed a psychosocial theory of development in which he tried to synthesize Freud's drive theory with various aspects of ego psychology and object relations theory (see Chapter 1). He merged these into a task-oriented psychology that is intuitively easy to grasp and very useful for clinicians. Erikson conceptualized a series of chronologically age-related psychosocial crises. The first stage, basic trust vs basic mistrust, occurs during infancy. Children learn to rely on the sameness and continuity of care providers, and they learn to trust themselves and the capacity of their bodies to cope with the vicissitudes of their instinctual urges. Successful resolution of this stage depends on the quality rather than the quantity of caretaking. Caretakers tend to create a sense of trust by combining sensitive care of needs with a firm sense of personal trustworthiness. For example, a mother brings her temperamentally difficult infant into the office and asks the physician what to do. Based on this framework (and others), the physician should say, "Just try to be calm and be as available as you can be. Things will eventually get better."

Many of the early tasks of infancy focus on basic regulation and development of gross motor skills. Much of this development is correlated with myelination of brain regions important for that skill (birth of neurons and migration is prenatal). Rolling over occurs at 4 months and sitting up with assistance at 6 months. It is typical for development to occur with relative plateaus and discontinuous leaps in development at approximately 2 months, 6 months, 12 months, and 18 months. However, the experience of most parents is that their children learn new things every day or week during this period.

A 1-year-old child typically says a few single words other than "mama" or "dada." (Children typically say "dada" first because the ability to say 'd' predates the ability to say 'm.') See Table 2-2 for an overview of language development steps. Children at this age

TABLE 2-2 Language Development Steps

1. Crying—relatively undifferentiated at birth, then becomes more differentiated (eg, hungry, wet)

2. Cooing and vowel sounds

3. Consonants and babbling (5 months)

4. Words (9–12 months)

5. Sentences (two words) (24 months)

usually take their first steps without holding on. They have passed a period of stranger anxiety during 6–10 months and are in a period of enjoying their developing mobility. At this time, they have typically attained object permanence (the ability to know that an object does not go away just because it has disappeared under covers). They are also developing behavioral independence, but this is usually not a time during which they have large struggles over autonomy. A key issue related to the development of motor skills is that places where dangerous household products (eg, kitchen cleaners, medication) could be safely stored are now accessible to the child.

The next shift occurs as language development begins to accelerate at 18–24 months. During this critical period for the development of new capacities in symbolic development and language, the child often begins to struggle for more autonomy. The term *terrible two's* doesn't give justice to the pleasure parents get when their child gains many more skills and learns to enjoy the world. For healthy psychological development, it is important for parents to be relatively patient concerning power struggles, which inevitably develop. These struggles can often be handled by simplifying complex choices so as to allow the child a limited choice between two safe alternatives. The most important thing is for parents to assert their control in situations relating to safety or basic health, rather than situations in which the child is struggling for his or her own sense of needing to feel more autonomous.

The separation/individuation phase described by Margaret Mahler and others occurs between 6 months and approximately 3 years of age. This period is marked by increased physical and cognitive development, which allows the child to function more independently. The first subphase is called *hatching,* which refers to the process whereby a child turns attention to the outward world, away from the self and the mother. During the second subphase, *practicing,* which begins at approximately 12 months of age, the newly mobile child actively explores the environment. She takes great joy in exercising new capacities, such as walking and talking. Basically, she is unaware of physical separation until she encounters an obstacle, at which point the child looks back to the mother for emotional refueling. If the mother is calm and supportive during these moments, the child continues her healthy exploration. During the last 18 months of the separation/ individuation process, referred to as *rapprochement,* the child struggles emotionally to come to terms with her increasing ambivalence about leaving the security of her dependent relationship with her parents. This ambivalence is no doubt fueled by the child's growing cognitive capacity, which allows her to more realistically understand her various capacities.

The latter part of this period is referred to as the anal period in Freud's theory of psychosexual development. This is because the child is gaining control over excretion, which is an expectation of others during this phase. Also, much of the struggle over control is symbolized by withholding or giving, which is inherent in a child who is gaining continence of bowel functions. Few parents would consider this their favorite time with children, although at the end of this period (usually at about 3½ years of age) the child feels enough mastery of the world to enjoy his or her newly found competence.

Between the ages of 2 and 4, children struggle with the Eriksonian issue of autonomy vs shame and doubt. Muscular development leads to the capacity to either hold on or let go. The anal zone is the modal zone for retention and elimination at this point in development. The concept of shame refers to the intense embarrassment children experience when they are somehow exposed before they are ready to be visible. Doubt has to do with a fear of hidden vulnerability or outside control. Good parenting is characterized by firmly setting limits that provide children with the sense that others, stronger and wiser than they, will prevent them from making unfortunate decisions. An example would be for the physician to counsel parents not to get into power struggles with their 2-year-old over toilet training.

John Bowlby's attachment theory is based on the idea of attachment as an enduring emotional bond uniting one person with another in space over time. This type of bond is especially relevant, from an evolutionary point of view, to protection of the young. In practical terms, attachment is commonly manifested as an effort to seek proximity to, and contact with, an attachment figure who is typically older, wiser, and more competent than the other member of the attachment pair. Healthy attachments, which develop after 4 or 5 months of age, are relatively discriminating and specific. Children can form more than one attachment, but attachment figures should be people with whom the child has a great deal of familiarity. Children who have had multiple foster placements, eg, are often indiscriminate in their predisposition to form relationships. Ultimately, Bowlby proposed that through their various interpersonal experiences, people generate working models of self and other and of patterns of interaction that characterize these relationships. Other examples include a child becoming anxious about starting school, a child getting homesick at camp, or a teenager being devastated when a friendship ends.

Bowlby asserted that attachment tendencies are most prominent during periods of stress. Since the basic predisposition to seek out attachments supersedes the basic drive to explore and master the environment under challenging conditions, it is normal and healthy for people to seek emotional support from attachment figures. Thus, regressive behavior in the face of difficult circumstances should not be considered pathological. This is especially relevant to the medical setting because patients may appear to be regressed during periods of physical stress, when in fact what they are really doing is simply searching out healthy attachment figures.

PRESCHOOL (AGES 4–6; OEDIPAL/ELEKTRAL)

Ages 4 to 6 are often the most enjoyable for parents who delight in creative play. The play of children at this age is often quite elaborate, and the magical quality of preoperational thought does not place as many constraints to adhere to reality as that of the older child. Language has developed to allow the use of complex words as an accompaniment to play.

Because a child at this age does not have a full sense of the difference between fantasy and reality, he or she is often quite stereotypic in his or her roles. For example, during this period it is difficult to engage most boys in doll play and most girls in playing superheroes. This is not to say that the absence of stereotypic play represents any kind of psychopathology. It also does not mean that the child who loves play with aggressive themes will grow up to live a macho stereotype. However, this is why reference to sex-specific Greek plays, *Oedipus Rex* and *Elektra,* is used to define this stage psychosexually. In addition, from an interpersonal standpoint, this phase is inherently triadic (involving three persons in the core conflict) as opposed to the dyadic (two-person relationship) quality of the earlier oral and anal periods.

During this period, children struggle with the Eriksonian task of initiative vs guilt. The oedipal configuration presupposes an intrusion, initiated by the child, into the psychological space occupied by the parents. At a more practical level, children need to take initiative as they enter school, start to make friends, and begin to participate in various extracurricular activities. At this point in their lives, most children are not terribly socialized. Consequently, they take a great deal of pleasure in attack and conquest. However, if they are too harshly punished, they may develop a hypertrophied capacity for guilt (a harsh superego) over acts initiated or goals contemplated. A clinical example would be when a father notes that his son seems to resent his time with his wife. In this instance, the physician can suggest that this is normal and that the father set some limits but try not to get too angry.

SCHOOL AGE (AGES 6–12; LATENCY)

For those who love the creativity of the 4- to 6-year-old child, it may appear that someone pulled the curtain down on imagination during the next period of development. Latency implies that this is a period of relative calm in emotional development between the excitement of the previous phases and puberty, which ushers in adolescence.

Once children enter school, their radius of significant interpersonal relationships widens significantly. As they compete with other children, they confront the crisis of industry vs inferiority. Erikson referred to this as a stage of outer hindrances. There is a strong focus on academic and social accomplishments, and children begin to identify themselves as differentially successful in comparison to their peer group. One danger of this period is that the child's sense of identity will remain fixed on being a "good little worker" or student in the eyes of others, such that he or she may never enjoy pleasure and pride in work or accomplishment for its own sake.

Latency

Secular trends have influenced latency in the current cultural environment. Often, this period is not emotionally quiescent due to divorce, parent loss, or domestic or community violence; and the idea that grade-school children are less sexually preoccupied than oedipal or adolescent children predates media flooding with what would be considered more adult sexual themes. In addition, puberty is occurring progressively earlier during the 20th and early 21st centuries, thus encroaching on the time of late latency from an earlier era.

Although school-aged children continue to look to their parents as a source of strength and idealized stability (even in the case of severe abuse by the parents), by about age 9 children begin to have romance fantasies of having a better life (and better parents) elsewhere (eg, the typical Disney movie scenario of being raised by a cruel stepparent is not an accident but responsive to the interests of school-aged children). During this time, development is often much more linear, as opposed to that of the first 36 months of life.

Another interesting element of latency for school-aged children is that this is what most adults recall about their childhood, with most memories before about age 5 being lost in a process that is not fully understood.

Cognitive Development

Much of our thinking about cognitive development derives from the work of Jean Piaget and his followers. Piaget, a development psychologist, was interested in explaining a wide variety of thinking episodes by positing a small set of underlying mental operations (structures). Much of his work involved close observation of small samples of children, including his own.

Piaget's theory relies on the concept of stages (see Table 2-3). He asserted that children move through various stages and in an invariant sequence, although not necessarily at the same speed. Thus, he attached little importance to the ages associated with various developmental stages. He felt that each stage derives from the previous stage and incorporates and transforms that stage so as to prepare for the next stage. Piaget's first stage, which lasts from birth until approximately 2 years of age, is called the *sensorimotor period.* The sensorimotor stage is divided into six substages.

Between 2 and 7 years of age, children are in the preoperational stage. Their judgment is dominated by their perception, and they can attend to only one perceptual attribute of a situation at a time. The concept of time is not available to preoperational children. They are generally egocentric, unable to perceive or think about events from any viewpoint other than their own. When a 3-year-old comes into your office, she simply assumes that you know everything about her life and experience. She does not bother to explain that Billy is her brother, Monica is her friend, or Susan is her teacher. Between 4 and 7 years of age, children are engaged in the process of decentration, the progressive transition from a strictly egocentric point of view to a more reality-based, consensual point of view. This development then serves as the basis for operational thinking.

Between the ages of 7 and 11, children are in the concrete operational stage. They develop the capacity for some logical reasoning. Their thinking is no longer strictly bound by their perceptual experience. They can take into account more than one variable of a perceptual experience, eg, height and depth rather than just one or the other. They begin to master the concepts of conservation of quantity, weight, volume, number, etc. They can begin to apply the principles of logic to at least their own concrete experiences. Often, children seem to be extremely rule-bound, with a strong focus on fairness. Then, during adolescence, some children move into the formal operational stage. They can think systematically about more abstract concepts. This capacity for cognitively generating and testing hypotheses is the ability that allows us to succeed academically. It is also the quality that predisposes teenagers to become passionately involved in political or social movements.

TABLE 2-3 Stages of Cognitive Development

- Sensorimotor Stage (birth to 18–24 months)

    Primary circular reactions: 1–4 months, action occurs by chance, continued for own sake

    Secondary circular reactions: 4–10 months, actions to make interesting sights continue, eg, remove blanket partially covering a toy

    Coordination of means and ends: 10–12 months, will remove blanket covering a toy but not persist with two covers

    Tertiary circular reactions: 12–18 months, discovery of means

    Beginning of representational thought: 18–24 months, will remove layers of covers to find object = object permanence

- Preoperational Stage (2 to 7 years)—closely linked to the development of language

    Symbolic activity and make-believe play (2–4 years): reasoning symbolically rather than motorically, limited by perceptions rather than use of deduction, generally can attend to one perceptual dimension at a time, egocentric (only able to view events from her own perspective)

    Decentration (4–7 years): gradually increasing accommodation to reality, progressive decentering from the child's point of view, related to social development and expectations

- Concrete Operational Stage (7–11 years)

    Can symbolically test a given action before carrying it out

    Can precorrect behavior through mental trial and error

- Formal Operational Stage (11 or 12 through older adulthood)

    Can make theoretical statements independent of specific content (abstraction)

    Mental operations completely free from original observations

Latency-aged children move into concrete operations and leave preoperational thinking behind. Of course, they are capable of imaginative play and stories, and it is only a relative change in emphasis across stages. Peer relationships become more important to children at this age; at the end of this time, they start to shift to believing that peer relationships are almost central to their sense of self relative to their relationships with their parents. The reading and math skills that develop between ages 5 and 8 lead to progressively more challenging school tasks. Children will move from counting skills at age 5 to relatively complex multiplication at age 8 and simple division 1 year later.

Moral Development

Lawrence Kohlberg's theory of moral development is related to Piaget's stages of cognitive development. Kohlberg refers to the earliest level of morality, until the age of 6 or 7, as preconventional. During this period, children tend to define morality strictly in terms of the consequences of their behavior. Children who are obedient and avoid punishment are "good," and children who are punished are "bad." Kohlberg's second stage, from ages 8 or 9 through early adolescence, is termed *conventional morality*. At this developmental level children begin to appreciate that there is more than one way to look at a moral question. This understanding corresponds with their growing ability for operational thinking. They believe that others should live up to expectations of the family and community, maintaining good relations so as to obtain the approval of others. Eventually, conventionally moral children come to appreciate the various social and legal institutions that maintain morality. Thus, at the highest level of moral functioning, post-conventional morality, late adolescents and young adults develop a greater appreciation of the social contract. They recognize that moral principles are justified by a larger social good but that the morality of individual principles of conscience may override the larger social contract.

ADOLESCENCE (AGES 11–20)

The onset of puberty dates the beginning of adolescence. Anticipatory guidance for the onset of the physical changes of adolescence is useful. Although parents are in the best position to provide such support, pediatricians and family physicians can assure families that adolescence is proceeding by discussing relevant issues with the parents and children during office visits.

Erikson described the adolescent years (11–20) as the stage of identity vs role diffusion. The main task at this stage is to firm up an emerging personal sense of identity, ie, knowing who one is and where one is going in the world. There is often a sense of inner solidarity with the ideas and values of one or more particular social groups, often peers. These identifications may shift over the developmental period, at times resembling a "trying on" of various identities until the right fit is found. At times identity is influenced by attempts to differentiate one's self from one's family values and ideals. During these processes, ethical systems develop and occupational choices (or at least trajectories) are generally made. Failure to successfully navigate these identity issues can lead to problematic behaviors such as running away, criminality, suicidality, drug use, or joining cults.

Research has shown that normal adolescence is not the brew of incessant turmoil that forms the basis of stereotypes. There are, however, more vicissitudes than are seen during latency because of the need to develop so many different features of personal identity. Some of these are listed in Table 2-4. Distress about these aspects or conflict within the family unit over them may lead to consultation with the physician.

ADULTHOOD (AGE 20 AND OLDER)

Development is often naively assumed to stop with the end of physical maturation, which occurs toward the end of adolescence. Clearly, psychosocial issues and tasks remain after the body moves from maturation to gradual physical decline. Adulthood is sometimes divided into three stages, based on the Eriksonian model:

- *Intimacy vs isolation* occurs during young adulthood (20–40). Individuals face the developmental task of forming intimate relationships with others. Erikson describes intimacy as finding oneself yet losing oneself in another. If the young adult forms healthy friendships and an intimate relationship with another individual, intimacy will be achieved. If not, isolation will result.

- *Generativity vs stagnation* occurs during middle adulthood (40–65). By "generativity" Erikson refers to the adult's ability to look outside himself or herself and care for

TABLE 2-4 Aspects of Identity in Adolescents

- Dress, grooming (body adornment, hair, jewelry, etc)

- Sleep-wake schedule

- Language usage—vocabulary, grammar, syntax

- Food choices

- Cliques/social networks

- Musical preferences

- Cultural, ethical, spiritual values

- Relation to authority

- Sexual orientation

- Communication styles—indirect (to parents) vs direct (to peers)

- Risk-taking behaviors, experimentation (sex, drugs, and rock & roll)

others, eg, through parenting. A chief concern is to assist the younger generation in developing and leading useful lives. Generativity reflects the need to create a living legacy. The feeling of having done nothing to help the next generation is stagnation. Existential issues (eg, the meaning of one's life in the greater scheme of things) often come to the fore, particularly as familial and career responsibilities wane.

- *Integrity vs despair* occurs during late adulthood (65+). This period is a time to reflect on one's own life and its role in the larger scheme of things, seeing it filled with pleasure and satisfaction and/or disappointment and failure. If the person has achieved a sense of fulfillment about life and a sense of unity within herself, she will accept death with a sense of integrity. Just as the healthy child will not fear life, said Erikson, the healthy adult will not fear death. George Vaillaint, who has written extensively about healthy adult development, highlights ongoing social ties and a sense of excitement and purpose as important factors that promote healthy mental and physical aging.

SUMMARY

Human psychosocial development is a process that begins during intrauterine growth and continues throughout life. One's early years are tremendously influenced by the developing brain and body; later development has a trajectory that is more independent of one's physical self. Development occurs along a series of parallel lines (cognitive, language/ communication, interpersonal, etc), which shape and influence one another in complex ways. Each stage of life can be seen as a series of tasks and challenges that all people undergo but that occur in each individual in a unique way.

ADDITIONAL READINGS

Ainsworth MD, Blehar M, Waters E, Wall S. *Patterns of Attachment*. Hillsdale, NJ: Lawrence Erlbaum Associates, Inc; 1978.

Bronfenbrenner U. *The Ecology of Human Development*. Cambridge, Mass: Harvard University Press; 1979.

Crain W. *Theories of Development: Concepts and Applications*. Upper Saddle River, NJ: Prentice-Hall; 2000.

Flavell JH. *Cognitive Development*. Englewood Cliffs, NJ: Prentice-Hall; 1985.

Gardner H, Kornhaber M, Wake W. *Intelligence, Multiple Perspectives*. Fort Worth, Tex: Harcourt Brace; 1996.

Goldsmith HH, Buss AH, Plomin R, et al. Roundtable: What is temperament? Four approaches. *Child Development*. 1987;58:505-529.

Hetherington EM, Parke RD. *Child Psychology, a Contemporary Viewpoint*. New York, NY: McGraw-Hill; 1999.

Lamb ME. *The Role of the Father in Child Development*. New York, NY: John Wiley & Sons; 1996.

Lewis MV, Volkmar FR. *Clinical Aspects of Child and Adolescent Development: An Introductory Synthesis of Developmental Concepts and Clinical Experience*. 3rd ed. Philadelphia, Pa: Lea & Febiger; 1990.

Main M, Kaplan N, Cassidy J. Security in infancy, childhood, and adulthood: a move to the level of representation. *Monogr Soc Res Child Development*. 1985;50:66-104.

Sameroff AJ, Chandler, MJ. Reproductive risk and the continuum of caretaking casualty. Review of child development research. In: Horowitz FD, Hetherington M, Scarr-Salapatek S, Siegel EG, eds. *Review of Child Development Research*. Vol 4. Chicago, Ill: University of Chicago Press; 1975.

Sameroff AJ, Emde RN, ed. *Relationship Disturbances in Early Childhood: A Developmental Approach*. New York, NY: Basic Books; 1992.

Sroufe LA. *Emotional Development: The Organization of Emotional Life in the Early Years*. New York, NY: Cambridge University Press; 1996.

Stern D. *The Interpersonal World of the Infant: A View from Psychoanalysis and Developmental Psychology*. New York, NY: Basic Books; 1985.

Vaillant G. *Aging Well*. Boston, Mass: Little, Brown & Co; 2002.

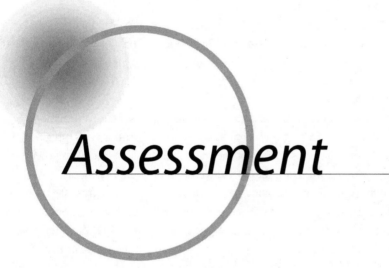

Chapter 3

Assessment

Steven Cole, MD
Mack Lipkin Jr, MD

Approximately 25% of all primary care patients suffer from significant mental disorders. Anxiety and depressive disorders are the most common. More patients with these disorders turn to their primary care physicians rather than to providers in the specialty behavioral health sector. These disorders are associated with excessive medical utilization and costs. When they co-occur with other general medical conditions, they contribute to increased morbidity and mortality. Because patients with mental disorders can be difficult to diagnose and manage, they also cause frustration for the physician. Despite the frequency of these illnesses, 30% to 50% of these mental disorders are not diagnosed and not treated optimally in primary care.

The first section of the chapter discusses barriers to assessment, including a brief presentation of the biopsychosocial model of illness. This approach can provide physicians with a framework for conceptualizing assessment and management of mental disorders and can also assist in evaluating the psychosocial variables important to the etiology and outcome of virtually all medical conditions.

Functional and structural models of the medical interview are presented to provide an overview of the interviewing process, which can be useful to the primary care physician. Assessment skills relevant to each segment of the medical interview (including the mental status exam) are discussed in detail. Rapport-development skills in general, including suggestions to help physicians respond to patients' emotions, are presented and discussed, with particular reference to the assessment of mental disorders (though these skills, again, remain relevant for all patients, not just those with mental disorders). For this latter group of conditions, however, rapport-development skills can be critical in overcoming resistance and stigma and in developing a working partnership as patients begin treatment.

With these models of the interview in mind, the elements of the history that are most important in assessing mental disorders are discussed in detail. The most pertinent elements of the examination are then summarized, including the mental status examination, which is relevant to this assessment task. Finally, the roles of the laboratory, radiologic studies, and psychological testing for actual or suspected mental disorders are reviewed.

THE MEDICAL INTERVIEW

With respect to assessment, the primary care physician's challenge occurs on many levels. In some cases, a physician may be aware that a patient showing symptoms of emotional distress probably suffers from a mental disorder. The assessment challenge then expands to clarifying the diagnosis and evaluating the severity of the problem. In most primary care cases, however, the psychiatric condition is masked by the presenting physical problem. The physician's task then becomes considerably more complex and subtle, one of uncovering hidden psychiatric morbidity. Even after hidden psychiatric morbidity has been detected, diagnosed, and evaluated for treatment selection, the stigma of mental illness creates additional educational challenges for physicians who must persuade reluctant patients to accept proper treatment. This chapter presents assessment approaches oriented to these tasks, ie, routine procedures to increase sensitivity for the detection of hidden psychiatric morbidity and focused assessment approaches to clarify the diagnosis and evaluate the severity of the condition.

Regardless of the task, application of basic interviewing skills remains the most important assessment tool available to the primary care physician. Development and use of optimal interviewing techniques for general medical care is necessary for improving the detection and management of mental disorders in primary care.

Do data exist that show that the interviewing skills of primary care physicians are not optimal? If they are not optimal, is it known if interviewing skills can be improved? The answer to both these questions is yes. A generation of research now exists documenting inadequacies in the medical interview process, including inadequate skills in collecting data, dissatisfied patients, and inadequately educated patients. Dozens of studies in the last decade document that interviewing skills can be learned. This chapter therefore focuses on the key elements of the interview that can make the difference between detection and accurate assessment compared to nondetection and/or inaccurate assessment of mental disorders in the primary care setting.

Barriers to Assessment

Educators and health service researchers have long questioned the sources of under-recognition and undertreatment of mental disorders in primary care. Although it is maintained in this chapter that improved communication skills are necessary for better detection and diagnosis of mental disorders in primary care, they are insufficient in themselves to change outcome.

At least 10 different barriers to the process of identifying and treating mental disorders in primary care have been identified (Table 3-1). These include the culture of medicine, the fear of opening Pandora's box, the fallacy of good reasons, inadequate reimbursement, other sources of discrimination, problems of inadequate knowledge, inadequate skills, ingrained habits of behavior, and financial and ecological barriers. Note that these barriers include factors that are intrinsic to the patient (and family), the physician, the patient-physician dyad, and the broader medical care delivery system.

TABLE 3-1 Barriers to Recognition and Treatment of Mental Disorders

- Inadequate physician knowledge
- Inadequate physician skills
- Ingrained physician habits
- Culture of medicine (mind-body dualism)
- Pandora's box (time pressure)
- Fallacy of good reasons (rationalizing emotional distress)
- Inadequate reimbursement for the physician
- Inadequate coverage for the patient
- Other discrimination (insurance coverage, workplace, etc)
- Financial and ecological barriers

The culture of medicine has been largely biomedical rather than biopsychosocial. That is, physicians and patients alike tend to divide the mind and the body into separate domains, allocating the body to the medical system and carving out the mind—or psychological issues—from the purview of medicine. The biomedical model implies dualism, or separation of mind and body, as well as reductionism, or the approach that suggests that medical problems can be best understood by smaller and smaller levels of analysis, ultimately relying on molecular explanations for diagnosis and treatment. Within a purely biomedical model, psychological problems and mental disorders get relegated out of "real" medicine. This relates to the stigma associated with mental disorders, in that patients do not want to be labeled as mentally ill because of the negative impact the diagnosis carries within medicine as well as the rest of society. Adequate attention to mental disorders and overcoming stigma require widespread adoption of the conceptual framework of the biopsychosocial model of illness.

As managed care intrudes further into the patient-physician relationship, time becomes more precious to the busy practitioner. Most physicians are feeling increasing pressure to see more patients in less time, which is leaving even less "flexible" time to assess and manage mental disorders that are perceived to require even more focused time and attention. It is small wonder that physicians say they often avoid psychiatric issues, even when they know they are present, for fear of opening a Pandora's box that they cannot gracefully close in a short period of time. In actuality, primary care physicians who learn improved interviewing skills increase their rate of detecting mental disorders without increasing the time they spend with patients.

Even when emotional symptoms are recognized and discussed in the medical interview, the fallacy of good reasons often operates as both physician and patient collude in avoiding a psychiatric diagnosis. Typically, a patient (or physician) might remark, "Well, I'm (or he's) certainly very depressed, but who wouldn't be depressed with. . . . " Physicians and patients need to increase their understanding of the syndromal nature of psychiatric disorders; they are distinct entities that warrant focused assessment and management. Without treatment, these disorders contribute markedly to impaired quality of life, morbidity, mortality, and health resource utilization. Even when there are good reasons for a sad or anxious mood, the presence of an anxiety, depressive, or other mental disorder should be rigorously evaluated and considered a complication of a concurrent life stress or physical illness, one that warrants specific treatment in its own right.

Many health insurance plans do not reimburse primary care physicians for the assessment or management of mental disorders. Many plans also have highly reduced benefits for mental disorders as compared with "medical" ones. Life and disability insurance companies and employers also discriminate against people with past histories of mental illness. These social barriers also operate against the routine evaluation and treatment of mental disorders in primary care.

Finally, many primary care physicians have not received adequate training to accurately diagnose and manage mental disorders. A change in their practice requires new knowledge, new skills, and the routinization of behaviors, which can increase the likelihood of diagnosing psychiatric problems when they are present.

The Biopsychosocial Model of Illness

In contrast to the biomedical model of illness, the biopsychosocial model of illness posits that a dynamic interaction of biological, psychological, and social variables accounts for the predisposition, onset, course, and outcome of all illness (mental, as well as other illnesses). With awareness that the assessment and management of psychosocial variables play an integral role in the medical care of all illness, it becomes obvious that interviewing strategies that encompass these domains must become a core process of all medical care.

Application of the biopsychosocial model of illness to general medical practice requires integrating several specific new dimensions into the interview (Table 3-2). In each case, the data collected are incorporated into the broader framework.

Three Functions of the Medical Interview

The patient interview consists of both functional and structural elements. As described elsewhere (see Cole and Bird 2000; Lipkin et al 1994), the interviewing process can be usefully understood as comprising three central functions:

* Building rapport (responding to the patient's emotions)
* Assessing the patient's problem (gathering information)
* Managing the patient's problem (education and maximizing adherence)

Although it may initially seem that only data-gathering skills are important for the assessment process, it is important to realize that the efficient collection of information from the patient also depends on the two other functions: developing and maintaining rapport (ie, responding to the patient's emotions during the interview whenever they become apparent) and educating the patient when necessary. If adequate rapport does not develop between the patient and the physician, the physician will not be able to be efficient, or perhaps even accurate, in the data collection process. The patient who is angry, sad, or anxious will not be able to participate as an effective partner in the interview

TABLE 3-2 Incorporation of the Biopsychosocial Model Into Assessment

* *History of present illness.* This section of the medical history should include an assessment of the psychological and social variables that may relate to the etiology, onset, course, and outcome of an illness (or presenting problem).

* *Elicitation of the patient's expectations for the visit.* This is essential because patients do not always present their true wishes to the primary care physician. Determining the nature of the patient's desires can save the physician considerable time and energy.

* *Evaluation of the impact of the patient's symptoms on his or her quality of life.* This type of questioning has been shown to relate to the physician's ability to detect mental distress in his or her patients.

* *Family and social history.* A significant focus must remain on the patient's stressors. Recent life stresses, as well as current sources of support, should be evaluated.

* *Mental status examination.* At least a screening mental status examination should be part of every general medical assessment.

process if he or she does not feel an empathic connection with the physician. Similarly, if the physician does not provide adequate patient education throughout the interview process, the patient will feel his or her needs are not being adequately addressed and also will not be optimally cooperative during the interview process. Regardless of their contribution to the data collection process, rapport development and education stand as independent, critically important functions of the medical interview.

Function one: building rapport (responding to the patient's emotions). Rapport between the physician and the patient is essential to the entire interview process and outcome. Without rapport, the patient will not cooperate with efficient data gathering. Similarly, without rapport the patient will not be educated properly and will not adhere to management recommendations. With particular respect to the assessment of mental disorders, rapport is central to the detection process. Patients who do not feel comfortable with their physicians generally will not reveal the private parts of their lives that most often contain the early clues of mental distress.

Some physicians and other observers maintain that rapport-building skills are simply innate and are not inherently teachable or learnable. Nothing could be further from the truth. Emerging data confirm that these skills are indeed teachable. Although there may be many ways for physicians to develop and maintain rapport with patients, specific types of interventions seem to be common and effective. Attention to key nonverbal behaviors is important, eg, maintaining eye contact, maintaining open posture, keeping body position at the same level of the patient, etc. Appropriate use of touch is also central to good patient care.

Five specific types of verbal interventions have been shown to be quite useful and effective in primary care (Table 3-3). Reflection refers to statements that bring attention to the patient's observed emotion, eg, "I can see that you are feeling pretty upset right now, Mr Brown." Legitimation refers to statements that point to the physician's empathy with the patient, eg, "I can certainly understand why you feel so upset about the current situation." Support means use of personal statements that confirm the physician's availability to personally help the patient, eg, "I want you to know I am here to help you." Partnership expresses the collaborative partnership between patient and physician, eg, "Let's you and I together try to come up with a plan that has a better chance of working." Finally, respect refers to statements praising the patient for coping as well as he or she has, eg, "I am impressed with how well you have been managing under the circumstances."

Function two: assessment (gathering information). By using a specific skill set, physicians can collect information efficiently and effectively. These skills are summarized in Table 3-4.

Questioning is central to the assessment process. Physicians must ask patients questions in order to receive information that can be used in the assessment process.

TABLE 3-3 Verbal Interventions Used for Rapport

- Reflection
- Legitimation
- Supportive statements
- Partnership statements
- Respect

TABLE 3-4 Data Collection Skills
• Use of appropriate forms of questions (open vs closed)
• Facilitation
• Surveying
• Summarization

Appropriate questioning can make the difference between an efficient interview process that arrives at the correct diagnosis or an interview that is unnecessarily long or fails to detect an underlying mental disorder. In general, the most efficient form of questioning entails open-ended questioning at the beginning stages of the interview, and then uses progressively more focused questions until the physician uses closed questions to complete a specific line of investigation.

Open-ended questions are questions that cannot be answered with one word. For example, the typical opening question "What can I do to help you today?" is a representative open-ended question that most physicians use. Unfortunately, physicians on average move from this exemplary opening question to closed questions *within the first 18 seconds* of the interview! When this occurs, physicians typically interrupt patients and may not find out about other problems and may not collect the most relevant information. That is, most patients come to the physician with more than one problem. When the physician interrupts the patient to follow the physician's agenda, it is quite possible that time may be spent on evaluating a problem that is not central or that other key problems are ignored. Furthermore, closed questioning is not the most efficient way to obtain the most relevant information for any particular complaint.

The recommended approach to questioning can be thought of as an open-to-closed cone. Skillful interviewers maintain a relatively open interview as they progressively narrow the focus. For example, when a patient complains of chest pain, early requests for information may include "Please describe the pain," "Tell me what situations make the pain worse," "Describe the last episode in some detail from beginning to end," "Tell me what other symptoms you have with the chest pain." This approach is more efficient for assessing symptoms than is use of closed questions like, "Does it radiate to your back?" "Do you get short of breath?"

Skillful interviewers use facilitation frequently. Facilitation refers to interviewing behaviors that keep an interview flowing in a relatively open-ended manner. Examples of facilitation include head-nods, attentive silence, saying "uh-huh" or "tell me more," etc. These techniques allow the patient to describe his or her problems in his or her own words, which in turn allows the physician to increase the efficiency of the interview.

Surveying is another core data-gathering technique. This refers to asking the patient "What else is bothering you?" early in every interview. This question can become extremely cost efficient in helping physicians to avoid the end-of-the-interview questions like "Oh, by the way doctor . . . ," which tend to occur in about 20% of medical interviews. Physicians who learn to let patients complete their opening statements (this usually takes about 90 seconds) and also learn to survey the patient's problems by asking "what else" are generally able to ascertain most patients' problems without consuming excessive time and energy.

Finally, summarization has special utility as a data-gathering skill. Skillful interviewers use summarization during segments of the interview and also at the conclusion of the data-gathering process. At any point in the interview, physicians can and should tell patients they wish to summarize what has been said, eg, "I'd like to take a few moments now to summarize what I believe you have told me so far." The summarization process serves several useful functions. On the most basic level, it allows the patient the opportunity to correct any misunderstandings the physician may have developed. It also allows the patient the opportunity to add important information that he or she may not have communicated earlier, and it allows the physician the opportunity to identify items in the history that may need clarification. Finally, summarization builds rapport because the patient realizes during the summarization process that the physician has been listening to his or her problems.

Function three: managing the patient (educating the patient and maximizing adherence). Educating the patient and maximizing adherence are critically important to the interview. Up to 50% of all medical patients either do not understand their illness and its treatment or do not follow the physician's recommendations. Many lawsuits against physicians arise from patients who feel their physicians did not adequately explain their illnesses or treatments to them.

The key strategies for patient education and adherence maximization include eliciting the patient's prior understanding, presenting information in small bundles, responding to the patient's emotion, and developing a true partnership with the patient to negotiate management decisions. A sequence of five steps (the "five what's") is recommended for purposes of brief education and motivation interventions:

1. *What* do you understand about your illness and its treatment? (eg, What do you understand about the relationship of smoking to your heart problem?)
2. *What* are you willing to do to manage this illness? (eg, What are you willing to do now about smoking? Are you willing to make any commitment?)
3. *What* problems do you anticipate in meeting this goal? (eg, What will you do when you feel the need for another cigarette?)
4. *What* can I do to be of help to you in achieving this goal? (eg, Would you be interested in hearing about a nicotine patch that may help you with withdrawal symptoms?)
5. *What* are you willing to commit to now? (eg, What is it you will be doing now to help care for your illness?)

When patients indicate a lack of adequate understanding about key elements, the physician can and should provide relevant information. When patients demonstrate emotions, eg, anxiety, grief, irritation, the physician should immediately respond to these emotions.

To achieve informed consent concerning medications or a procedure, the mnemonic **PREPARED** can be used to ensure all relevant informational domains have been covered (see Gambone and Reiter 1994):

- **P**rocedure or plan (Let me explain this procedure/plan to you. . . .)
- **R**easons (The reasons I am making it are. . . .)

- **E**xpectations the patient should have (If you go ahead with this plan, I think you have good reason to expect. . . .)
- **P**robability of success (If you go ahead with this plan, the chances that you will achieve success is. . . .)
- **A**lternatives (If you do not want to go ahead with this plan, the alternatives are. . . .)
- **R**isks associated with the proposed intervention (If you go ahead with this plan, the risks are. . . .)
- **E**xpense (The cost of this plan is. . . .)
- **D**ecision (Do you know what you want to do, or do you need some more time or more information to be able to make this decision?)

TAKING THE PATIENT HISTORY

Eliciting a history to make a psychiatric diagnosis is fundamentally no different from general medical history-taking. The same elements are used, although the elements are based on the knowledge of particular common symptoms and syndromes seen in mental disorders. For example, patients complaining of depressed mood should, among other things, be asked about sleep, appetite, energy level, suicidal ideation, etc. Generally, there are three steps in assessing a possible mental disorder: (1) thinking to include it in the differential diagnosis, (2) eliciting a relevant history to see if the patient has a particular syndrome, and (3) in some cases, undertaking further investigation to see if the syndrome can be explained by a general medical condition or drug-related problem.

Very early in the history-taking process, most physicians begin to compile a differential diagnosis. Perhaps the most important element in subsequent history-taking is to include relevant mental disorders in the differential diagnosis early in the process. As is done with other medical conditions, specific questioning may rapidly rule in or rule out a mental disorder. As an example, one reason why so many patients with panic disorder receive unnecessary cardiac, neurologic, or gastrointestinal workups is that the full clinical picture was not elicited during the history-taking process. A young patient presenting with chest tightness, few cardiac risk factors, recurrent nonexertional spontaneous panic attacks, phobic avoidance, and a family history of panic disorder can have a diagnosis made quite confidently at initial assessment instead of making the diagnosis after an expensive and fruitless hunt for, at least in this case, what amounts to "zebras."

Chief Complaint and History of Present Illness

The physician usually begins taking the patient's history by eliciting a chief complaint and investigating the history of the present illness. Often there will be more than one complaint. In this case, the physician must evaluate the history of each of the patient's significant complaints. The best skill for elaborating the history of the present illness is the ability to let the patient tell his or her own story, facilitating the patient to develop a narrative thread of the illness experience. Once the physician identifies the initial development of the symptom, he or she should encourage the patient to discuss the emergence of the problem by asking questions like "And then what happened?" The skilled interviewer will briefly sidetrack the development of this narrative thread when new symptoms or other problems emerge. If any of the other symptoms or problems are identified, they should be briefly reviewed to get a sense of their relative importance. However, generally speaking, the physician should not be sidetracked to the point of losing the original narrative thread. These other issues should be noted and examined later in the interview.

As the patient recounts the history of his or her symptoms, the physician often notes the appearance of emotions. In most instances, it is important for the physician to let the patient know these emotions have been noticed and it is acceptable, even desirable, for the patient to talk about them. Although many physicians may think this focus on emotions takes excessive time, it actually saves time. For example, if a patient becomes sad when discussing a certain situation, the physician can acknowledge the emotion in many simple ways. A nonverbal touch, lowering the voice, or directly noting the emotion with a comment like "I can see this is distressing for you" can let the patient know the emotion has been observed and that it is acceptable to talk directly about the feeling. Once a patient realizes that the physician accepts his or her feelings as a legitimate dimension of the medical interview, the full biopsychosocial dimensions of a medical problem may emerge. Emergence of the emotional aspects of a patient's problem usually helps in assessing and managing the condition and will also help reveal an underlying or comorbid presence of a mental disorder.

If the patient's underlying emotional issues do not become apparent while taking the history of the present illness, the physician should inquire as to the impact of the patient's symptoms on his or her quality of life. The appropriate question for this investigation may be something like, "What impact has your problem had on your life (in general, at home, or at work)?" This type of question has been associated with improved detection of emotional distress in patients.

Past Psychiatric History

Many patients with mental disorders have had some history of treatment for a psychiatric condition. For new patients, a brief question about the history of the psychiatric disorder or treatment can effectively detect current disorders. It is important to ask explicitly about substance use disorders, not only because patients may be reluctant to bring them up spontaneously but because many people do not automatically think of them as psychiatric or mental disorders.

The nature of previous treatment should be clarified—knowing about hospitalizations, detoxifications, specific types of medication taken, or experiences with psychotherapy may clarify the picture. Even a previous evaluation or consultation may provide clues about prior occurrence of symptoms (and records of those assessments may help clarify a diagnosis).

Finally, even in the absence of prior treatment, a history of symptoms earlier in life may influence diagnosis and management. The onset of mania in middle age, eg, is quite unusual and would generally merit a fairly careful medical and neurologic investigation. Eliciting the history that this "has occurred every spring for many years, but it's just worse this time" might suggest such a workup is not necessary.

Family and Social History

In this part of the history, asking about current life stresses and social supports can be effective in uncovering emotional distress and underlying mental disorders. High social stress and low social support have been shown to be risk factors for most general medical

TABLE 3-5 Psychosocial Areas of Potential Stress

- Relationship(s) with current or former intimate partner(s)
- Relationship(s) with family of origin
- Relationship(s) with children
- Relationship(s) with friends, neighbors
- School, job, career situation or transitions (eg, retirement)
- Relationship(s) with classmates or coworkers
- Financial issues
- Religious, spiritual matters
- Legal difficulties
- Reproductive issues (eg, fertility problems, pregnancy, childbirth)
- Health, disability of self or loved ones

disorders as well as for mental disorders. Learning about these risk factors is important when evaluating all medical disorders and can be effective for revealing mental disorders as well. These issues may be asked about in a fairly open-ended way or in a more structured manner by addressing different areas of life and functioning (Table 3-5). It is most important to ask about *changes* in life rather than stress or problems because even positive life events (eg, marriage, new job, or promotion) require adaptation and may precipitate illness.

This is also the time to ask about family history of mental disorders, alcohol or other drug problems, and treatment. Such illnesses may represent stresses or affect the patient's views about mental disorders. More important, many mental disorders run in families, ie, relatives with a particular illness place the patient at higher risk. Other times, several illnesses may run together. For example, those with somatization disorder are more likely to have first-degree relatives with alcoholism, antisocial personality disorder, or depression, as well as somatization disorder itself. It is worth noting that suicide runs in families, above and beyond the presence of specific disorders, ie, families that experience depression and suicides are probably genetically different from those that experience depression without suicides. Finally, treatment-response clues may be obtained from a family history. The fact that a close relative with depression "did really well on drug X" may be a factor in selecting a medication for a patient.

Review of Systems

Key elements of a mental health review of systems must be performed on all new patients to ensure that important mental illness is not overlooked. The US Preventive Health Services Task Force now recommends that all primary care patients be screened for depressive disorders. Two questions have demonstrated a high sensitivity for the detection of depression. These are:

In the last 2 weeks:

1. Have you been sad, down, depressed, or blue?

Yes ___ No ___ , and

2. Have you lost interest or pleasure in your usual activities?
Yes ___ No ___.

A positive response to either question requires follow-up with a more formal assessment for the presence of major depression. It is recommended that physicians use the patient health questionnaire (PHQ-9) as an aid to assessing depression in patients who screen positive on the two-question screener (see attached instrument in Appendix 1 and scoring guide in Appendix 2). The PHQ-9, a nine-item self-administered tool for assessing major depression, has been shown to have high sensitivity and specificity for the diagnosis of major depression in primary care. By deriving a quantitative score of severity, physicians can follow the course of a patient's depression and its treatment.

In addition to the two-item screener for depression, which should be used with all new patients, all patients should also be screened for anxiety disorders with questions like, "Have you been under a lot of stress lately?" "Have you had any problems with anxiety?"

In addition to screening all new patients for anxiety and depression with three or four brief questions, primary care physicians must remain highly suspicious for development of new psychiatric disorders. Because physicians cannot screen all patients for anxiety and depression at every visit, it is recommended that they screen those "red flag" patients most at risk of having a psychiatric disorder. Red flag patients include those with unexplained somatic complaints, previous history of psychiatric disorders, severe psychosocial stressors, chronic physical illness (diabetes, cardiac disease, etc), and an appearance of sadness or anxiousness.

Table 3-6 lists some of the more common symptoms of mental disorders. Some of this material can be incorporated into an initial patient questionnaire or into a focused review during history-taking. Once it is clear that a mental disorder is present, the physician must gather information specific to that disorder. This information is reviewed in subsequent chapters, focused on the diagnosis and treatment of specific disorders.

When patients report evidence of depression or anxiety, physicians must develop an understanding of the impact of these symptoms on the patient's functioning and quality of life. The most important indicators of function include the patient's ability to carry out normal activities at home and at work. Typical questions to determine this include, "In what ways have these symptoms affected your functioning at work? . . . or at home?" The more impairment reported by the patient, the more crucial is immediate clinical attention to the problem.

TABLE 3-6   Key Symptoms in Mental Disorders

- Loss of control over drinking, drug use; alcohol or drug cravings; morning shakes or need for drink; failed attempts at reducing or stopping use

- Sleep disturbance (difficulty falling asleep, middle-of-the-night awakening, early morning awakening, hypersomnia)

- Appetite disturbance (anorexia, overeating, carbohydrate craving)

- Memory impairment, forgetfulness, trouble concentrating, loss of acquired abilities

- Decreased energy, interest, pleasure in usual activities

- Hopelessness, guilt, self-criticism, low self-esteem, suicidal ideation

- Diminished need for sleep, excess energy, racing thoughts, irritable mood

- Panic attacks (panicky feeling, racing heart, dyspnea, chest discomfort, paresthesias, feeling of impending doom)

- Anxiety, restlessness, agitation, muscle tension

- Doubting, checking, ruminations, rituals

- Nightmares, flashbacks, easy startling, emotional numbing

- Hearing voices; seeing things that others don't; unusual smells, tastes, tactile sensations

- Suspiciousness, loss of ambition or motivation, social withdrawal

- Tics, tremors, bradykinesia, muscle stiffness, restlessness, seizures, gait disturbance, change in personality

- Preoccupation with weight, body image, binge eating, forced emesis, laxative, diuretic abuse, amenorrhea or irregular menses

- Falling asleep during the day, fitful sleep, sleepwalking, irregular sleep-wake pattern, nocturnal leg movements or discomfort

- Impaired interest in sex, arousal, ability to reach orgasm; pain during intercourse

- Preoccupation with illness, appearance, frequent unexplained physical symptoms, implausible or exaggerated physical complaint(s)

PHYSICAL AND MENTAL STATUS EXAMINATIONS

In addition to the medical interview, the physician can gain important information for assessment and treatment in the process of the physical and mental status examination.

General Physical Examination

The way in which a physician conducts a general physical examination is no different than the way he or she conducts an examination when mental disorders are suspected (with the exception of psychotic patients who need to be examined with the utmost sensitivity and caution). Certain physical findings that might confirm the presence of particular disorders (perforated nasal septum in cocaine abuse, enlarged parotid gland in bulimia nervosa) should be sought. Other findings may be germane because they suggest the presence of a general medical condition that might explain a particular syndrome. It is for this reason that in most cases a careful neurologic exam should be conducted as part of the assessment, particularly if the history suggests cognitive impairment or psychosis. Examples of abnormalities on physical examination and their associated mental illnesses are shown in Table 3-7.

Mental Status Examination

Many physicians erroneously think that the mental status exam refers only to assessment of cognitive functioning. It refers instead to a complete evaluation of the patient's behavior, thinking processes, and emotional state, in addition to the cognitive elements (Table 3-8).

The mental status exam generally falls into five dimensions, which should be covered in all full general medical evaluations as well as specific psychiatric evaluations. A

TABLE 3-7 Examples of Physical Findings in Mental Disorders

Finding	Might Indicate
Cachexia	Depression, anorexia nervosa
Hypertension	Alcohol, stimulant, or cocaine abuse; anxiety
Constricted pupils	Opiate use
Dilated pupils	Stimulant or cocaine use, anti-muscarinic drugs
Perforated nasal septum	Intranasal cocaine use
Swollen parotid glands	Bulimia nervosa
Calluses on dorsum of hand	Bulimia nervosa
Tremor	Alcohol, stimulant, cocaine abuse; Parkinson disease
Abnormal gait	Parkinson, normal-pressure hydrocephalus, neurosyphilis
Wrist scars	Depression, borderline personality disorder
Multiple surgical scars	Somatization disorder, factitious illness
Extra-ocular nerve palsies	Wernicke encephalopathy
Asterixis	Delirium
Bald spots	Trichotillomania (obsessive-compulsive disorder)

behavior statement will point out the patient's level of activation and note any abnormal motor behaviors; it might also include observations about interpersonal behavior directed at the physician, such as seductive behavior or excessive complaining. A statement about speech/language should point to problems in the patient's communication style. Is the language understandable? Is speech slurred, rapid, incoherent, disjointed, tangential, or circumstantial (ie, unfocused)? The patient's affect should be evaluated; affect refers to the emotions demonstrated during the interview. This needs to be evaluated in terms of the predominant affect, the appropriateness of the affect to what is being discussed, and the variability of the affect (ie, is there a fixed mood state or does the patient shift affect?). Thought refers to the patient's concerns, the presence of psychotic thinking (delusions), the organization of thoughts, and the presence of suicidal or homicidal ideation.

Cognition/sensorium refers to the patient's orientation to person, place, and situation; attention; and overall cognitive function. The brief screening evaluation for cognitive function should include an assessment of immediate memory (ability to repeat three words after the examiner), recent memory (ability to remember three words in 3 minutes), and remote memory (ability to recall events that occurred years ago). The brief screen for cognitive function should also include evaluation of concentration and some cognitive operation that involves higher cortical functioning, eg, subtraction of serial 7s ("Subtract 7 from 100 and keep going until I tell you to stop."), repeating numbers forward and backward, drawing the numbers on a clock, etc. The Mini-Mental State Examination (MMSE) is a 5-minute structured assessment of cognitive function that is widely used. Patients with some evidence of cognitive impairment should be administered the MMSE routinely (see Table 3-9).

TABLE 3-8 Outline of the Mental Status Examination

Behavior
- Abnormal motor activity (tremors, tics, choreiform movements, etc)
- Level of activation (agitation, retardation)
- Stereotypical movements, compulsive behaviors, rituals

Speech
- Amount (spontaneous, when prompted)
- Volume
- Clarity (dysarthria, etc)
- Rate
- Evidence of aphasia (trouble speaking or understanding)

Thought
- Quantity (poverty of thought, racing thoughts)
- Content (delusions, guilt, grandiosity, paranoia, etc)
- Form (looseness of associations, tangentiality, flight of ideas, circumstantiality)
- Suicidal, homicidal ideation
- Preoccupations, concerns

Affect
- Predominant affective state
- Responsiveness of affect to different topics
- Appropriateness of affect to content

Cognition/sensorium
- Attention, orientation
- Fund of knowledge
- Memory (immediate, short-term, long-term)
- Calculations, naming
- Abstraction, insight, judgment
- Praxis, prosody, construction

TABLE 3-9 Mini-Mental Status Examination °

This 30-point exam measures the following cognitive components:

Measure	Possible Points
1. Repetition of a sentence	1
2. Comprehension of three commands	3
3. Reading a short sentence	1
4. Writing a sentence	1
5. Copying a design drawing	1
6. Time orientation	5

Measure	Possible Points
7. Place orientation	5
8. Registration of three words	3
9. Serial 7s (attention/concentration)	5
10. Recall of three words	3
11. Naming of common objects	2
Total	30

Interpreting the patient's score: 30 points is the maximum score. Scores below mid-20s suggest some cognitive impairment, with lower scores generally suggesting greater degrees of impairment. The patient's effort, environment, and educational level can influence the exact interpretation of the degree of impairment.

Source: Folstein MF, Folstein SE, McHugh PR. *J Psychiatr Res.* 1975;12:189–198, Elsevier Science Ltd, Oxford, England.

LABORATORY, PHYSIOLOGICAL, RADIOLOGICAL, AND PSYCHOLOGICAL TESTS

In addition to the history, physical, and mental status examination, the physician or other mental health provider often needs additional corroborating (or not corroborating) evidence from numerous available sources. These sources include general laboratory and radiologic tests, as well as a referral to a psychologist experienced in the assessment and management of chronic pain.

Use of the Clinical Laboratory

The history and the mental status examination usually provide sufficient data for clinicians to arrive at the appropriate diagnosis. Appropriate use of laboratory and radiological data is occasionally necessary to confirm a diagnosis, provide prognostic information, and evaluate general medical disorders that may cause psychiatric syndromes. Biologic investigations relevant to psychiatric disorders can be anatomic (magnetic resonance imaging [MRI], computerized tomography [CT], angiography), functional (electroencephalogram [EEG], evoked potentials, single photon emission computed tomography [SPECT], positron emission tomography [PET]), or diagnostic (cerebrospinal fluid [CSF]/serum Venereal Disease Research Laboratories [VDRL] test, serum toxicology, antinuclear antibody [ANA], tissue culture). Recent developments in psychopharmacology often require quantitative measures of medication levels. Some of the most common investigations are described below.

Toxicology screen. Serum or urine tests for toxic substances are crucial for patients presenting with confusional states of any kind. Substances that should be considered for toxic screening include: pain medications (opiates, etc), alcohol, sedative-hypnotics and anxiolytics (benzodiazepines, barbiturates), anticonvulsants, stimulants (methylphenidate, cocaine, amphetamines), hallucinogens (LSD [lysergic acid diethylamide], PCP [phencyclidine], THC [tetrahydrocannabinol]), atropinic agents (tricyclic antidepressants, anti–Parkinson agents, phenothiazines), and heavy metals (arsenic, lead, mercury).

Serum chemistry, hematology, and other related studies. A serum chemistry evaluation should be considered when evaluating confusional states or cognitive impairment of any kind. Abnormalities of any of the following are associated with cognitive disorders: sodium, calcium, magnesium, creatinine, blood urea nitrogen (BUN), glucose, and arterial blood gases. Abnormalities in bilirubin, protein, lactic acid, liver transaminase, erythrocyte sedimentation rate, and ceruloplasmin can be markers for conditions that can also cause mental disorders. Thyroid assessments are important for many patients; several mental disorders may be due to thyroid abnormalities, and lithium and carbamazepine use are associated with hypothyroidism.

The chemistry laboratory is also important for monitoring serum levels of numerous psychotropics, especially tricyclic antidepressants, lithium, valproate, and carbamazepine. Antipsychotic and benzodiazepine levels may need to be assessed. There is no well-established relationship between serum levels of newer antidepressants (selective serotonin reuptake inhibitors [SSRIs], venlafaxine, nefazodone, bupropion, mirtazapine) and therapeutic response. Drugs generally have a minimum level for likely therapeutic action, although some exhibit a window, with decreasing efficacy above certain levels. Most adverse effects tend to increase with increasing serum levels (at least until receptor sites are saturated). See Chapter 19 for more information about drug monitoring.

Antigen and antibody tests. Serum and CSF/VDRL tests for syphilis are important, as is the fluorescent treponemal antibody absorption (FTA-ABS) test to assess the presence and significance of syphilis. A variety of other antigen and antibody tests are available to assess connective tissue disease in the central nervous system (CNS) or periphery that may relate to abnormal mental status, seizures, motor disorders, or strokes. These include CSF IgG (immunoglobulin G), IgG synthesis rate, oligoclonal bands, cryptococcal antigen, and direct antigens against specific microbes, antiphospholipid antibody, anticardiolipin antibody, and lupus anticoagulant. HIV testing is essential for many abnormal mental states.

Dexamethasone suppression test. It has been found that many, but not all, depressed patients demonstrate a failure to suppress cortisol production after the administration of exogenous dexamethasone. Because of the high number of false negatives as well as false positives, DST is not widely used in clinical practice at this time.

Thyrotropin-releasing hormone stimulation test. Normal patients respond to exogenous thyrotropin-releasing hormone (TRH) by producing thyroid-stimulating hormone (TSH). Many, but not all, depressed patients demonstrate a blunted response of TSH to exogenous TRH. Like DST, this test produces many false positives as well as many false negatives. It is primarily a research tool at this time and has not found a place in the clinical setting.

Lumbar puncture. A lumbar puncture (LP) is critical in evaluating suspected CNS infection and helpful in assessing cancer, motor disorders, connective tissues disorders, dementia, demyelinating disorders, and other conditions. When possible, a computerized tomography (CT) should be ordered before an LP to rule out increased intracranial pressure, which could lead to brain herniation.

Physiological Testing

Electrocardiogram. A baseline electrocardiogram (ECG) is important in patients who are starting on certain psychotropic medications, some of which can cause tachycardia, conduction delay, or arrhythmias. Abnormal cardiac rhythm can at times cause psychiatric symptoms, especially anxiety or lethargy.

Electroencephalogram. Many patients with seizure disorders suffer from comorbid psychiatric disorders and vice versa. A large group of patients suffer from pseudo-seizures; some also suffer from true seizures. An electroencephalogram (EEG), sometimes in conjunction with video monitoring, may clarify diagnostic issues.

Many types of epilepsy can mimic psychiatric conditions, especially complex partial seizures (temporal lobe epilepsy). Such seizures can cause confusional states, anxiety episodes, loss of consciousness, hallucinations, delusions, abnormal affect, etc. Provocative maneuvers such as sleep deprivation, sleep, photic stimulation, and nasopharyngeal leads are often helpful in producing frank seizures or clear dysrhythmias. However, epilepsy remains primarily a clinical diagnosis, and patients can have multiple "normal" EEGs with clinical epilepsy, and abnormal EEGs can be found in patients without clinical epilepsy.

The EEG can also be useful in evaluating patients with delirium. With the exception of patients in alcohol or sedative withdrawal delirium, which is characterized by excessive fast wave activity, most patients with delirium have generalized slowing on the EEG, which reverses as the delirium improves. Certain disease states produce characteristic EEGs: hepatic or renal disease may cause triphasic waves, Creutzfeldt-Jakob disease causes periodic spike and high-amplitude slow waves, periodic lateralizing epileptiform discharges (PLEDS) are seen in diseases like herpes encephalitis, and frontal epileptiform rhythmic delta activity (FERDA) is seen in diffuse cerebral vascular disease or diencephalic mass lesions.

Finally, the EEG along with other physiologic measures comprises a polysomnographic examination for the evaluation of sleep disorders (see Chapter 11).

Radiological Studies

Computerized tomography. A CT scan of the head allows the clinician to view serial sections of brain. The scan identifies abnormal structures and indicates their nature (CSF, air, bone, blood, brain tissue). The CT scan (or MRI) is essential in evaluating all patients with suspected dementia and, in some cases, those with delirium. Relevant findings on CT include generalized or focal degeneration, acute or chronic subdural hematomas, infarctions, tumors or other space-occupying lesions, or normal pressure hydrocephalus.

Magnetic resonance imaging. The MRI offers superior resolution of brain anatomy (compared to CT). It is preferred for investigating most CNS conditions, with the exception of a suspected acute intracranial hemorrhage (for which a noncontrast CT should be ordered). The use of contrast (gadolinium) in the MRI can increase resolution further.

Positron emission tomography, functional magnetic resonance imaging, and single photon emission computed tomography. PET, fMRI, and SPECT assess CNS metabolic function (as opposed to CT or MRI, which assesses structure). PET involves the use of radioactive glucose (or another tracer), which is injected by vein and followed radiographically through the CNS. Many psychiatric and neurologic conditions, including schizophrenia, depression, obsessive-compulsive disorder, dementias, strokes, motor diseases, and epilepsy, demonstrate characteristic abnormalities on functional imaging examinations. Because of its high cost and noncoverage by most insurance plans, PET scanning has been limited primarily to research settings. SPECT and fMRI, like PET, represent other vehicles for assessing CNS function. Though typically offering less definitive resolution, SPECT and fMRI scanning are less costly than PET studies and are now covered by many insurance plans, making their use more widespread in the clinical setting.

Psychological and Neuropsychological Assessment

Psychological testing can be helpful when assessing personality disorders as well as general mental disorders. Such testing provides objective assessments of patients' symptoms and functioning and can assist the diagnostic process. The Minnesota Multiphasic Personality Inventory (MMPI) and the more recent version (MMPI-2) is a 567-item true/false test that can provide an objective assessment of a patient's profile. Other objective tests include the California Psychological Inventory (CPI) and the Millon Clinical Multiaxial Inventory-II (for personality disorders). Projective tests provide more detail about a patient's style and form of thinking and require complicated scoring and interpretation by evaluators. The Rorschach Test and thematic apperception test (TAT) require the subject to report what he or she sees in inkblots or to tell a story about a picture of people. These and related tests are not substitutes for clinical assessment, cannot yield a diagnosis when used alone, and generally play a very limited role in primary care settings.

Neuropsychological testing has become prominent as a way to measure and assess cognitive function and higher mental processes, such as language, thinking, attention, concentration, psychomotor abilities, etc. These tests are particularly valuable for assessing dementias, other cognitive disorders, and learning disabilities. The Halstead-Reitan and Luria-Nebraska batteries are commonly used neuropsychological assessment batteries. Other tests measure specific intellectual or executive functions.

Neuropsychological testing may play a valuable role in assessing dementia, particularly when a distinction needs to be made between normal aging and early dementia. Serial testing may suggest an illness course trajectory or, in contrast, the stability over time that is seen when no illness is present.

Specific cortical functions may need to be assessed if there has been localized brain damage, eg, post-CVA (cerebrovascular accident) or following traumatic brain injury. Chapters 10 (Cognitive Disorders) and 18 (Geropsychiatry) discuss these topics in depth.

SUMMARY

Adequate assessment for mental disorders requires the same skills that are applied in most medical encounters. These skills include an interviewing technique that is sensitive to process and obtains critical content; a history that is structured in the same way as the general medical history; a physical examination with particular attention paid to the neurologic and mental status exams; and, increasingly, judicious use of relevant laboratory studies.

ADDITIONAL READING

Cole S. Mental and behavioral disorders in primary care: bridging the gap. In: Nobel J, ed. *Primary Care Medicine*. 2nd ed. St Louis, Mo: Mosby-Yearbook; 2001.

Cole S, Bird J. *The Medical Interview: The Three-Function Approach*. 2nd ed. St Louis, Mo: Mosby; 2000.

Cole S, Raju M. Making the diagnosis of depression in the primary care setting. *Am J Med*. 1996;101:6A,10s-17s.

Cole S, Raju M, Dietrich A, Barrett J, Gerrity M. The MacArthur Foundation Depression Education Program for Primary Care Physicians: Rationale, Participants' Workbook, and Facilitators' Guide. *Gen Hosp Psychiatry.* 2000;22:299-358.

Coyne JC, Schwenk TL, Fechner-Bates S. Non-detection of depression by primary care physicians reconsidered. *Gen Hosp Psychiatry.* 1995;17:3-12.

Gambone J, Reiter R. *The Prepared Provider: A Guide for Improved Patient Communications.* Beaverton, Ore: Healthcare Works; 1994.

Higgins ES. A review of unrecognized mental illness in primary care: prevalence, natural history, and efforts to change the course. *Arch Fam Med.* 1994;3:908-917.

Lipkin M Jr, Putnam SM, Lazare A, eds. *The Medical Interview: Clinical Care, Education, and Research.* New York, NY: Springer-Verlag; 1994.

Regier DA, Narrow WE, Rae DS. The de facto US mental health and addictive disorders service system. Epidemiologic Catchment Area prospective study. *Arch Gen Psychiatry.* 1993;50:85-94.

Roter DL, Hall JA, Kern DE. Improving physicians' interviewing skills and reducing patients' emotional distress. *Arch Intern Med.* 1995;155:1877-1884.

Appendix 1

Patient Health Questionnaire (PHQ-9)

Name _____ Physician _____ Date _____

Over the *last two weeks*, how often have you been bothered by any of the following problems?

	Not At All (0)	Several Days (1)	More Than Half the Days (2)	Nearly Every Day (3)
1. Feeling down, depressed, or hopeless?	☐	☐	☐	☐
2. Little interest or pleasure in doing things?	☐	☐	☐	☐
3. Trouble falling or staying asleep, or sleeping too much?	☐	☐	☐	☐
4. Feeling tired or having little energy?	☐	☐	☐	☐
5. Poor appetite or overeating?	☐	☐	☐	☐
6. Feeling bad about yourself—or that you are a failure or have let yourself or your family down?	☐	☐	☐	☐
7. Trouble concentrating on things, such as reading the newspaper or watching television?	☐	☐	☐	☐
8. Moving or speaking so slowly that other people could have noticed? Or the opposite—being so fidgety or restless that you have been moving around a lot more than usual?	☐	☐	☐	☐
9. Thoughts that you would be better off dead or of hurting yourself in some way?**	☐	☐	☐	☐

10. If you are experiencing any of the problems on this form, how **difficult** have these problems made it for you to do your work, take care of things at home, or get along with other people?

☐ Not difficult at all   ☐ Somewhat difficult   ☐ Very difficult   ☐ Extremely difficult

11. In the past two years, have you felt depressed or sad most days, even if you felt okay sometimes?

☐ Yes   ☐ No

**If you have had thoughts that you would be better off dead or of hurting yourself in some way, please discuss this with your physician, go to a hospital emergency room, or call 911.

Source: Adapted with permission from the Primary Care Evaluation of Mental Disorders Patient Health Questionnaire (PRIME-MD® PHQ-9). PRIME-MD® is a trademark of Pfizer Inc. Copyright© 1999 Pfizer Inc. For research information, contact Dr Spitzer at RLS8@columbia.edu.

Appendix 2

How to Score the Patient Health Questionnaire

The patient health questionnaire (PHQ-9) can assist in diagnosing depression, as well as planning and monitoring depression treatment. There are three components to scoring the PHQ-9: number of depressive symptoms, severity score, and functional assessment. The number of depressive symptoms is used to aid in making the diagnosis of depression. The PHQ-9 severity score and functional assessment are measured at initial assessment and regularly after treatment begins to determine the severity of depression and to evaluate patient progress.

Number of Depressive Symptoms (Diagnosis)

1. For questions 1 through 8, count the number of symptoms the patient checked as "more than half the days" or "nearly every day." For question 9, count the question positive if the patient checks "several days," "more than half the days, or "nearly every day."
2. Use the following interpretation grid to diagnose depression subtypes:

0–2 PHQ symptoms	Not clinically depressed
3–4 PHQ symptoms*	Other depressive syndrome
5 or more PHQ symptoms*	Major depression

* PHQ items 1 or 2 must be one of the symptoms checked.

Severity Score

1. Assign a score to each response by the number value under the answer headings (not at all = 0; several days = 1; more than half the days = 2; and nearly every day = 3).
2. Total the values for each response to obtain the severity score.
3. Use the following interpretation grid:

0–4	Not clinically depressed
5–9	Mild depression
10–14	Moderate depression
15 or greater	Severe depression

Functional Assessment

The final two questions on the PHQ-9 ask the patient how emotional difficulties or problems impact work, things at home, or relationships with other people and if this has caused difficulty for 2 years or more. Patient responses can be one of four: "not difficult at all"; "somewhat difficult"; "very difficult"; or "extremely difficult."

- If the patient selects one of the last two responses, "very difficult" or "extremely difficult," his or her functionality at work, at home, or in relationships with other people is significantly impaired.
- If the patient has had difficulty with these problems for 2 years or more, consider the diagnosis of dysthymia (chronic depression).

Source: Adapted with permission from the Primary Care Evaluation of Mental Disorders Patient Health Questionnaire (PRIME-MD® PHQ-9). PRIME-MD® is a trademark of Pfizer Inc. Copyright© 1999 Pfizer Inc. For research information, contact Dr Spitzer at RLS8@columbia.edu.

Chapter **4**

Psychiatric Emergencies

Jeffrey I. Bennett, MD
Larry S. Goldman, MD

Evaluating and treating psychiatric disorders is integral to patient care in the primary care clinic or office setting. Psychiatric emergencies, which do occur from time to time, can generally be handled in the appropriately prepared outpatient setting, although they may require more specialized resources for successful management. Ready access to psychiatric consultation, emergency rooms, or inpatient psychiatric facilities can make the task easier to accomplish, even in a busy medical practice setting. However, not all of these resources need to be available on the premises (eg, certain medications). This chapter outlines the processes, requirements, and boundaries of office-based primary care emergency psychiatry.

BACKGROUND

Little information is available regarding the rate of presentation of psychiatric emergencies to primary care settings, but some data are available. A 1995 survey found that 3.3% of an urban primary care population had suicidal ideation during the previous year. Epidemiological studies of the pathways followed by patients with mental disorders indicate that 60% to 96% of those who receive care visit a primary care setting first. Occurrence rates of common mental disorders in primary care populations are quite high. For example, major depressive disorder, substance-related disorders, and anxiety disorders are found in the aggregate in about 25% of primary care patients and borderline personality disorders in 6%. Limited availability of specialized mental health care has led to increasing referrals of patients with severe mental disorders, such as bipolar disorder and schizophrenia, into primary care management. Because many of these conditions can present emergently, the prudent practitioner must be vigilant for and able to manage the emergency presentation of disorders involving suicidality, acute psychosis, severe depression, anxiety, aggression, and confusion. The pressure on primary care settings to handle these problems is likely to increase if the current trend to close US emergency departments continues, thus shifting the burden of many acute problems elsewhere.

Psychiatric emergencies generally arise from the presence of a psychiatric condition or present with neuropsychiatric symptoms in which urgent intervention is necessary for the prevention of injury, further severe morbidity, or death. Common situations that may require consideration for psychiatric admission for further evaluation and treatment include suicidality in any context, acute psychosis, violence or aggressive ideation, severe agitation, and severe psychomotor retardation or catatonia that interferes with proper and safe self-care. Other less common emergencies include the presence of a severe, untoward reaction to psychotropic medications; delirium; substance intoxication or withdrawal; or acute exacerbation of a medical condition presenting with neuropsychiatric symptoms.

Each condition requires verbally engaging the patient to calm, reassure, and assess in order to look for the underlying causes of the presentation and enable treatment planning. It is often necessary to provide for the safety of the patient and the safety of others while arrangements for transfer to an emergency room or inpatient facility are being made. Examples include continuously observing the patient by staff (sitter), searching a patient's belongings for dangerous objects, removing objects with which the patient could harm himself (by cutting, ingestion, or hanging), and restricting a patient's potential wandering or elopement.

PRINCIPLES OF ASSESSMENT AND MANAGEMENT

As the availability of inpatient and outpatient mental health care diminishes, providers of more routine care will be faced with the evaluation and management of more psychiatric acuity in their patients. The approach to the patient must be designed to provide adequate triage of psychiatric emergencies to the resources that they require. This need requires that history-gathering, ancillary sources, laboratory, and psychiatric consultation be used in the most effective manner. Below are guidelines in such an approach.

Patient History

The emergency psychiatric evaluation is a time-limited and focused process. It shares with routine psychiatric evaluation the common goals of facilitating the collection of data, clarifying the presenting problem, arriving at a differential diagnosis, obtaining further diagnostic studies, and executing an appropriate treatment plan in a safe and efficient fashion. Advantages to conducting an emergency evaluation in the primary care setting include the tendency for a treatment relationship to preexist with already-obtained knowledge of the patient, the patient's medical history, and, at times, the patient's family and other support systems. Disadvantages involve the relative rarity of psychiatric emergencies and thus the absence of heightened staff awareness, security resources, medical-legal knowledge, and appropriate medications and restraint equipment should the need arise.

Although patient safety is always a consideration during any emergency evaluation, emergency psychiatric evaluation and treatment also implies attention to ensuring the safety of others. The major elements of the assessment include the following:

- Conducting interviews in a controlled and low-stimulus environment
- Having an aware and prepared, trained staff available in the event that crisis intervention, emergency seclusion, or restraint becomes necessary
- Having tranquilizing medication on hand
- Having access to an emergency room or inpatient psychiatric setting for further safe observation, evaluation, and treatment

Components of the emergency psychiatric interview and examination (Table 4-1) should be performed and documented. The use of additional informants such as family members, friends, or acquaintances is usually helpful, particularly if the patient is too confused, disorganized in thought, or emotionally overwhelmed to give an adequate narrative. History-gathering should focus on the specific reasons for the acuity of the presentation with elaboration of the accompanying symptoms, the patient's experience of psychosocial or other precipitants, ongoing stressors, and their relevance to the presentation. A thorough understanding of any medical condition that may suggest a specific neuropsychiatric etiology to the presentation is important and should be accompanied by information about any recent medication use or changes, substance use, and recent central nervous system trauma.

TABLE 4-1 Components of the Emergency Psychiatric Interview and Exam

Interview

- Specific reason(s) for acute presentation

- Focused history of symptom development

- Psychosocial precipitants and concomitants

- Ongoing medical condition symptoms and exacerbations as they relate to the timing of the psychiatric symptoms

- Medications and medication changes over past 3 months

- Past or present substance use including over-the-counter herbals, hypnotics, analgesics, or nutritional supplements; alcohol; tobacco; illicit substances including intravenous use

- Past psychiatric history

- Family medical and psychiatric history

- Review of systems emphasizing those that may result in psychiatric symptoms

Examination

- General appearance, demeanor, and psychomotor activity

- Speech and language with emphasis on the narrative quality

- Mood and affect

- Thought process and content including rate; latency; presence or absence of aberrant ideas such as suicidal, homicidal, self-referential, or persecutory ideas regarding others toward self; thought broadcasting or insertion

- Perceptions such as illusions or auditory, visual, tactile, olfactory, or taste hallucinations and their interpretation

- Insight (knowledge of current abnormal state of mind) and judgment (impulse control, willingness to participate in and adhere to treatment plan)

- Cognitive function including attention and orientation, immediate and short-term memory, confrontation naming, construction, writing ability, ability to organize complex alternating motor sequences (fist-ring-palm alternations), verbal fluency tasks, mental trails (consecutive alternations between the numeric and alphabetic sequences within 30 seconds, eg, 1-A, 2-B, 3-C, …), response-inhibition tasks

Past psychiatric history and past patterns of symptom exacerbations can be critical to defining the nature of the current complaints. Although the mental status examination takes place concomitant to the interview, explicit cognitive testing should generally be performed to the extent possible. Screens such as the Mini-Mental State Exam (MMSE) and Frontal Assessment Battery (FAB) are particularly sensitive to and useful for detecting cortical and subcortical pathology, respectively.

Examination and Laboratory Studies

A thorough history along with physical, neurologic, and mental status examinations should guide subsequent laboratory testing. This strategy can be critical in the evaluation of possible general medical causes in the presentation of the patient. It is critical to note

TABLE 4-2 Useful Laboratory Tests in Emergency Psychiatric Presentations

- Urine or serum toxicological screen
- Serum drug level (eg, lithium, tricyclic antidepressant)
- Blood alcohol level
- Serum electrolytes, blood urea nitrogen (BUN), creatinine
- Serum glucose
- Serum calcium, magnesium
- Complete blood count (CBC) with differential and platelet count
- Thyroid stimulating hormone
- Pulse oximetry, arterial blood gas
- Head computerized tomography (CT) scan

that not all mood, cognitive, or behavioral abnormalities are from so-called functional psychiatric disorders; many general medical conditions, prescribed medications, and nonprescribed drugs can cause such "psychiatric" symptoms.

Of one group of emergency physicians surveyed (Broderick et al 2002), 52% endorsed having one or more laboratory tests done, regardless of the clinical presentation during a psychiatric medical screening exam. However, there is a wide range of opinion in this area. The yield of clinically significant abnormalities also varies depending on the population served. Laboratory screening without the benefit of a proper history and examination has very low yield in the setting of emergency psychiatric complaints. Due to the lack of availability of these tests in many offices, it may be necessary to transfer the patient to an emergency room setting where these tests can be performed. Common tests that may be required in emergency evaluations are listed in Table 4-2.

Management

The primary care physician should quickly establish the need for transfer of an at-risk, acutely ill patient to an emergency room or to an inpatient treatment facility where observation and more longitudinal evaluation can proceed. Once the need for transfer is established and arrangements are made, the physician is responsible for ensuring the patient's safety during the interim. This responsibility usually requires the following:

- Maintaining a low-stimulus environment to the degree possible for the acutely agitated or suicidal patient
- Establishing an environment free of dangerous items that might be used by an agitated or suicidal patient to harm himself, herself, or others
- Ensuring that the patient cannot elope through the use of a staff member or (preferably) a security office if available
- Ensuring stabilization of any acute medical problem while awaiting transfer
- Use of restraints if necessary and available
- Use of appropriate tranquilizing medications if indicated and available (see Table 4-3)

TABLE 4-3 Tranquilizing Medications in Emergencies

General Principles
- The goal is not to oversedate the patient but to facilitate cooperation and reduce agitation to enable an evaluation to proceed.

- A combination of lorazepam and antipsychotic has been found to work more effectively than either alone.

- Dosing must be adjusted for the elderly for all medications.

- Caution must be exercised for the use of antipsychotics in those with alcohol intoxication or recent abuse, hypokalemia, hypomagnesemia, and hypocalcemia, and in those with prolonged QT interval on electrocardiogram.

- Many antipsychotics can be used, but those of low potency (eg, chlorpromazine) should be avoided due to the risk of hypotension.

Drug and Dosing Specifics
- Haloperidol: 2-5mg (0.5-2.0 mg in the elderly) orally (PO) or intramuscularly (IM) with repeat every 45 to 90 minutes as needed (must monitor for acute dystonic reactions, hypotension, excessive sedation).

- Lorazepam: 1-2 mg PO or IM with repeat every 45 to 90 minutes as needed (must monitor for excessive sedation, respiratory compromise).

- Risperidone (liquid concentrate): 2-4 mg PO with repeat every 1 to 2 hours as needed.

- Ziprasidone: 10 mg IM every 2 hours or 20 mg IM every 4 hours to a maximum of 40 mg IM in any 24-hour period (for use in those with known diagnoses of schizophrenia or schizoaffective disorder).

- Appropriate paperwork according to the local mental health code to document the necessity of emergency transfer for evaluation or hospitalization

Referral and Consultation

According to their own experience and knowledge, most primary care providers are able to provide emergency psychiatric services on their own. However, having access to and using a psychiatric consultant (see Table 4-4) can be critical to successful management of a case. These consultants have knowledge of the procedures and laws regarding management of psychiatric patients, are experienced with these types of clinical emergencies, and provide expert opinion to the clinical decision-making process. Although relatively few

TABLE 4-4 Indications for Psychiatric Consultation

- Suicidal ideation
- Violent or homicidal ideation
- Acute mania or other agitation
- Acute psychosis
- Acute mental status changes, confusion, disorganization
- Medical and legal uncertainty

primary care settings have on-the-spot consultants immediately available, experienced colleagues can be made available to offer advice over the phone in these often charged situations. By making advance arrangements with colleagues to help out (perhaps with a promise of reciprocal availability), the physician can provide better care and reduce physician and office staff stress.

Medical-Legal Issues

Three main issues arise when handling psychiatric emergencies: involuntary commitment, use of restraints and involuntary medications, and the so-called Tarasoff duty to protect and warn.

All states have statutes concerning the *involuntary commitment* of patients to psychiatric facilities under certain circumstances. In general, patients must have a mental illness and meet one of three conditions. They must be an imminent danger to themselves, be an imminent danger to others, or be unable to adequately care for themselves. Some states allow commitment of patients under other circumstances. In these instances, documentation generally requires a petition attesting to the patient's potential dangerousness, which can often be completed by anyone who has witnessed the dangerous threats or behaviors, and a certificate by a physician or other qualified professional attesting to the mental illness and corroborating the potential dangerousness. There are often special rules or procedures for children, adolescents, those already under guardianship, and those with special types of advance directives about their psychiatric care. Information and forms can usually be obtained from local state's attorneys' offices, community mental health centers, emergency rooms, and psychiatric facilities or units. Transfer of an unwilling patient to an emergency room or psychiatric facility may require completion of these forms.

Many states also have regulations concerning the seclusion or physical restraint of patients in medical settings as well as provisions for giving tranquilizing medications to a nonconsenting patient. Imminent danger to the patient or others (eg, office staff) is usually adequate justification for overriding the patient's objections, but there should be clear documentation of the clinical situation and rationale for the intervention.

Most jurisdictions have either statutory or court case–based expectations that health care professionals will adequately protect potential victims who may be harmed by patients examined by the professional. In general, the clinician must know or have a reasonable basis for believing that a specific individual or individuals will be harmed by the patient. This duty can generally be discharged by admitting patients to a hospital where they are restricted from contact with their potential victims. If the patient is not hospitalized, the clinician must warn the intended victim or the local police about the threat. If the potential victim is a child or adolescent, the local child protective services agency should be contacted.

SPECIFIC EMERGENCY SITUATIONS

Aggression against the self and others confronts the primary care provider with serious and relatively common crises that must be evaluated and managed within the framework of available resources. Knowing what resources may be necessary enables the provider to be prepared for specific situations that may arise requiring more than the usual resources.

Described below are specific psychiatric problems that typically present as crises to the office-based provider including suicidality, violence, acute anxiety, grief, and catatonia. Each requires an approach as outlined above that provides for the safety of all, evaluation for underlying medical etiology, and management of a psychiatric syndrome through the use of immediate and longer term intervention.

Suicide and Self-Harm

Suicide is the ninth leading cause of death in the general population; the third leading cause of death in children, adolescents, and young adults ages 10 to 24; and the second leading cause of death in young adults ages 25 to 34. The rate of suicide in the US population as a whole has not varied much from between 11 to 12 per 100,000 annually over the last 10 years, yet the annual burden of parasuicide (intentional nonfatal self-injury) including both suicide attempts and acts without suicide intent is estimated at about 300 persons per 100,000. In 1996, there were 30,903 completed suicides and more than 650,000 emergency room visits for the treatment of attempted suicides. Of all suicides completed in the United States, 90% occur in whites, 17% in females, and 73% in males, with completion rates increasing with age to as high as 72 per 100,000 for males age 85 and older. Although the findings vary, more than half of all suicide victims have visited their primary care physician during the month prior to completing their suicide. Today's elderly population is particularly prone to make less use of mental health care providers as conduits of psychological care, which in turn increases the need for recognition of suicidal acuity by primary care providers.

Although the chief risk factor for completed suicide is the presence of one or more psychiatric disorders, particularly unipolar and bipolar depression, schizophrenia, and alcohol abuse or dependence, marked situational stressors should heighten the concern for detection by the primary care physician. A previous history of a suicide attempt increases the risk significantly. For those patients hospitalized after previously attempting suicide, the first 6 months to 1 year post-discharge is a particularly high-risk period. Table 4-5 lists patient types and circumstances when inquiries about suicide are especially appropriate.

Patients with suicidal ideation or plans will seldom spontaneously state their concerns and so need to be queried. There is no evidence that asking a patient about suicide places him or her at higher risk for completing it, and most patients will use the opportunity to talk about their concerns when suicidal ideas have been or are present. Those at risk should be asked about general stressors in life, evaluated for depression, and screened for alcohol misuse using the CAGE questions (see Chapter 7).

Patients should be asked about suicide using questions with progressively more focused content regarding suicidal ideas and risk (see Table 4-6). Risk of suicide should be assessed into imminent risk (within 48 hours), short-term risk (days to weeks), and long-term risk (months to years). The patient who has a cogent plan, access to lethal means, hopelessness about the future, and few social supports should be considered at imminent risk and requires immediate hospitalization. She or he should not be left alone and should be transported to a nearby psychiatric inpatient facility by ambulance or police. The care should not be entrusted to friends or family members because they may minimize the danger or harbor ambivalent feelings about the patient.

TABLE 4-5 Characteristics of Patients Who Should Be Asked About Suicidal Ideation

- New patients
- Depressed (currently undergoing treatment or previous episode)
- History of suicide attempt
- Recent (6 months to 1 year) discharge from psychiatric hospitalization
- HIV positive, especially if recent diagnosis
- Diagnosis of bipolar disorder, major depressive disorder, alcohol or substance abuse or dependence, schizoaffective disorder, or schizophrenia
- Borderline personality disorder
- Antisocial personality disorder
- Recent divorce, unemployment, loss of significant relationship
- Other overwhelming stressor or loss
- Recent diagnosis of terminal or chronic disease
- Patients who ask about death or dying

TABLE 4-6 Questions to Ask About Suicidal Ideation

- Do you feel hopeless about your situation?
- Have you ever felt that life was not worth living?
- Do you ever have thoughts of wanting to end your life?
- How far have these thoughts gone?
- Have you thought of ways that you might end your life?
- What plans have you made?
- Have you ever attempted to harm yourself or end your life? When and how?
- Do you have access to the means to end your life? How?
- Do you have access to a gun at home or elsewhere?

Case Vignette

A 20-year-old college student is brought to the student health service by his roommate because of concerns about his poor self-care. The student had been depressed for 2 months since the breakup of a relationship; he has been eating little, sleeping a great deal, staying in his room, and skipping classes. He has also been drinking heavily. He was treated for depression as a high school sophomore following an intentional overdose of acetaminophen. The roommate notes that the patient has been talking lately about the futility of life; he has also been giving away his favorite books. Examination reveals a disheveled young man with marked psychomotor retardation who speaks softly and sparsely. He expresses the belief that his "whole life had been a lie" and that his family and friends turn on him as they figure this out. He admits to hoping that he would get meningitis and die as a former classmate had, but he denies any plan to harm himself actively.

This situation should be regarded as a high risk because it involves an adolescent male with a major depression, the presence of alcohol misuse, a prior suicide attempt, hopelessness, and possible psychosis (guilty delusion); the absence of expressed suicidal intention or plan should not mislead the examiner. Psychiatric consultation and hospitalization are almost certainly necessary.

Violence Against Others

Violence against others is generally evaluated along lines similar to the assessment for self-harm. A past history of violence, impulsivity, paranoia, irritability, psychosis, cluster B personality disorders, and substance use disorders (especially involving alcohol, stimulants, cocaine, and phenylhexylarylamines such as phencyclidine) are all significant risk factors. The questions in Table 4-6 can be adapted to address violence toward others. Physicians should not hesitate to ask such questions directly and neutrally. Patients often appreciate the opportunity to discuss such thoughts, especially if they are unwanted. All states include some variation on "dangerousness to others" as grounds for involuntary psychiatric hospitalization or hold for further observation. Once a patient is assessed as a significant risk to others, the physician is responsible for preventing elopement until a secure care setting can be provided. If hospitalization is not arranged, the physician may have a duty to protect a specifically identified victim.

Panic Attacks and Acute Anxiety

Panic attacks represent a psychological emergency for which many patients seek help and reassurance that theirs is not a life-threatening emergency. Since acute anxiety can be part of the presentation of many potentially serious medical problems, possible medical etiology cannot be overlooked (see Table 4-7 and Chapter 8). Reassurance, having the patient focus on his breathing, having the patient concentrate on a previously experienced calming scene, and the judicious use of minor tranquilizers can successfully alleviate the symptoms and restore some measure of confidence that although the attacks are distressing, they can be managed.

Grief, Psychological Trauma

Responses to acute trauma, including physical trauma, assault, and significant and sudden loss, are common in emergency settings. These responses often are addressed by lay professionals such as police, firemen, clergy, and other nonphysician staff who perform such interventions regularly. Five steps (see Table 4-8) based on a cognitive approach may be helpful in the initial evaluation and management of patients suffering overwhelming, acute psychological stress.

Catatonia

Kahlbaum first described catatonia (motor immobility with catalepsy or stupor alternating with purposeless motor activity, mutism, or negativism, peculiarities of voluntary movement, echopraxia, or echolalia) in 1874 for 11 patients, several of whom had demonstrable underlying medical disease believed to give rise to this syndrome. The constellation of symptoms (Table 4-9) can fluctuate significantly over the course of

TABLE 4-7 Medical and Psychiatric Causes of Acute Anxiety or Panic Attacks

- Myocardial infarction

- Arrhythmia

- Pulmonary embolus

- Asthma

- Pulmonary edema

- Pneumothorax

- Pheochromocytoma

- Hyperthyroidism

- Esophageal tear

- Aortic aneurysm

- Pancreatitis

- Acute withdrawal from alcohol, benzodiazepines, barbiturates

- Intoxication from cocaine, LSD (lysergic acid diethylamide), MDMA (methylenedioxymethamphetamine), phencyclidine

- Adjustment disorder with anxiety

- Grief

- Posttraumatic reexperiencing

- Dissociative disorder

- Situational and nonsituational panic attack

- Phobic reaction

TABLE 4-8 Interventions for Acute Grief or Stress

- Establish sense of safety (reassurance, family and friends to provide comfort, low-dose benzodiazepines).

- Provide information (convey information about the event, fate of others, patient's own medical condition).

- Correct misattributions (help patient recognize catastrophizing, reduce tendency to blame self, talk about their perspective).

- Restore and support effective coping (educate patient, family, and acquaintances about normal responses to abnormal situations; have patient participate in further planning and decision making about the future).

- Ensure social support (referral to community agencies, self-help groups, outpatient mental health care; ensure provision of shelter, food, and protection).

minutes, hours, and days and can vary with environment, further complicating its recognition. Although schizophrenia and major mood disorders (both depression and mania) can give rise to catatonia, until demonstrated otherwise, catatonia must be considered of medical etiology and, like delirium, be approached as a potentially life-threatening

TABLE 4-9 Features of Catatonia

- Negativism or motiveless resistance to all instructions

- Mutism

- Excessive motor activity that is apparently purposeless

- Hypokinetic movement abnormalities (waxy flexibility, catalepsy)

- Language abnormalities (verbigeration, echolalia)

- Bizarre posturing or prominent grimacing, stereotypies, or mannerisms

emergency. In addition to a thorough history of medical and psychiatric symptoms concomitant to the development of the presentation, diagnostic studies are often required. Virtually all of the conditions that can give rise to delirium can also cause catatonia, so a similar approach is warranted (see Chapter 10).

Case Vignette

A 55-year-old woman with no previous psychiatric history is brought to the physician's office by her family because she has not been eating or speaking for the past 48 hours. Her family attributes her change to the death of an aunt to whom the patient was very close; the death occurred 2 weeks ago. The patient has had mild asthma for many years, using only a prn sympathomimetic inhaler. On examination, her temperature is 38.5°C, heart rate 110/minute, blood pressure 132/68 mm Hg, respiratory rate 16/minute. She resists physical examination, and it is not possible to do an adequate neurological examination. Her lungs are clear and her cardiac examination is unremarkable. The patient is awake and alert, but she stares at the physician, occasionally echoing back her questions instead of answering them. She picks repeatedly at the buttons on her blouse in a stereotypic fashion. At times she looks off into the corner of the room and mumbles to herself as if responding to internal stimuli.

A middle-aged patient whose presentation is strongly suggestive of catatonia is more likely to have a medical or neurological disorder than a primary psychiatric illness (eg, psychotic depression) that is beginning at this age. The stressor should be regarded as a red herring for the time being, and this situation should be regarded as a serious medical emergency. She needs transfer to an emergency department or admission to a medical floor for blood tests, toxicological analysis, neuro-imaging, and a lumbar puncture.

Approaches to the management of catatonia include the initial use of parenteral anxiolytics, such as lorazepam or amobarbital, and the use of electroconvulsive therapy with subsequent or ongoing treatment of underlying medical or psychiatric disorders. Careful attention must be paid to adequate hydration, the risk of thromboembolism from immobility, and the risk of cardiovascular collapse from exhaustion in the agitated catatonic patient, especially if elderly.

OTHER EMERGENCIES

Substance-induced emergencies (intoxication, withdrawal from drugs of abuse) are discussed in Chapter 6. Psychotic disorders are covered in Chapter 9, and adverse reactions to psychotropic medications are discussed in Chapter 19.

SUMMARY

Primary care physicians are increasingly being called on to evaluate and manage psychiatric emergencies. A focused history and examination can often determine whether the patient's behavior represents a serious immediate threat to his life, his general health, his functioning, or the well-being of others. Physicians working in primary care settings must have plans in place to arrange for more extensive emergency department evaluations, timely psychiatric consultations, and hospitalization with suitable precautions for behavioral emergencies. They must also be aware of some of the critical medical-legal issues that apply to the handling of such cases.

ADDITIONAL READING

American College of Emergency Physicians. Emergency Medicine Statistical Profile. Available at: www.acep.org/3,381,0.html. Last updated December 13, 2001.

American Psychiatric Association. *Diagnostic and Statistical Manual of Mental Disorders*. 4th ed. Primary Care Edition. Washington, DC: American Psychiatric Press, Inc; 1995.

Broderick KB, Lerner B, McCourt JD, Fraser E, Salerno K. Emergency physician practices and requirements regarding the medical screening examination of psychiatric patients. *Acad Emerg Med*. 2002;9:88-92.

Dubois B, Slachevsky A, Litvan I, Pillon B. The FAB: a frontal assessment battery at bedside. *Neurology*. 2000;55(11):1621-1626.

Folstein MF, Folstein SE, McHugh PR. "Mini-Mental State": a practical method for grading the cognitive state of patients for the clinician. *J Psychiatr Res*. 1975;12:189-198.

Hirschfeld RMA, Russell JM. Assessment and treatment of suicidal patients. *N Engl J Med*. 1997;337(13):910-915.

Linehan MM. Behavioral treatments of suicidal behaviors: definitional obfuscation and treatment outcomes. In: Maris RW, Canetto SS, McIntosh JL, Silverman MM, eds. *Review of Suicidology, 2000*. New York, NY: Guilford Press; 2000:84-111.

Maris RW, Berman AL, Silverman MM. *Comprehensive Textbook of Suicidology*. New York, NY: Guilford Press; 2000.

McCaig LF, Ly N. *National Hospital Ambulatory Medical Care Survey: 2000 Emergency Department Summary*. Advance data from vital and health statistics; no 326. Hyattsville, Md: National Center for Health Statistics; 2002.

Office of the Surgeon General. *National Strategy for Suicide Prevention: Goals and Objectives for Action*. Rockville, Md: US Department of Health and Human Services, Public Health Service; 2001.

Olfson M, Marcus SC, Druss B, Elinson L, Tanielian T, Pincus HA. National trends in the outpatient treatment of depression. *JAMA*. 2002;287:203-209.

Olshaker JS, Browne B, Jerrard DA, Prendergast H, Stair TO. Medical clearance and screening of psychiatric patients in the emergency department. *Acad Emerg Med*. 1997;4(2):124-128.

Ustun TB. Unmet need for management of mental disorders in primary care. In: Andrews G, Henderson S, eds. *Unmet Need in Psychiatry*. Cambridge, Mass: Cambridge University Press; 2000:157-171.

Chapter **5**

Child and
Adolescent
Disorders

Alan Ravitz, MD

It has been estimated that approximately 10% of the child and adolescent population in the United States suffers from some form of psychiatric disorder. Child and adolescent psychopathology differs from adult psychopathology in a couple of ways. First, psychiatric illness in childhood is typically densely embedded in a psychosocial context. Because primary care physicians are often most familiar with and comfortable using pharmacological therapeutics, this chapter emphasizes specific pharmacological treatments of various disorders. In good clinical practice, however, it is often vitally important to attend to familial, peer, and educational issues. Thus, assessment of multiple domains of function may help the clinician plan comprehensive treatment. It is especially important to attend to psychosocial and environmental problems in planning treatment for children and adolescents.

Second, comorbidity is the rule rather than the exception in younger patients. Each psychopathological entity has developmental consequences related to the development of self-esteem, interpersonal relationships, and educational achievement. These elements then have a profound impact on the patient's ability to sustain an effort in the face of life's inevitable obstacles. Children with untreated attention deficit hyperactivity disorder, eg, have a high risk for developing conduct disorders. Children with major depressive disorder are at increased risk for school failure. Consequently, the best treatments take into consideration the child's larger psychosocial context.

This chapter highlights a few key elements of assessment that are specific to children and adolescents. It then outlines the various disorders of infancy, childhood, and adolescence, which are presented in the diagnostic categories outlined in the *Diagnostic and Statistical Mental Disorders*, fourth edition (DSM-IV). Pharmacologic treatment for these disorders is described, and other treatment modalities, often of a psychotherapeutic or educational nature (and thus less likely to be available within primary care settings), are mentioned as well.

ASSESSMENT

Assessing children and adolescents is often complicated, especially because these patients are frequently relatively unwilling participants in the diagnostic process. Therefore, information should be obtained from several sources, including parents and schools as well as the patients themselves. Confidentiality issues complicate the process, especially with adolescents; it is one thing to obtain information and another to disseminate it. The clinician must balance privacy with comprehensiveness. Although it is usually a good idea to explain in advance to teenagers what information can be held in confidence and what cannot, it is also important to obtain as much information as possible from collateral sources in the interest of painting a complete and accurate picture of the patient.

Diagnostic interviews of the patient and his or her caretakers are by far the most important procedures for accurate assessment. These interviews should focus on the following:

- Presenting problem and its impact on individual, family, school, and community functioning

- A history of previous therapeutic attempts, including a detailed and complete description of pharmacologic interventions (What worked? What did not? What doses? What duration? Why were medications stopped?)
- An inquiry into neurologic diagnostic procedures such as electroencephalograms (EEGs) or various brain scans
- A description of previous psychological, neuropsychological, and psycho-educational testing
- A careful family history of psychiatric and/or neurological disorders

This interview is in addition to a basic physical examination, a developmental history, and a social history.

The areas that should be part of the mental status examination are listed in Table 5-1.

TABLE 5-1 Characteristics to Assess in a Mental Status Examination

Physical/Motor Function
- Appearance
- Posture
- General coordination
- Fine and gross motor control
- Motor activity
- Abnormal movements

Affect
- Mood
- Range
- Appropriateness
- Depth
- Precipitants
- Modes of regulation
- Vegetative signs and symptoms

Anxiety
- Manifestation
- Intensity
- Modulation
- Precipitants
- Developmental level

Cognition
- Intelligence
- IQ
- Synthetic capacity/creativity

TABLE 5-1 (continued)

Cognition—(continued)
- Understanding of contextual expectations

- Piagetian stage (age appropriateness)

- Reality testing

- Attention/distractibility

- Organization/flow/associations

- Content/theme

- Fantasy life/dreams (when called into service)

- Insight and judgment

Communication
- Language

- Nonverbal

- Directness

- Mutuality

Social/Interpersonal/Object Relations
- Quality and stability of attachment

- Object constancy (stability of relations)

- Sense of self/self-esteem (demoralization)

- Family

- Peers

- Relatedness to examiner

Impulse Control
- Flexibility

- Mechanisms for modulation

- Drives/defenses

- Libido

- Aggression

- Defense mechanisms

- Superego function

- Integration of thoughts and emotions

Competency/Mastery
- Adaptation

- Ego strengths

- Mastery drives

- Self-esteem maintenance

TABLE 5-1 (concluded)

Environmental Manifestations
- Family

- Peers

- Other significant adults

- School behavior

- Academic performance

- Leisure activities

CHILD-SPECIFIC PHARMACOLOGICAL ISSUES

Many childhood disorders respond to medication, although the use of medication is not as well established in children as it is in adults. Medications should be administered only after completing a thorough diagnostic evaluation. This caution cannot be emphasized enough. The process should include a full psychiatric assessment, a physical examination, and relevant laboratory studies.

Note that children metabolize most medications much more efficiently than adults and therefore may require greater (rather than lesser) doses of medication on a milligram-per-kilogram basis than adults. Children often have higher peak plasma concentrations as well as lower trough plasma concentrations because of the efficiency of their metabolic machinery; therefore, certain medications, such as tricyclic antidepressants, require multiple rather than once-daily dosing.

DISRUPTIVE BEHAVIOR DISORDERS

Disruptive behavior disorders are characterized by poor social relationships with peers, family, and authority figures due to extremes of aggressiveness, non-normative risk-taking behaviors, lying, defiance, irritability, externalization of blame, cruelty, stealing, destructiveness, and anger. These problems, which typically are associated with poor academic performance and a higher risk of substance abuse, often result in referrals for psychiatric and/or psychological treatment.

Attention Deficit Hyperactivity Disorder

Attention deficit hyperactivity disorder (ADHD) is the most common child psychiatric disorder. Its prevalence is between 3% and 5% of school-age children. Patients with this condition typically experience significant social and academic dysfunction. The most typical presentation includes problems with inattention, hyperactivity, and impulsivity. However, many children may be primarily hyperactive while others are primarily inattentive. The clinician should identify a child as predominantly inattentive type, predominantly hyperactive-impulsive type, or combined type.

Case Vignette

Jenny is an 8-year-old second-grade student who is brought to the physician's office by her mother at the urging of Jenny's teacher, who notes she is a smart girl but doesn't live up to her potential. The mother describes Jenny as a lively, bright girl who has always been "a bit of a daydreamer" with "trouble staying on task" at preschool, school, and in family and social interactions. She is easily distracted by external events when reading, watching television, or even playing with her friends. She often misplaces or loses school supplies, toys, and articles of clothing such as hats and gloves. There have been no recent stressors or family changes, and the mother describes Jenny as happy and calm most of the time. There is no history of aggression, impulsivity, or cruelty toward others, but Jenny is regarded as somewhat "out of step" with her peers socially and, although she has friends, she is by no means particularly popular. Her developmental milestones have been normal, and there have been no previous significant health problems. Physical examination is unremarkable. Jenny sits calmly throughout the interview with her mother, but she seems bored and looks around a lot. When the physician talks with her and examines her, she is cooperative. The physician obtains Jenny's school records: her performance evaluations have all been average to above average, but there are comments from several teachers about her wandering attention and distractibility from kindergarten on. A school psychologist did a Wechsler Intelligence Scale for Children (WISC), which revealed a verbal IQ of 110, performance of 102, full-scale 104. The physician diagnoses attention deficit disorder, primarily inattentive type, and recommends a trial of sustained-release methylphenidate.

Children are typically brought in to physicians because of complaints about difficult behavior and/or academic problems noted by the school. It is less common for the parents themselves to note problematic behavior at home or with peers. It is important to note that ADHD is fundamentally a clinical diagnosis, based on careful history-taking from patient, parents, and teachers. Currently, laboratory investigations, including neuroimaging studies, are investigational rather than of established clinical value. Using only school or parental observations is not an adequate means to establish the diagnosis. Relying excessively on a child's behavior in the physician's office is equally limited for several reasons:

- Even the most hyperactive child may be able to stay still for a short office visit.
- Inattention may be difficult to elicit in a mental status exam.
- Inattention and/or hyperactivity may be due to causes other than ADHD.

The symptoms of ADHD include at least six signs of inattention and/or six signs of hyperactivity/impulsivity for a 6-month period or longer. These symptoms are listed in Table 5-2.

In moderation, all of the behaviors noted above may be typical of normal children, especially boys. The DSM-IV notes that the pattern of behavior in diagnosed children should be more frequent and/or severe than that observed in other children at the same age or developmental level. Diagnosis of ADHD requires that the symptoms be present before the age of 7 years, although in clinical practice, many children are diagnosed at a later age. This is likely due to the fact that ADHD symptoms do not interfere with day-to-day functioning until various interpersonal and educational expectations reach a certain level of sophistication. While obtaining histories from children who present at an older

TABLE 5-2 Symptoms and Signs of ADHD

Symptoms of Inattention
- Failure to pay close attention to details, which may manifest itself in careless mistakes in schoolwork, work, or other activities

- Difficulty sustaining attention in various tasks and play activities

- Failure to listen when spoken to directly

- Difficulty following through on instructions, which manifests itself as a failure to finish schoolwork, chores, or various workplace duties

- Difficulty organizing tasks and activities

- Avoidance of tasks that require sustained mental effort, such as schoolwork or homework; tendency to lose things necessary for tasks and activities, such as toys, school assignments, pencils, books, or tools

- Easy distractibility by extraneous stimuli

- Forgetfulness in daily activities

Symptoms of Hyperactivity
- Tendency to fidget or squirm while sitting

- Inability to sit still, which manifests itself in hyperactivity in the classroom or in other situations in which remaining seated is expected

- Tendency to run or climb excessively or to experience subjective feelings of restlessness

- Difficulty playing quietly

- Tendency to be seen as on the go or driven by a motor

- Tendency to talk excessively in situations where this behavior is inappropriate

Symptoms of Impulsivity
- Blurting out answers before questions have been completed

- Difficulty awaiting turn

- Tendency to interrupt or intrude on others

age, it is usually clear that the symptoms have been present for some time before the patient presented for diagnosis and treatment.

To make the diagnosis, the various symptoms must manifest themselves across situations and they must be noted in at least two settings, such as school *and* home. If there is a great deal of environmental disorganization, such as a chaotic, neglectful, or abusive home, it is difficult to make the diagnosis of ADHD.

Epidemiology and course. Boys are affected more frequently than girls are, with the ratio ranging from 3:1 to 9:1 depending on the population studied. Family studies have indicated a strong genetic component in susceptibility to ADHD. There appears to be an approximately five- to sixfold increase in the frequency of ADHD among first-degree relatives when compared with the general population. Twin studies have estimated the heritability of ADHD to range from 39% to 91% for various symptoms of the disorder.

Symptoms of ADHD often persist into adolescence and adulthood. Although motor hyperactivity may diminish, the tendency toward inattention and impulsivity remains.

This compromises educational and vocational achievement as well as interpersonal adjustment. Therefore, treatment often continues into adulthood.

Treatment. Medication is unquestionably the first line of treatment for ADHD. There is a 70% to 80% response rate to psychomotor stimulant medications, which include methylphenidate, dextroamphetamine, and various amphetamine salts (see Table 5-3).

TABLE 5-3 Pharmacological Treatments for ADHD

Drug	Trade Names	Duration of Action (hours)	Typical Dose (mg)
Stimulants			
Methylphenidate			Approximately 1mg/kg
Short-acting*	Ritalin	3–5	10 tid–20 bid
Intermediate-acting (sustained release)*	Ritalin SR Metadate ER Methylin ER	3–8	40 qam
Long-acting (sustained release)	Ritalin LA Metadate CD Concerta	8–12	40 qam 40 qam 36 qam
Dexmethylphenidate	Focalin	6	10 bid
Dextroamphetamine sulfate			Approximately 0.5 mg/kg
Short-acting*	Dexedrine	4–6	5 tid–10 bid
Intermediate-acting*	Dexedrine spansule	6–8	20 qam
Mixed amphetamines			
Regular*	Adderall	4–6	10 bid
Sustained release	Adderall XR	10–12	20 qam
Pemoline	Cylert	8–12	56.25 qam
Norepinephrine reuptake inhibitor			
Atomoxetine	Strattera	8	1.2 mg/kg/day
Alpha-2 agonists†			
Clonidine	Catapres	6–8	4-5 mcg/kg/day in two divided doses
Guanfacine	Tenex	12	0.5 mg tid
Antidepressants†			
Desipramine*	Norpramin	24	1–3 mg/kg
Bupropion extended release	Wellbutrin XR	12	2–4 mg/kg/day in two divided doses

* Available as generic formulation.
† Not approved by the Food and Drug Administration for treatment of ADHD in children.

Typical side effects include insomnia, decreased appetite, mood changes, motor tics, headache, abdominal pain, and, very rarely, paranoia and/or psychosis. Within the last several years, a number of long-acting medication preparations have been developed. In general, once-daily dosing is preferable to multiple-daily dosing. Not only is it easier to comply with a medication regimen that requires the patient to take medication only once a day, but many ADHD patients feel stigmatized by being required to take medication during school hours. If a long-acting medication is taken in the morning before school, the patient avoids the teasing and demoralization that may occur as a consequence of visiting the nurse during the school day for medication administration.

The exact dosing regimen should be based on a variety of factors. At times, when decreased appetite is especially problematic, children need to take short-acting psychomotor stimulants because they benefit from brief windows of time during which their appetites improve. Other patients may require a long-acting medication in the morning before school and then a short-acting medication after school. Keep in mind that the symptoms of ADHD occur 24 hours a day, 7 days a week, 52 weeks a year. The purpose of prescribing medication is not simply to control behavior during the school hours but, rather, to improve general functioning.

For some younger children who are unable swallow pills, there are liquid preparations of some psychomotor stimulants, although all are of the shorter-acting variety. Some drug companies have recently developed longer-acting preparations in "sprinkle" form. These should be seriously considered for children who have difficulty swallowing pills and who need a sustained-release medication.

Although all psychomotor stimulants have the same general mechanism of action, children respond differently to different medications. Before giving up on this general class of agents, the child should have a trial of both short- and long-acting methylphenidate, both short- and long-acting dextroamphetamine, and both short- and long-acting amphetamine salts. Many patients will respond to all of the agents, but some respond only to a specific agent and/or preparation.

When psychomotor stimulants are ineffective or cannot be tolerated because of side effects, second-line agents should be used. The most common are antihypertensive medications such as clonidine and guanfacine. The side effects of these medications include sedation, depression, and rebound hypertension. Because of their sedating side effects, both agents can be used as adjuncts to psychomotor stimulants when insomnia is a problem. Tricyclic antidepressants and bupropion (sustained release is preferable) may also be used to treat ADHD. Tricyclics have been shown to be quite effective; however, because there are electrocardiogram (ECG) changes with tricyclic antidepressants, every patient who begins one of these types of medication should have an ECG prior to beginning treatment.

At times, behavioral therapy plays an important role in the management of ADHD. Many children will have developed adjustment, self-esteem, and other psychological reactions to the adverse academic and interpersonal consequences of their ADHD. Cognitive-behavioral psychotherapy (generally conducted by a mental health professional trained to provide this) as well as family education and counseling are often important in such cases. Comorbidities, including learning disorders, conduct disorders, mood disorders, and in adolescents, substance use disorders, are fairly common. Most children with ADHD and a comorbid condition will benefit from specialist referral.

Conduct Disorder

Children with conduct disorder (CD) demonstrate a repetitive and persistent pattern of behavior that violates the rights of others and/or of societal norms and rules. They present to primary care physicians largely through complaints from schools, typically after serious disciplinary actions for misbehavior. These types of behaviors include:

- aggression toward other people and/or animals;
- deliberate destruction of other people's property;
- deceitfulness;
- theft; and/or
- serious violations of parental and/or school rules.

To qualify for this diagnosis, patients must manifest at least one of the above symptoms during the 6 months prior to assessment. Typically, children with CD have severe impairments in social, academic, and/or vocational functioning that begin before the age of 13. Once patients are older than 18, the differential diagnosis should include antisocial personality disorder.

There are two subtypes of CD based on the age at onset of the disorder. Childhood-onset subtype is characterized by the onset of at least one symptom prior to 10 years of age. These are typically males who display physical aggression toward others, have disturbed peer relationships, and may have had oppositional defiant disorder during early childhood. These patients are often very difficult to treat, and many of them develop antisocial personality disorder. Adolescent-onset subtype is characterized by the absence of any diagnostic criteria prior to 10 years of age. Compared with childhood-onset type, these patients tend to display less aggressive behaviors and usually have more normative peer relationships. They are less likely to have persistent problems or to develop antisocial personality disorder.

The prevalence of CD has increased over the last several decades. It is likely that the incidence is higher in urban settings than in rural settings. Rates vary widely depending on the population sampled. There appears to be an earlier average age of onset for boys than for girls. Prognosis is worse with childhood-onset subtype. The prevalence rates reported for boys range from 6% to 16% and for girls from 2% to 9%.

It is difficult to treat CD because the problem is usually firmly set within a troubled familial and/or other psychosocial context. Typically, the problem is approached through behavioral therapy. Although there have not been double-blind placebo-controlled studies, many physicians who treat CD use low-dose neuroleptics such as risperidone or olanzapine. The risks with these medications are quite low, and the benefits may be substantial. It appears that neuroleptic medications decrease affective reactivity in this group of patients. Occasionally there are comorbid disorders such as ADHD or major depression. If this is the case, the co-occurring disorder should also be treated.

Oppositional Defiant Disorder

Children with oppositional defiant disorder (ODD) manifest a pattern of negativistic, hostile, and defiant behavior toward authority figures lasting at least 6 months. As with the other disruptive behavior disorders, school troubles are often the impetus to seek medical care, although parents of children with ODD may be quite distressed by their child's rebellious behaviors. The specific behaviors listed in the DSM-IV include:

- loss of temper;
- arguing with adults;
- active defiance of adult requests;
- deliberate annoyance of other people;
- externalization of blame for his or her mistakes or misbehavior;
- touchiness or easy annoyance;
- frequent anger and resentment; and/or
- frequent spitefulness or vindictiveness.

These behavioral disturbances cause clinically significant impairment in the social, academic, or occupational functioning of patients with the diagnosis. ODD is not diagnosed in the context of a mood or a psychotic disorder and it cannot be diagnosed if CD is also present.

Prevalence rates range from 2% to 16%, depending on the nature of the population sample and the methods of measurement. Prior to puberty, males suffer from this disorder more frequently than females. After puberty, the male:female ratio evens out. The disorder is usually evident prior to the age of 8; only infrequently is the commencement later than early adolescence. The oppositional symptoms usually first emerge in the home setting. Over time, symptoms may appear at school or in the community. The onset is usually gradual, occurring over a period of months to years. Approximately 25% of children diagnosed with ODD no longer meet the criteria after several years, but many others worsen and are eventually diagnosed with conduct disorder.

The treatments for ODD include: first, identification of any other comorbid disorder that can be treated pharmacologically; second, appropriate educational placement; and third, behavioral therapy that involves both the patient and his family.

MOOD AND ANXIETY DISORDERS

Mood disorders in children and adolescents are classified just as they are in adult populations (see Chapter 7). Depressive disorders include major depression and dysthymic disorder. Bipolar disorders include bipolar I disorder, which is defined by the occurrence of a full manic episode, or bipolar II disorder, which includes the occurrence of a hypomanic episode. As a general class, juvenile mood disorders tend to be more severe and more refractory to pharmacologic interventions than adult-onset disorders. It is likely that this has to do with various genetic and familial factors. The prevalence of both unipolar depression and bipolar disorder increases with age.

A number of different anxiety disorders affect children. According to the DSM-IV, however, only separation anxiety disorder is classified as a childhood-onset anxiety disorder. The other anxiety disorders, including obsessive-compulsive disorder (OCD), posttraumatic stress disorder (PTSD), social phobia, and generalized anxiety disorder, occur relatively frequently during childhood; they also occur in adulthood. However, separation anxiety disorder is exceedingly rare in adults.

Major Depression

Case Vignette

Roy is a 16-year-old boy, a high school sophomore, who is brought to the physician because of weight loss. He describes having no appetite for the past 3 months since he broke up with his first girlfriend, and he has lost 15 pounds. He denies abdominal pain, change in bowel habits, or a wish to lose weight. He has been irritable and moody during this time, and he has stopped seeing most of his friends; he spends most weekends sleeping. His concentration has been poor, and his grades, normally As and Bs, have fallen to Cs and Ds for the first time. He admits that he has been smoking marijuana daily during the past 3 months; he had only tried it a few times in the past. He has no previous psychiatric history, and he had been in good physical health throughout childhood. Physical examination is normal. Mental status examination reveals a disheveled adolescent who is sulky and minimally cooperative. He is very preoccupied with the breakup, and he castigates himself for not being attractive enough to his girlfriend. He admits that he sees little future for himself and believes that there is no point in living without the relationship. He has thought about running his father's car in the garage with the door closed while his parents are away.

The physician seeks specialty consultation because of the severity of the depression, the risk of suicide, and the substance abuse comorbidity. His parents are told that he is suffering from a major depression, and they are referred to see a child psychiatrist the next day. They are advised not to leave their son alone until he is evaluated further regarding his suicide risk and the need for psychiatric hospitalization; they are asked to remove any firearms from the home until he is better.

Major depression is characterized by a 2-week period with a depressed or irritable mood and/or a markedly diminished interest or pleasure in all, or almost all, activities. In children and adolescents, irritability is at least as common as sadness. Other depressive symptoms include:

- changes in appetite and sleep;
- psychomotor agitation or retardation;
- decreased energy;
- feelings of worthlessness or inappropriate guilt;
- decreased ability for concentration; and
- recurrent thoughts of death and/or suicide.

Depression may manifest itself as a decrease in academic performance, school refusal, somatic complaints, and/or aggressive or antisocial behavior patterns that are more common presenting complaints than the mood disturbance itself. If any symptom is accompanied by apparent changes in mood, the clinician must attempt to elicit signs and symptoms of major depression. Psychosis (delusions or hallucinations, generally congruent with the mood) may accompany depression.

The prevalence of depression ranges from approximately 0.3% in preschoolers to as high as 5% in adolescents. There is an equal male:female ratio until puberty, at which point the adult pattern of 3:2 female:male ratio emerges.

Treatment of depression, even in younger children, often includes administration of an antidepressant medication. Older children and adolescents who are sufficiently motivated may be treated with cognitive-behavioral therapy. Medications of choice include all of the selective serotonin reuptake inhibitors (SSRIs) as well as tricyclics and other atypical antidepressants such as venlafaxine. The side effects most relevant to children and adolescents include insomnia and/or hypersomnolence, gastrointestinal disturbances, and agitation, which may interfere with concentration.

There is no evidence that early administration of antidepressants is associated with developmental risk. As a matter of fact, there is an emerging body of literature to support the idea that the longer a person remains depressed, the more difficult it is to treat the depression and the more likely it is that the patient will have recurrences of depressive episodes in the future. This body of work, then, would argue for early, aggressive treatment of depression.

Juvenile Bipolar Disorder

Juvenile bipolar disorder is an extremely rare diagnosis. It is characterized by the same symptomatology as is seen in adults. Symptoms include:

- euphoric or irritable mood;
- grandiosity;
- decreased need for sleep;
- pressured speech;
- racing thoughts;
- extreme distractibility;
- hypersexuality; and
- extremely poor judgment.

An attempt must be made to differentiate juvenile mania from ADHD, CD, major depression, or other psychotic disorders that may mimic the symptomatology of mania. Additionally, keep in mind that comorbidity is the rule rather than the exception with child and adolescent psychopathology. At times, juvenile mania may coexist with another disorder such as ADHD.

The drugs most commonly studied in children with bipolar disorder are divalproex and lithium. Either drug could be considered as first-line treatment. Both agents have significant risks associated with them, and it is sometimes difficult to decide which medication is preferable. Both cause weight gain, some cognitive slowing, and various metabolic problems. Liver functions must be monitored with divalproex, and there is concern regarding polycystic ovarian syndrome along with possible effects on fertility and androgynization in adolescent females. With lithium, there are problems with enuresis, frequent urination, and hypothyroidism. Both medications require regular monitoring of blood levels. Generally, bipolar children and adolescents should be referred to a child psychiatrist for care if available.

Separation Anxiety Disorder

Separation anxiety disorder manifests itself as excessive anxiety concerning separation from the home or from people to whom the patient is attached. The anxiety is beyond that which might be expected at any given developmental level. The disturbance must last for at least 4 weeks and it must cause clinically significant distress or impairment in social, academic, and other important areas of functioning. Children with this disorder are usually brought to primary care physicians because of their refusal to attend school, although occasionally the parents are troubled by the reluctance of the child to let them leave the home. Specific symptoms include:

- excessive distress when separation from home or major attachment figures occurs or is even anticipated;
- persistent worries about harm befalling major attachment figures;
- excessive concerns about events that might lead to separation such as getting lost or being kidnapped;
- persistent reluctance or refusal to attend school;
- intense reluctance to be alone at home or in other settings;
- persistent reluctance or refusal to go to sleep by oneself;
- repeated nightmares involving the theme of separation; and
- somatic complaints related to real or anticipated separations from attachment figures.

Separation anxiety disorder occurs in approximately 4% of school-age children and approximately 1% of adolescents. It occurs equally in boys and girls. Treatment for separation anxiety includes cognitive-behavioral therapy as well as various medications, most commonly benzodiazepines and SSRIs. There is good clinical evidence that both agents are effective. Benzodiazepines have a more rapid onset of action, but the tendency to cause sedation and cognitive slowing as well as the risk of dependence limit their use. SSRIs are just as effective as benzodiazepines. Although they may not work as rapidly, there is no risk of dependence and they do not appear to interfere with cognitive function.

Obsessive-Compulsive Disorder

Obsessive-compulsive disorder (OCD) in children presents as recurrent and distressing ideas that intrude on one's thoughts. To avoid obsessional thinking, children and adolescents engage in various repetitive and purposeful behaviors, referred to as compulsions. The types of thoughts that plague children who suffer from OCD typically include:

- fears of contamination;
- feelings of self-doubt; and
- feelings of guilt.

Compulsive behaviors include:

- checking;
- counting;
- hand washing; and
- touching.

The prevalence of OCD is 1% to 2% in the adult population. The prevalence in childhood and adolescence is likely to be the same. As with separation anxiety, treatment includes cognitive-behavioral therapy, which is usually very effective, in conjunction with pharmacologic treatment with SSRIs. The onset of OCD is sometimes seen after the occurrence of a streptococcal infection.

Posttraumatic Stress Disorder

Posttraumatic stress disorder (PTSD) occurs when children experience or witness a traumatic event and then develop anxiety-related symptoms subsequent to that trauma. The traumatic event typically involves actual or threatened death or serious injury or a threat to the physical integrity of self or others. Child abuse is a too-common precipitant of this disorder. The emotions that accompany this experience include intense fear and helplessness. Children typically manifest disorganized and/or agitated behavior during the event. There are three types of specific symptoms of reexperiencing the trauma: (1) reexperiencing of the event, (2) autonomic arousal, and (3) avoidance of any stimuli associated with the trauma. Children with PTSD often engage in repetitive play or traumatic reenactments, or they have extremely upsetting dreams without any recognizable content. The specific symptoms are listed in Table 5-4.

TABLE 5-4 PTSD Symptoms

Reexperiencing Symptoms
- Recurrent thoughts or perceptions

- Recurrent distressing dreams

- A sense of reliving the experience with various illusions, hallucinations, or dissociative flashback episodes

- Actual trauma-specific behavioral reenactments in children

- Psychological distress related to traumatic reminders

- Physiological distress related to traumatic reminders

Avoidance Symptoms
- Efforts to avoid thoughts

- Feelings or discussions associated with the trauma

- Avoidance of activities, places, or people associated with the trauma

- An inability to recall various aspects of the trauma

- Markedly diminished interest or participation in significant activities

- Feelings of detachment or estrangement

- Decreased range of affective experience

- A sense of a foreshortened future

Arousal Symptoms
- Insomnia

- Irritability

- Angry outbursts

- Impaired concentration

- Hypervigilance

- An exaggerated startle response

Many PTSD victims recover spontaneously, although it may take as long as 3 or 4 years for the symptoms to resolve. At least one third of individuals diagnosed with PTSD will continue to have the diagnosis 5 years after the traumatic incident. Treatment includes a variety of psychotherapeutic interventions that focus on providing a sense of safety, clarifying reality, and identifying support. Pharmacologic treatment includes SSRIs, venlafaxine, benzodiazepines, and various mood stabilizers.

Social Phobia

Social phobia, which is sometimes referred to as social anxiety disorder or avoidant disorder of childhood, is characterized by an exaggerated and persistent fear of social or performance situations in which embarrassment may occur. In most instances, exposure to these situations provokes an anxiety response that may take the form of a panic attack. Typically, the social or performance situation is avoided, although it is often tolerated with dread. The diagnosis of social phobia should be made only if the avoidance or fear interferes significantly with the patient's daily routine, educational functioning, or social life. In children and adolescents, the symptoms must persist for at least 6 months before social phobia is diagnosed.

Children tend to exhibit their fears by crying or maintaining physical proximity to familiar adults. They often appear shy and on the periphery of social situations. Because children are required to attend school, they are often unable to avoid the situations that cause their anxiety and/or unable to identify the source of the anxiety, which may manifest itself as crying, tantrums, freezing, or shrinking from social situations.

The incidence of social phobia ranges from 3% to 13%. Typically, onset is in the mid-teens, although there is often a childhood history of social inhibition and shyness. Occasionally the onset acutely follows a stressful or humiliating experience, but more often it is insidious. Social phobia is typically a lifelong problem, although the severity may vary depending on life stressors and demands. As with the other anxiety disorders, SSRIs are the pharmacologic treatment of choice. Venlafaxine, which has serotonergic activity, is also effective. Older children and adolescents may be candidates for cognitive-behavioral therapy in addition to or in place of medication.

Generalized Anxiety Disorder

Generalized anxiety disorder (GAD) is characterized by excessive anxiety present for at least 6 months. Children frequently worry about their ability to perform academically, socially, or athletically. The anxiety may also be focused on various catastrophic events. Patients with this diagnosis suffer from restlessness, fatigue, difficulty concentrating, irritability, muscle tension, and disturbed sleep. Physical complaints may lead to presentation for medical care, but recognition of the disorder can obviate the need for an extensive and fruitless medical workup. The intensity and/or frequency of the anxiety are out of proportion to the actual likelihood or impact of the feared events. Children with GAD are often excessively perfectionistic and they frequently seek reassurance from others that they have done well.

The prevalence rate for GAD is between 3% and 5%. As with social phobia, GAD is a lifelong problem, although the symptoms may wax and wane in association with environmental stressors. Treatment interventions include cognitive-behavioral psychotherapy and SSRIs.

PSYCHOTIC DISORDERS

Psychosis accompanies a variety of different diagnostic entities. The term refers to impaired reality testing accompanied by abnormal behavior. Positive symptoms include delusions, hallucinations, bizarre behavior, and thought disorder. Negative symptoms include inattention, anhedonia, apathy, avolition, and poverty of speech.

It is often challenging to assess psychosis in younger children. The differentiation of normal fantasies from delusions is difficult. Additionally, the cognitive structure of preschool and younger school-age children is often directly perception-bound, unmediated by more sophisticated interpretive processes. In psychotic children, however, thinking is extremely disordered. The diagnosis of psychosis should therefore be reserved for those children who are unable, even on careful questioning, to distinguish between fantasy and reality.

Psychotic children have visual hallucinations more commonly than do adults, although they usually occur in conjunction with auditory hallucinations. They may also become paranoid or suffer from delusions, but these delusions typically are less fixed than are the delusions of adults.

Childhood schizophrenia is a very rare disorder. It occurs in approximately 1 out of 10,000 children. The onset is typically insidious, and parents often do not recognize the slow deterioration in reality testing. The male:female ratio ranges from 3:1 to 5:1. Most children with psychotic symptoms during childhood have an affective disorder rather than schizophrenia.

Treatment requires administration of antipsychotic medications. Atypical neuroleptics, given their lower risk of tardive dyskinesia, are unquestionably first-line treatments (see Chapters 9 and 19). Other medications should be used to treat comorbid disorders such as depression or bipolar disorder.

PERVASIVE DEVELOPMENTAL DISORDERS

Children with pervasive developmental disorders (PDDs) suffer from severe and pervasive impairments in multiple areas of development, such as reciprocal social interaction skills; communication skills; or the presence of stereotyped behaviors, interests, and activities (see Table 5-5). These impairments deviate significantly from the patient's developmental level or mental age. PDDs are usually evident in the first few years of life, and they are often associated with some degree of mental retardation.

Autistic Disorder

Children with autistic disorder have qualitative impairments in social interaction and communication. They also demonstrate restricted repetitive and stereotyped patterns of behavior, interests, and activities. The onset of autism occurs prior to 3 years of age. The prevalence is from 0.02% to 0.05%, with a male:female ratio of 4:1. Autism rates are increasing for unclear reasons; multiple well-designed studies have refuted the hypothesis that vaccinations are the cause. Approximately 75% of children with autism suffer from mental retardation.

Asperger Disorder

Asperger disorder is similar to autism in terms of the deficits in social interactions and restricted repetitive and stereotyped patterns of behavior, interests, and activities. In

TABLE 5-5 PDD Symptoms and Signs

Impairments in Social Interactions
- Deficits in the use of multiple nonverbal behaviors such as eye-to-eye gaze, facial expression, body posture, and other physical gestures to regulate social interaction
- Failure to develop peer relationships appropriate to developmental level
- Lack of spontaneous seeking to share enjoyment, interests, or achievements with other people
- Lack of social or emotional reciprocity

Impairments in Communication
- Delays, sometimes profound, in the development of spoken language
- In individuals with adequate speech, marked impairment in the ability to initiate or sustain conversation
- Stereotyped and repetitive use of language or idiosyncratic language
- Lack of varied, spontaneous, make-believe play or social imitative play appropriate to development level

Repetitive Behaviors and Interests
- Preoccupation with one or more stereotyped patterns of interest that is abnormal either in intensity or focus
- Inflexible adherence to specific, nonfunctional routines or rituals
- Stereotyped and repetitive motor mannerisms, such as hand-flapping or complex whole body movements
- Persistent preoccupation with parts of objects

contrast to autism, there is no delay in language or cognitive development. Additionally, there are no clinically significant delays in the development of self-help skills, adaptive behavior, or curiosity about the environment.

Rett Disorder

Rett disorder is similar to autism except that these individuals function normally until approximately 5 months of life. Between the ages of 5 and 48 months, head growth decelerates, previously acquired purposeful hand skills are lost, and characteristic stereotyped hand movements resembling hand-wringing or hand washing develop. Interest in the social environment diminishes in the first few years after onset of the disorder, although social interaction may develop later. Typically there are problems in the coordination of gait or trunk movements as well as severe impairments in expressive and receptive language and severe psychomotor retardation. Rett disorder is usually associated with severe or profound mental retardation. This is an extremely rare condition and has only been reported in females.

Childhood Disintegrative Disorder

Childhood disintegrative disorder is similar to autism except that the autistic symptoms develop after at least 2 years of apparently normal development. After the first 2 years and before age 10, there is a clinically significant loss of previously acquired skills in at least two of the following areas: expressive or receptive language, social skills or adaptive behavior, bowel or bladder control, play, or motor skills. Subsequently, patients with childhood disintegrative disorder look very much like children with autistic disorder; they have qualitative impairments in social interaction and communication and repetitive and stereotyped patterns of behavior, interests, and activities.

For all pervasive developmental disorders, treatment is typically multidisciplinary and should include behavioral, occupational, speech, and language therapy. Appropriate placement in an individualized school program is also vitally important. As with other child and adolescent psychiatric disorders, there is a great deal of comorbidity. The recognition and treatment of comorbid disorders is very important. Pharmacologic interventions should be targeted at specific symptoms. Atypical antipsychotics, SSRIs, and psychomotor stimulants have all been helpful.

OTHER NEURODEVELOPMENTAL DISORDERS

The disorders portrayed in this section are characterized by long-term difficulties with adaptation that result from various CNS abnormalities that have not been clearly identified.

Mental Retardation

The essential feature of mental retardation is significantly subaverage general intellectual functioning that is accompanied by significant limitations in adaptive functioning in at least two of the following areas: communication, self-care, home living, social/interpersonal skills, use of community resources, self-direction, functional academic skills, work, leisure, health, and safety. The onset must occur prior to 18 years of age.

General intellectual function is typically measured by IQ testing. Mental retardation is divided into the following categories based on severity:

- *Mild mental retardation* refers to IQs between 70 and approximately 50. Children with mild mental retardation are capable of developing social and communication skills, and they can function relatively normally as adults.
- *Moderate mental retardation* is defined by IQs between approximately 50 and 55 and 35 and 40. Children with moderate mental retardation have limited social awareness. They can be trained to care for most personal needs, but they will require sheltered job placements as well as moderate supervision during adulthood.
- Children with *severe mental retardation* have IQs between 35 and 40 and 20 and 25. Severely retarded children typically have slow motor development and very limited speech. They will require close supervision throughout their life span.
- Children with *profound mental retardation* have IQs below 20 to 25. They have very poor cognitive skills, almost no social capacities, and typically require help with activities of daily living. Profoundly mentally retarded individuals typically require almost constant supervision in special care settings.

Genetic factors as well as a variety of environmental agents during intrauterine development (infection, alcohol exposure, etc) are risk factors for the development of mental retardation. Mild mental retardation is by far the most common type. As the severity of retardation increases, its frequency diminishes.

There are no specific medications for mental retardation. Pharmacologic treatment should be targeted at specific behavioral symptoms or comorbid disorders such as ADHD, depression, mania, aggression, or psychosis.

Learning Disorders

In previous editions of the DSM, the category of learning disorders was referred to as *academic skills disorders*. Learning disorders are diagnosed when an individual's achievement in reading, mathematics, or written expression is substantially below that expected for age, schooling, and/or measured intelligence. The difference between achievement and IQ must be at least 2 standard deviations below the mean. Learning disorders are typically diagnosed during or after first grade when academic expectations increase. Learning disorders are important to identify because children with these disorders have a school dropout rate that is approximately 1.5 times the average. The prevalence of learning disorders ranges from 2% to 10%, with approximately 5% of all school-age children carrying a learning disorder diagnosis. Treatment involves appropriate educational interventions for the specific learning disability.

Reading disorder was previously called *dyslexia*. The prevalence of this disorder is approximately 4% of school-age children, with a male:female ratio of 4:1. Mathematics disorder has a lower prevalence; it occurs equally in males and females and is manifested by decreased skills in understanding, recognizing, copying, and following mathematical terms, symbols, figures, and operations. The prevalence of disorders of written expression is not known. All three learning disorders often occur simultaneously.

Communication Disorders

Disorders of communication interfere with academic achievement and/or social communication. Treatment typically includes appropriate school placement as well as speech therapy.

Expressive language disorder. Expressive language disorder is manifested by scores on standardized measures of expressive language development that are substantially below those obtained from measures of both intellectual capacity and receptive language development. As noted previously, these language difficulties interfere with academic achievement and social communication. The differential diagnosis includes pervasive developmental disorder, but children with expressive language disorder, despite their paucity of speech, typically have a normal capacity for reciprocal social interactions. Expressive language disorder is usually recognized by age 3; the outcome is variable. Approximately 50% of children appear to outgrow their problems; the other half has more long-lasting difficulties. Nevertheless, most children with this problem ultimately acquire normal language abilities by late adolescence, although subtle expressive deficits may persist.

There are two types of expressive language disorder: acquired type, in which the impairment occurs after a period of normal development as the result of a neurological or medical condition, and developmental type, in which the impairment is not associated with any obvious etiology. The prevalence for the developmental type is approximately 3% to 5%.

Mixed receptive-expressive language disorder. Mixed receptive-expressive language disorder combines the symptoms of expressive language disorder with a receptive language deficit. These individuals have difficulty expressing themselves as well as difficulty understanding words and sentences. This disorder is slightly less common than expressive language disorder. The prevalence is approximately 3%.

Phonological disorder. Children with phonological disorder have difficulty with speech production. The prevalence of moderate to severe symptoms is 2% to 3% in 6- and 7-year-olds, but by late adolescence the prevalence decreases to 0.5%.

Stuttering. Stuttering is characterized by disturbances in the normal fluency and time patterning of speech, ie, sound and syllable repetitions, sound prolongations, interjections, broken words, audible or silent blocking, circumlocutions (word substitutions to avoid problematic words), words produced with an excess of physical tension, and monosyllabic whole-word repetitions. Interestingly, patients who stutter when they talk can often sing fluently. The disorder begins between ages 2 and 7 with a peak at approximately 5 years of age. Most cases present before age 10. The prevalence of this disorder is approximately 1% in prepubertal children and 0.8% in adolescents. Males are more frequently affected, with a ratio of approximately 3:1.

The onset of stuttering is usually insidious, and children with this problem are usually not initially aware of it; over many months episodic, unnoticed speech dysfluencies become a more chronic problem. Initially, there are problems with repetition of initial consonants, words that are usually the first words of a phrase, or long words. The disorder typically waxes and wanes. Somewhere between 60% and 80% of individuals with stuttering recover either spontaneously or with speech therapy. There is evidence that genetics play a role in the etiology of stuttering. The risk among first-degree biological relatives is more than three times that of the general population.

Developmental Coordination Disorder

Developmental coordination disorder is characterized by a marked impairment in the development of motor coordination that interferes with academic achievement or activities of daily living. The coordination difficulties are not due to a general medical condition, and the criteria are not met for pervasive developmental disorder. Younger children are typically clumsy and may be delayed in achieving developmental motor milestones. Older children have difficulty with fine motor coordination, handwriting, building models, and participating in athletics. The prevalence has been estimated to be as high as 6% for children ages 5 through 11. The course of this condition is variable, and many individuals continue to have difficulty with coordination throughout adolescence and adulthood. Occupational and physical therapy are the treatments of choice.

FEEDING, EATING, AND ELIMINATION DISORDERS

Encopresis

Encopresis refers to the repeated passage of feces into inappropriate places either intentionally or involuntarily. These events must occur at least once a month for at least 3 months. The diagnosis is not made in children under the age of 4. Fecal incontinence must not be due to a medical condition. Encopresis can occur with or without constipation and overflow incontinence. Children with primary encopresis have never been toilet trained. Children with secondary encopresis have regressed after toilet training. The prevalence of this disorder is approximately 1% in 5-year-olds and then decreases with age. It is more common in boys than girls.

Treatment usually combines medical and behavioral interventions. When children have constipation and overflow incontinence, they typically require laxatives and/or enemas prior to beginning a course of treatment, which includes a high-bulk diet with various behavioral reinforcers.

Enuresis

Enuresis is characterized by repeated voiding of urine during the day or night into the bed or clothing. Most frequently, this is involuntary. To qualify for the diagnosis, the episodes must occur at least twice a week for at least 3 months, and children should be older than 5 years. Urinary incontinence due to physiological effects of medications or general medical conditions is not classified as enuresis. Enuresis may be nocturnal, diurnal, or both. As with encopresis, enuresis can also be primary or secondary. The prevalence of this disorder varies with age. Seven percent of 5-year-old boys and 3% of 5-year-old girls are enuretic. One percent of 18-year-old boys and less than 1% of 18-year-old girls are enuretic. Approximately 75% of all children with enuresis have a first-degree biological relative who has had the disorder. The concordance rate for this disorder is greater in monozygotic than in dizygotic twins.

Most children with enuresis become continent by adolescence. The rate of spontaneous remission is between 5% and 10% per year after the age of 5. Treatment includes both behavioral therapies and medication. The most common behavioral interventions use the bell-and-pad technique. Imipramine and vasopressin (ddAVP) have also been shown to be very effective, but the enuresis usually recurs when the medication is discontinued until there is a spontaneous, age-related remission. Nevertheless, pharmacologic interventions are often very helpful, especially in short-term situations such as sleepovers and/or summer camp.

Pica

Pica is the persistent ingestion of nonnutritional substances for at least 1 month. The behavior must be developmentally and culturally inappropriate. Pica is often associated with mental retardation, poverty, and nutritional deficiencies. Behavioral techniques are the treatments of choice.

Rumination Disorder

Rumination disorder involves the repeated regurgitation and rechewing of food, occurring for at least 1 month following a period of normal eating. This disorder is typically associated with neglect and/or developmental delay. It develops between the ages of 3 and 12 months and often remits spontaneously. Note that mortality rates as high as 25% have been reported for this disorder. This condition is extremely rare. Treatment should address the medical consequences of the illness, including dehydration and malnutrition, as well as the etiology (neglect and/or developmental delay).

Feeding Disorder of Infancy and Early Childhood

Feeding disorder of infancy and early childhood, also referred to as *failure to thrive,* is characterized by a failure to eat, which leads to an inability to gain weight or a significant loss of weight over a 1-month period. The disorder must be present before 6 years of age, but the usual presentation is during the first year of life. This disorder may be associated with problems in the infant-caregiver relationship, and treatment should address attachment issues.

TIC DISORDERS

Tics are rapid, recurrent, nonrhythmic stereotyped motor movements or vocalizations. They are categorized as motor or vocal and as simple or complex. A complex tic seems to be more purposeful and/or imitative than a simple tic. Although they are involuntary movements, tics can be voluntarily suppressed, at least for brief periods of time. Anxiety and stress typically exacerbate tics; sleep and engagement in interesting activities often lead to a decrease in these behaviors.

Tourette Syndrome

Tourette syndrome is characterized by multiple motor tics and at least one vocal tic at some point during the illness. The tics occur many times a day, usually every day, for at least 1 year. There is never a tic-free period of more than 3 consecutive months. Tourette syndrome leads to impairment in social and/or academic functioning. The prevalence of this disorder is approximately 0.05%. It is three times more common in males than females. Onset occurs before the age of 18, with a median age of onset of approximately 7 years. Motor tics usually present prior to vocal tics. Tourette syndrome is commonly associated with OCD, ADHD, and various anxiety disorders. The most effective treatments include atypical neuroleptics, clonidine, and guanfacine.

Chronic Motor or Vocal Tic Disorder

Chronic motor or vocal tic disorder is similar to Tourette syndrome except that the children have either motor or vocal tics, but not both. This disorder is somewhat more common than Tourette syndrome. It has a prevalence of 1% to 2% in school-age children, and it is more common in boys. In transient tic disorder, the symptoms are single or multiple motor and/or vocal tics that occur for at least 4 weeks but no longer than 12 months. Symptoms usually remit without treatment.

OTHER DISORDERS OF CHILDHOOD

Selective Mutism

Children who suffer from selective mutism will not speak in specific social situations even though their speech is fluent when they are at home with their families. In the uncomfortable social setting, communication usually occurs nonverbally, with eye contact and/or head nodding. To qualify for this diagnosis, the symptoms must be present for at least 1 month. Selective mutism is associated with anxiety and shyness. It is quite uncommon, occurring in less than 1% of children. Effective treatments include cognitive-behavioral therapy and the use of SSRIs.

Reactive Detachment Disorder

Reactive detachment disorder of infancy and early childhood is characterized by a disturbed and developmentally inappropriate ability to relate socially. There are two subtypes of this disorder. In the inhibited type, the child fails to initiate or respond to social interactions; in the disinhibited type, the child is indiscriminately social as manifested by diffuse, superficial attachments. The usual etiology is some form of pathological childcare, either emotional and/or physical neglect or repeated changes in the primary caregiver. The symptoms of this disorder present prior to 5 years of age. Treatment consists of establishing a consistent placement and then working with the caregiver and infant to establish a more secure attachment.

CHILD ABUSE AND NEGLECT

The congressionally mandated Third National Incidence Study of Child Abuse and Neglect, conducted in 1993 and based on a nationally representative sample of more than 5600 professionals in 842 agencies, found that there was a substantial increase in the incidence of child abuse and neglect between 1986 and 1993. Physical abuse nearly doubled, and sexual abuse more than doubled, as did emotional abuse, physical neglect, and emotional neglect. Hundreds of thousands of children are abused each year, primarily by a parent or close relative. Thousands are seriously injured.

From an epidemiological perspective, girls are at a three times greater risk for sexual abuse; boys are at greater risk for emotional neglect and serious physical injury. Children of single parents had a 77% greater risk of physical abuse, an 87% greater risk of harm by physical neglect, and an 80% greater risk of serious injury or harm than children living with both parents. Because the likelihood of abuse varies directly with the severity of psychosocial stressors, it is not surprising that children from families with annual incomes below $15,000 were between 22 and 25 times more likely to experience some form of maltreatment than children from families with an annual income greater than $30,000. Additionally, children from the lowest income families were 18 times more likely to be sexually abused.

Those who survive are likely to be emotionally scarred by their experiences. Many suffer from PTSD, but many others do not manifest the full clinical syndrome. Instead, victims of physical abuse may manifest a wide variety of problems with self-esteem, sexual acting-out, deficits in the capacity to trust other people, aggressive behavior, anger and rage, self-injurious behavior, extreme passivity, anxiety and various fears, depression, school refusal or failure, flashbacks, nightmares, or substance abuse. Victims of sexual abuse may show an unusual preoccupation with (or avoidance of) sexual topics, seductiveness, statements that their bodies are dirty or damaged, physical complaints related to the genital or anal area, secretiveness, social withdrawal, school refusal, or many of the signs and symptoms associated with physical abuse.

Early recognition and treatment are important to minimize the long-term effects of physical or sexual abuse. However, such maltreatment is often difficult to recognize because: (1) victims are reluctant to come forward for fear of increasing their own risk of further harm; (2) victims have ambivalent feelings about the perpetrator, who is frequently a family member; and (3) the emotional damage often does not surface until adolescence or even adulthood. Given the reluctance of victims to come forward, the clinician must make a special effort to help the child feel safe so that he or she can talk freely. In every case, the primary care provider must keep in mind that he or she is a "mandatory reporter." This means that he or she is legally mandated to report any suspicion of abuse to the local child protective authorities so that they can conduct a comprehensive investigation.

The first step in treatment is to recognize the abuse and then take measures to protect the child from further harm. The most reasonable thing to do is refer the child and family to a mental health professional who can provide additional assessment and symptomatic treatment with medication, individual psychotherapy, and family therapy. With protection and appropriate treatment, abuse victims can regain a sense of self-confidence and trust.

SUMMARY

Childhood psychiatric disorders are very common. Their evaluation typically requires historical information from several sources (child, parents, school, etc) as well as a careful, developmentally mindful examination of the child. Treatment planning must take into account the differences in drug handling between children and adults and the critical importance of the child's psychosocial system in his life. Many common disorders can be managed in primary care settings. However, less common illnesses, the presence of comorbid conditions, or increased severity of illness often warrant coordinated care between the primary care physician and a specialist.

ADDITIONAL READINGS

American Academy of Child and Adolescent Psychiatry. Practice parameters for the assessment and treatment of children, adolescents, and adults with attention-deficit/hyperactivity disorder. *J Am Acad Child Adolescent Psychiatry*. 1997;36(Oct suppl):85S-121S.

American Academy of Child and Adolescent Psychiatry. Practice parameters for the assessment and treatment of children and adolescents with anxiety disorders. *J Am Acad Child Adolescent Psychiatry*. 1997;369(Oct suppl):69S-84S.

American Academy of Child and Adolescent Psychiatry. Practice parameters for the assessment and treatment of children and adolescents with schizophrenia. *J Am Acad Child and Adolescent Psychiatry*. 2001;40(July suppl):4S-23S.

American Psychiatric Association. *Diagnostic and Statistical Manual of Mental Disorders*. 4th ed. Washington, DC: American Psychiatric Press; 2000.

Dulcan M, Lizarralde C, Dubovsky S, eds. *Helping Parents, Youth, and Teachers Understand Medications for Behavioral and Emotional Problems: A Resource Book of Medication Information Handouts*. 2nd ed. Washington, DC: American Psychiatric Press; 2002.

Klykylo WM, Kay J, Rube D. *Clinical Child Psychiatry*. Philadelphia, Pa: WB Saunders Co; 1998.

Kutcher S, ed. *Practical Child and Adolescent Psychopharmacology*. New York, NY: Cambridge University Press; 2002.

Lewis M. *Child and Adolescent Psychiatry: A Comprehensive Textbook*. Baltimore, Md: Lippincott Williams & Wilkins; 2002.

Chapter **6**

Addictive Disorders

Robert M. Swift, MD, PhD
Norman S. Miller, MD
David C. Lewis, MD

Alcohol and drug abuse and dependence are common problems in American society. The Epidemiological Catchment Area Study, a community survey of mental health and substance abuse disorders in nearly 20,000 adult Americans, identified a 13.5% lifetime prevalence of alcohol abuse or dependence and a 7% prevalence of drug dependence. The high prevalence of alcohol, tobacco, and drug use is associated with considerable morbidity and mortality. Each year, alcoholism is estimated to cause 100,000 excess deaths; illicit drug abuse, 19,000 excess deaths; and tobacco, 400,000 excess deaths. Alcohol dependence and drug dependence are responsible for many psychological and social problems, including family dysfunction, domestic violence, and child abuse. Alcohol use and drug use are major causes of accidents and violent crime. Approximately 50% of motor vehicle fatalities are alcohol related.

The economic impact of drug and alcohol use is substantial and compares to that of diabetes and stroke. It is estimated that the total yearly cost to the US economy from alcohol and drug abuse and dependence is $276 billion. Of this, almost $40 billion are attributed to direct health care costs of hospitals, treatment centers, nursing homes, and professional services. Alcoholism and drug dependence are associated with 25% to 50% of all general hospital admissions and 50% to 75% of psychiatric admissions and contribute to complications and increased costs in those admitted to hospitals for other reasons. A government survey of treatment programs found more than 940,000 persons are in active treatment in specialized alcohol and drug treatment programs on any given day: 37% are in treatment for alcoholism, 25% for drug addiction, and 38% for both.

Like many chronic illnesses, addictive disorders are characterized by exacerbations and remissions. However, clinical outcome studies confirm that treatments for alcohol and drug addiction can be as effective as treatments for other medical disorders. The treatment of addictive disorders is also cost effective and can result in significant savings in total health care costs. Approximately $7 are saved for every dollar invested in treatment.

For all of these reasons, it is imperative for primary care physicians to correctly diagnose and treat addictive disorders in their patients. The best way to reduce the medical, social, and economic impact of substance abuse and dependence is through prevention and treatment. Treatment requires the ability to properly assess and diagnose substance abuse and dependence, knowledge about therapies for the acute management of intoxicated or withdrawing patients, and knowledge regarding long-term treatment and rehabilitation. A treatment plan that is practical and based on well-established principles should be negotiated with the patient.

Optimally, treatment should be individualized and match the patient to the best treatment for his or her problem type and severity, although realistically, such services may not be available due to lack of resources. Because substance abuse and dependence are chronic, relapsing disorders and treatment often require several treatment episodes before a successful outcome is achieved; primary care physicians and other health care providers must be aware of the most effective interventions and treatments for their patients.

This chapter discusses the diagnosis and treatment of substance abuse and dependence in the primary care setting, first reviewing aspects common to all addictive disorders and then examining issues pertinent to specific drug classes.

GENERAL PRINCIPLES

All medical disorders, including addictive disorders, should be considered as having a biopsychosocial etiology. For both addictive disorders and classic "medical" disorders, such as diabetes and hypertension, genetically determined biological influences and psychosocial influences determine the onset and course of a disorder in a specific individual. Unfortunately, the biological basis of addictive disorders is often minimized, and addictive disorders are not seen as true medical illnesses by some.

Dependence, Tolerance, and Addiction

The concept of addictive disorders is complicated by philosophical questions of whether use of potentially addictive substances constitutes a medical or a moral condition. Although many psychoactive substances (eg, alcohol) are used for medicinal, social, recreational, and religious purposes, established diagnostic principles and practices delineate where acceptable use ends and disordered use begins. Individuals using psychoactive substances to excess, in an uncontrolled fashion, in situations that are not socially approved, or to the detriment of physical and mental health should be considered to have a substance use disorder.

The language used to describe substance use disorders can be misleading because words applied to addiction are used to describe other conditions. The commonly used term *abuse* is pejorative and implies unethical conduct and does not necessarily connote a disease state, as such. *Dependence*, a term derived from pharmacology, describes the withdrawal that occurs after cessation of chronic drug use. *Tolerance* refers to the process by which the physical or behavioral effects of a constant dose of a drug decrease over time or when a greater amount of the substance is required to produce the same effect. Dependence and tolerance occur with many pharmacological agents (eg, beta-blockers, antidepressants), in addition to addictive substances. The term *addiction* is preferred by organizations such as the American Society of Addiction Medicine (ASAM) and the American Academy of Addiction Psychiatry (AAAP) to describe the loss of control over the use of alcohol and drugs that is generated by neurobiological changes produced by alcohol and drugs.

To address these issues, organizations such as the American Psychiatric Association (APA) and the World Health Organization (WHO) have applied specific diagnostic criteria to problem psychoactive substance use and consider them to be medical disorders. The criteria for substance-related disorders in the APA's *Diagnostic and Statistical Manual of Mental Disorders*, fourth edition, Text Revision (DSM-IV-TR), and the *International Classification of Diseases*, version 10 (ICD-10) of the WHO represent the manifestations of addictive use of alcohol and drugs and include psychological and social dysfunction, in addition to tolerance and dependence.

Classification of Addictive Disorders

The DSM-IV classifies the acute and chronic effects of psychoactive substances under two major categories: substance use disorders and substance-induced disorders. The two substance use disorders are substance dependence and substance abuse. The diagnostic criteria for conditions are shown in Table 6-1.

Substance-induced disorders include the behavioral and neurological effects of acute and chronic drug use. These are substance intoxication, substance withdrawal,

TABLE 6-1 Classification of Addictive Disorders

Substance dependence: A maladaptive pattern of substance use with the association of substance use with uncontrolled use or with use in spite of adverse consequences. Abuse is a residual category that describes patterns of drug use that do not meet the criteria for dependence.

Substance abuse: A maladaptive pattern of substance use that causes clinically significant impairment. This may include impairments in social, family, or occupational functioning, in the presence of a psychological or physical problem or in situations where use of the substance is physically hazardous, such as driving while intoxicated.

Diagnosis: Diagnosing substance dependence requires the occurrence of at least three of the following conditions over a 12-month period of time:

- Tolerance, ie, the need for increased amounts of the substance in order to achieve in-toxication or other desired effect, or markedly diminished effect with use of the same amount of substance.

- Characteristic withdrawal symptoms (may not apply to cannabis, hallucinogens, or PCP) or the use of the substance (or a closely related substitute) to relieve or avoid withdrawal.

- Substance often taken in larger amounts or over a longer period of time than the person intended.

- Persistent desire or one or more unsuccessful attempts to cut down or to control substance use.

- A great deal of time spent in activities necessary to get the substance (eg, theft), taking the substance (eg, chain-smoking), or recovering from its effects.

- Important social, occupational, or recreational activities given up or reduced because of substance use.

- Continued substance use despite knowledge of having a persistent or recurrent social, psychological, or physical problem that is caused by or exacerbated by use of the substance.

Adapted with permission from: *Diagnostic and Statistical Manual of Mental Disorders.* 4th ed, text revision. Copyright 2000. American Psychiatric Association.

substance-induced psychotic disorder, substance-induced mood disorder, substance-induced anxiety, substance-induced sleep disorder, substance-induced persisting demen-tia (and amnestic) disorders, and substance-induced sexual dysfunction. These disorders are described in Table 6-2.

Eleven distinct classes of psychoactive substances are designated by DSM-IV: alcohol; amphetamine or related substances; caffeine; cannabis; cocaine; hallucinogens; inhalants; opioids; nicotine; phencyclidine or related substances; and sedatives, hypnotics, or anxi-olytics. Each class is associated with both an organic mental disorder and a substance use disorder. Under the category of substance use disorders, 10 classes (all but nicotine) are associated with abuse and dependence; dependence only is defined for nicotine. Polysub-stance dependence is defined as using three or more substance categories. A category for other substance use disorders includes use of anabolic steroids, nitrate inhalants, anti-cholinergic agents, and other substances.

TABLE 6-2 Classification of Substance-Induced Disorders

- *Substance intoxication.* Reversible, substance-specific physiological and behavioral changes due to recent exposure to a psychoactive substance. Produced by all substances.

- *Substance withdrawal.* A substance-specific syndrome that develops following cessation of, or reduction in dosage of, a regularly used substance. Occurs with chronic use of all substances, except perhaps cannabis and hallucinogens.

- *Substance-induced delirium (confusion, psychosis).* Occurs with overdose of many substances.

- *Substance-induced psychotic disorder (psychosis).* May occur with PCP and hallucinogens, stimulants, cannabis, and alcohol.

- *Substance-induced mood disorder (depression, mania) or anxiety.* Common with many substances, especially alcohol and stimulants. Disorder must be distinguished from primary psychiatric disorder that preceded drug use.

- *Substance-induced sleep disorder.* A sleep disturbance attributable to acute or chronic substance use. Common with alcohol, sedatives, and stimulants.

- *Substance-induced persisting dementia (and amnestic) disorders.* A substance-specific syndrome of cognitive dysfunction that persists after acute intoxication or withdrawal abates.

- *Substance-induced sexual dysfunction.* Alcohol, benzodiazepines, and opioids commonly reduce sexual responsiveness and performance.

The Causes of Addictive Disorders

Studies of individuals with addictive disorders or at risk for developing the disorders have identified many factors that foster the development and continuance of substance use. Genetic, familial, environmental, occupational, socioeconomic, cultural, personality, life stress, psychiatric comorbidity, biological, social learning, behavioral, and conditioning factors have all been proposed to influence the development of addictive disorders. The relative contributions of any of these factors vary from individual to individual, and no single factor accounts for all of the risk; ie, there is no "addictive personality," nor are all addicts seeking to treat underlying psychiatric disorders.

The influence of genetic factors in addiction is elucidated best for alcohol. The children of alcoholics (especially males) are several times more likely to become alcoholic than are the children of nonalcoholics. The increased risk of alcoholism exists regardless of whether children are raised by their biological parents or by nonalcoholic foster parents, indicating the importance of genetic factors. Children of alcoholics are also more susceptible to other drug dependence. A genetic predisposition for alcoholism also is supported by twin studies; the concordance for alcoholism among monozygotic twins is twice that for dizygotic twins. However, it should be emphasized that environmental factors also influence the development of alcoholism; 30% of identical twins of male alcoholics do not become alcoholic.

Factors proposed to account for the genetic predisposition for alcoholism include genetic variations in the rate of metabolism of ethanol and acetaldehyde; differences in brain electrophysiology; differential sensitivity to the intoxicating effects of alcohol; and altered cell membrane properties. The identification of specific genes that predispose or protect one from developing alcoholism is actively being investigated. Some genetic marker studies suggest that alcoholism is associated with the presence of a certain sub-type of the dopamine receptor D2; other studies suggest associations with genes control-ling serotonergic and neuropeptide Y systems.

DIAGNOSING ADDICTIVE DISORDERS

Studies of physician behavior consistently show that physicians diagnose addictive disor-ders at rates much lower than the prevalence of these disorders in the population. As discussed at the beginning of this chapter, undiagnosed addictive disorders lead to con-siderable morbidity and social costs. Thus, correctly diagnosing addictive disorders is important to identify substance abuse problems that require intervention and treatment. A proper diagnosis is also necessary in order to obtain authorization for treatment and payment for treatment from third-party payers.

Taking a Substance Use History

All patients should be screened for alcohol, drug, and tobacco use as part of the routine medical history and examination. Although some patients present with a chief complaint of substance use, most present with medical or surgical problems and only later reveal a substance use disorder. Some patients are unaware of the problematic nature of their sub-stance use, and others are reluctant to report drug and alcohol use out of shame or fear of consequences. In severe dependence there is often resistance by the patient and those affected by the patient to consider that drugs and alcohol can be problematic.

A supportive, therapeutic relationship is the best way to elicit accurate information. In the context of this relationship, the physician should conduct a detailed alcohol and drug history and a physical and mental status examination, order and interpret necessary labo-ratory tests, and meet with family or significant others to obtain additional information. To obtain information about the patient's alcohol and drug use, many clinicians routinely ask questions about quantity and frequency of use of psychoactive substances, such as How much? and How often? Although this type of question can be effective for detecting substance abuse or dependence in mild to moderate use pattern, it is less effective in heavy users. A more effective method explores whether the patient has experienced dele-terious social or behavioral consequences from psychoactive substances or has poor con-trol of use. Several formalized interviews have been developed that discriminate alcoholism using these criteria.

The CAGE questionnaire is a simple four-item test that uses the letters C-A-G-E as a mnemonic for questions about alcohol use (Table 6-3). A positive answer to more than two questions is considered suspicious for alcohol abuse. The CAGE may be a better predictor of alcoholism in medical patients than laboratory tests. It is often adapted to drug use, as well.

Several other screening instruments are available to the primary care physician. The Michigan Alcohol Screening Test (MAST) is a widely used 25-item scale that assesses for alcohol and drug use through social and behavioral consequences. A shortened 10-item test, the Brief MAST, has similar efficacy in diagnosing alcoholism. Another screening in-strument for alcohol use is the Alcohol Use Disorders Identification Test (AUDIT), devel-oped by the WHO for a multinational project; it is effective in screening patients and

TABLE 6-3 The CAGE Screening Tool
• Have you ever felt the need to **C**ut down on drinking (or drugs)?
• Have you ever felt **A**nnoyed by criticisms of drinking (or drugs)?
• Have you ever had **G**uilty feelings about drinking (or using drugs)?
• Have you ever taken a morning **E**ye opener (or used drugs to get going in the morning)?

nonpatients for problem drinking. An interview that addresses the behavioral consequences of drug abuse is the Drug Abuse Screening Test (DAST).

Other items in the medical history that should increase suspicion about substance use include divorce, problems at work (job loss, tardiness, absenteeism, and work-related injuries), injuries (falls, auto accidents, and fights), arrests, driving while intoxicated, leisure activities involving drugs or alcohol, and financial problems. Having an alcohol- or drug-abusing biological parent or spouse increases the risk for substance use.

In obtaining a history of alcohol intake and related consequences, a careful screen for other drugs and, vice versa, alcohol use in a history of drug intake is mandatory. Studies indicate that a high percentage of alcoholics, particularly those under the age of 30, use at least one other drug regularly, excluding nicotine. The harmful use of alcohol by the drug addict is also common—50% to 75% of heroin addicts, 80% of cocaine addicts, and 40% of cannabis addicts are heavy users of alcohol.

The Physical and Mental Status Examination

The physical examination provides important information about the presence of substance use and its medical complications. There are many physical stigmata of substance use specific to the drug used or the route of administration. These include a necrotic nasal septum from cocaine abuse, peripheral neuropathy from solvent inhalation, signs of liver disease or gastrointestinal bleeding from alcoholism, tachycardia and weight loss from chronic stimulant use, and tremor and agitation from caffeine use. Heavy users of alcohol, sedatives, opioids, cannabis, and stimulants may show general physical debilitation. Smokers of cocaine, nicotine, and cannabis may manifest respiratory and oropharyngeal problems. Intravenous drug users may show track marks from intravenous injection and signs and symptoms of HIV-related illnesses and hepatitis B or C. Repeated trauma, especially to the head, is strongly suggestive of substance abuse.

All patients should receive a mental status examination to assess cognitive and psychiatric function. Psychiatric disorders such as mood, anxiety, attention deficit, and personality disorders frequently coexist with substance abuse disorders. Mental status testing can elicit deficits in memory, concentration, and abstract reasoning. If abnormalities are found, formal neuropsychological testing can quantify deficits in attention, cognition, and performance.

Laboratory and Toxicological Screening for Substance Use

Serum and urine toxicological screens have an important role in assessing and treating patients with substance use disorders. Physicians must be aware of how to properly conduct testing and interpret test results. Informed consent should be obtained for all drug testing. Because substances may be differentially distributed in body fluids, the laboratory should be queried as to whether urine or serum should be collected. To minimize collection errors, obtain all samples under direct observation. Positive test results should be confirmed by a second test using a different analytical method, because chemically similar compounds in foods or medications may yield false-positive results under certain analytic methods. A positive test suggests use of a psychoactive substance but may not indicate the extent of use, when it occurred, or whether there was behavioral impairment.

Because alcohol has a short half-life (approximately 1 ounce of ingested alcohol is metabolized per hour), it is difficult to detect unless patients are currently intoxicated. Breath, blood, or saliva tests can quantitate current intoxication. Laboratory tests can be used as markers to detect heavy drinking in the past several days. These tests include mean corpuscular volume (MCV) and liver function tests such as aspartate aminotransferase (SGOT) and gamma glutamyl transferase (GGT). However, medical illnesses, such as liver disease and nutritional deficiencies, may produce abnormal results. In the past decade, several biochemical tests have been proposed to detect alcohol use. The most promising of these, carbohydrate deficient transferrin (CDT), has been found to be effective in discriminating heavy drinking. The test is based on the observation that alcohol inhibits the addition of sialic acid to glycoproteins, such as serum transferrin. The CDT test was recently approved by the US Food and Drug Administration as a test for heavy alcohol use.

OVERVIEW OF TREATMENT OF ADDICTIVE DISORDERS

The most effective way to reduce the medical, social, and psychological impacts of addictive substances is through effective treatment. Addiction treatment may be defined as the use of medical, psychological, and/or social interventions to reduce or eliminate the harmful effects of psychoactive substances (drugs and alcohol) on the individual, his or her family and associates, and others in society. Treatment usually consists of the following components:

- *Intervention:* initiation of treatment and/or referral
- *Detoxification:* removal of alcohol or drug from the body and treatment of withdrawal
- *Rehabilitation:* medical, psychological, and social measures to help avoid the use of psychoactive substances in the future
- *Aftercare:* processes to assist in maintaining a sober or drug-free state

Treatment for substance abuse and dependence ranges from low-cost, less intensive methods (eg, brief advice to stop drinking or using drugs and self-help programs) to high-cost, more intensive methods, including referral to specialized treatment and other community programs (eg, inpatient detoxification and rehabilitation programs). For patients with substance dependence, the goals of treatment are to establish a drug- or alcohol-free state. If total abstinence is not obtainable, a significant reduction in harmful drug or alcohol use will still be of some benefit. For patients with substance abuse, the goal is to reduce harmful drug or alcohol use. The assessment and treatment of underlying psychiatric symptoms, medical illness, and pain are important because the need for self-medication may be reduced. Individual and group psychotherapy can be useful for understanding the role of the drug in the individual's life, improving self-esteem, and relieving psychological distress. Although most treatment can be provided in an outpatient setting, halfway houses, therapeutic communities, and other residential treatment situations may be necessary to ensure a drug-free environment. Self-help groups, such as Alcoholics Anonymous (AA), Narcotics Anonymous (NA), AL-ANON, and Rational Recovery, provide treatment, education, social support, and hope to patients and their families.

Intervention

After identifying substance abuse or substance dependence, the clinician should provide feedback on diagnosis and treatment options and assess the individual's readiness to engage in treatment. Historically, physicians have felt ill prepared to contend with substance abuse and dependence. However, several methods have been developed to help physicians successfully intervene with patients. *The Physician's Guide to Helping Patients With Alcohol Problems*, recently released by the National Institute on Alcohol Abuse and Alcoholism (NIAAA), presents several useful intervention methods.

The transtheoretical model is a widely accepted model of human behavior that explains behavioral change in addiction. This model posits that behavioral change is a series of stages. These stages include the following:

- *Precontemplative stage:* not even thinking about changing
- *Contemplative stage:* thinking about changing
- *Action stage:* making efforts toward change
- *Maintenance stage:* maintaining the change

By understanding the patient's stage, the physician can better optimize the intervention. For example, a patient in the precontemplative stage would benefit most from education about the disorder and its consequences; a patient in the action phase would benefit most by learning skills to help avoid substances. The goal of the intervention is to move the patient from precontemplation into contemplation or from contemplation into action (treatment).

Brief interventions conducted in a supportive manner have been shown to be extremely effective in enhancing entrance into alcoholism treatment. Such interventions can consist of one or more sessions in the physician's office, during which education about substance use and dependence is provided and a plan for cutting down or eliminating substance use is negotiated. Together the patient and physician should develop a written contract that defines the treatment and intervention plan. A formal assessment of effectiveness and follow-up should be part of the plan. Motivational interviewing (MI) identifies and motivates patients to use their own treatment resources and is effective in reducing the use of addictive substances.

Case Vignette

Mr Billis is a 38-year-old man who has been followed by his primary care physician, Dr Ladd, for several years. At the initial assessment, Dr Ladd screened Mr Billis with a CAGE questionnaire; Mr Billis scored 2 out of 4 (he had tried several times to cut back on his drinking and he had blown up at his wife when she suggested the same thing). Mr Billis asserted then that his drinking was not a problem. Over the next few office visits, Dr Ladd made a point of asking him about his drinking and gently expressed several concerns about the potential effects on his health and marriage. When Mr Billis acknowledged that he was becoming concerned about his wife's emotional withdrawal and the amount of time he had missed work because of hangovers, Dr Ladd asked him how he wanted to get some help. Mr Billis said he thought he could control things himself, and Dr Ladd challenged him to abstain from drinking for a week to "see whether he was controlling his drinking or his drinking was controlling him." Mr Billis returned 2 weeks later and confessed that he had had no luck at all avoiding alcohol for more than 2 days. He agreed to attend three AA meetings over the next 3 weeks and report back. He later reported that he had attended the meetings and that he had come to feel that his drinking problem was worse than he had realized. He then readily accepted referral to an outpatient evening (after-work) intensive alcohol treatment program.

When a patient is referred to a specialized addiction treatment program or an addiction treatment professional, the primary care clinician must remain in contact with the patient, the family, and the other clinicians in order to maintain continuity of care and help coordinate treatment.

Detoxification and Treatment of Withdrawal

The goal of detoxification is a drug-free state and minimization of any withdrawal-associated morbidity. Withdrawal, which is a distinct physiological and/or behavioral state, follows cessation or reduction in the amount of drug used. In general, the signs and symptoms of withdrawal are the opposite of those that the drug produces (eg, withdrawal from depressants produces excitation). The proposed neurobiological mechanism for withdrawal is a change in the number of postsynaptic neurotransmitter receptors or in receptor sensitivity that occurs with chronic drug use. Withdrawal is not specific to addictive substances; a withdrawal syndrome may follow discontinuation from medications such as beta-adrenergic blockers, antihistamines, antiarrhythmics, and antidepressants.

Ideally, patients with substance dependence undergo a supervised detoxification. This may be accomplished in an outpatient, inpatient, or residential setting, depending on the drug used, the level of dependence, and the presence of coexisting medical and psychiatric problems. Criteria, such as the ASAM's patient placement criteria, are helpful in matching a patient's severity to the setting. General approaches to detoxification are shown in Table 6-4.

TABLE 6-4 General Approaches to Detoxification

- Controlled administration of the drug, with a slow taper in the daily drug dose.
  Example: Tapering nicotine gum or patch in nicotine dependence.

- Administration of a cross-tolerant agent that is slowly tapered over time.
  Example: Chlordiazepoxide in alcohol withdrawal; methadone in opioid withdrawal.

- Administration of an alternate agent to suppress signs and symptoms of withdrawal.
  Example: Clonidine hydrochloride in opioid withdrawal; atenolol in alcohol withdrawal.

- Nonpharmacological detoxification with supportive care.
  Example: Social setting detoxification in alcohol dependence.

Aftercare Approaches

The hallmark of addictive disorders is that they readily respond to effective treatment interventions. Abstinence is the goal in treatment and recovery; both short- and long-term abstinence can be achieved with the proper treatment methods. Standard treatment practices have indicated that abstinence-based treatment methods are effective in inducing and maintaining abstinence from alcohol and drugs. The abstinence-based method, which is used to treat the diseases of alcohol and drug addiction, uses cognitive-behavioral techniques and referral to 12-step recovery programs such as AA and NA.

Withdrawal alone is usually insufficient to provide sustained abstinence from the use of alcohol or drugs. Additional addictions treatment concurrently with or following treatment of withdrawal is indicated to prevent relapse. Treatment outcome studies have found that at 1 year postdischarge from abstinence-based treatment programs, 60% of patients had continuous abstinence from alcohol or drugs. Participation in continuing care and/or attendance at AA meetings following treatment program discharge can substantially improve abstinence and reduce use of medical care.

TREATMENT OF ADDICTION TO SPECIFIC SUBSTANCES

Alcohol

Pharmacology. Alcohol is a drug that affects several neurotransmitter systems in the brain. Gamma-aminobutyric acid (GABA) is the major inhibitory neurotransmitter in the central nervous system (CNS). When GABA binds to its receptor, an associated membrane chloride channel opens and hyperpolarizes or inhibits neurons from firing. Alcohol, at physiologically relevant concentrations, facilitates GABA-induced inhibition. Barbiturates, anticonvulsants, and other sedatives also appear to facilitate chloride channel opening and neuronal inhibition. Glutamate is a major excitatory neurotransmitter in the CNS. When glutamate binds to its receptors, an ion channel opens and stimulates the neuron or makes it more likely to fire. Low doses of alcohol strongly inhibit the glutamate receptor and inhibit neurons. The combined effect of alcohol on these two neurotransmitter systems is to inhibit neurons and produce sedation. With chronic alcohol use, brain GABA receptors adapt to become less inhibitory, and the glutamate receptors adapt to become more excitatory. Then, if alcohol is stopped, the adapted GABA receptors are less able to inhibit neurons, and the adapted glutamate receptors are more excitatory. The brain shows the excitation characteristic of alcohol withdrawal.

Medical consequences of alcohol use. Gastrointestinal disturbances occur commonly in alcohol use. The diagnosis of esophagitis (heartburn) and peptic ulcer disease are suggestive of regular alcohol consumption. Also, abdominal discomfort, diarrhea, constipation, heme-positive stools, and gastric cancer are associated with acute and chronic alcohol use. Laënnec cirrhosis of the liver occurs in about 5% to 10% of all alcoholics. If present, transient elevations of liver enzymes, such as alkaline phosphatase, SGOT, and GGT, can be used to indicate recent alcohol use. Persistent elevation of liver functions can suggest continued drinking or the presence of liver disease, such as hepatitis C.

Hypertension and tachycardia are common sequelae of alcohol ingestion and withdrawal. An elevation in the first 24 to 72 hours of 20 mm Hg to 30 mm Hg in systolic blood pressure and 10 mm Hg to 20 mm Hg in diastolic blood pressure over that of baseline is typical for mild to moderate alcohol withdrawal. Alcohol-related hypertension usually reverts to normal, although elevated blood pressure may be sustained for weeks, after cessation of chronic alcohol use. Individuals presenting with hypertension should be screened for alcohol use before prescribing antihypertensive medication.

Cardiac problems, such as alcohol cardiomyopathy, atrial fibrillation, and other cardiac arrhythmias, can follow chronic alcohol use. Congestive heart failure may be precipitated or aggravated by a combination of the toxic effects of alcohol on the heart and the hypertension and tachycardia induced by stimulation of the sympathetic nervous system in response to alcohol withdrawal.

Heavy alcohol use is associated with a number of reversible, hematological abnormalities. Alcohol use can lead to bone marrow suppression, producing thrombocytopenia or pancytopenia. An elevated mean corpuscular volume (MCV) of the peripheral blood erythrocytes indicates regular alcohol use but may also be due to a folate- or B_{12}-deficient state. Diabetes mellitus can be significantly aggravated by regular alcohol use. Intoxication is associated with poor dietary compliance and weight control. Alcohol may directly produce hypoglycemia during and shortly after intoxication. The toxic effects of alcohol may also produce chronic pancreatitis with insulin deficiency and subsequent glucose intolerance. Several cancers have been associated with chronic alcohol use, including carcinomas of the oral pharynx and gastrointestinal tract (esophagus, stomach, and liver).

Because alcoholics frequently smoke cigarettes (80%), lung cancer is common among alcoholics, as is chronic obstructive pulmonary disease such as chronic bronchitis and emphysema. Regular drinkers who smoke often have a productive cough in the morning, sometimes associated with nausea. These individuals also show a predilection for pneumonias, particularly *Streptococcus pneumoniae* and *Klebsiella*, and tuberculosis.

An array of dermatologic abnormalities may be present in heavy alcohol users. These include decrease in hair; gynecomastia; increased flushing or vascularity of the face; livedo reticularis (reddish-blue mottling); multiple contusions, abrasions, and cuts in various stages of healing; nicotine stains in fingers; palmar erythema; rhinophyma; poor personal hygiene; spider angiomas; and edema.

Neurological complications such as dementia syndrome, amnestic state (blackouts), Wernicke encephalopathy, seizures, hallucinosis, and peripheral neuropathy are relatively common in chronic alcohol consumers. Cognitive impairment, including reduced concentration, memory, and abstraction abilities, also occurs frequently. Some cognitive deficits may be reversible with complete abstinence from alcohol.

Trauma frequently is associated with alcohol use because intoxication impairs coordination and mental judgment. Visible evidence of trauma includes bruises, new and old wounds, and fractures. Alcohol suppresses certain clotting factors and platelets, which increases susceptibility to bruising and bleeding.

Treatment of alcohol intoxication. The treatment of alcohol intoxication is essentially supportive and includes support of vital functions, maintenance of physiological homeostasis, and prevention of behavioral problems. Patients using alcohol should always be medicated with thiamin and other B-vitamin supplements to prevent development of Wernicke-Korsakoff syndrome due to thiamin deficiency. This condition is characterized by ocular disturbances (nystagmus and sixth nerve ophthalmoplegia), ataxia, and mental status changes. Its presence is a medical emergency because delay in treatment diminishes its reversibility. Patients should receive 25 to 100 mg intramuscular or oral thiamin daily for 3 days to ensure proper dosing. Patients with neurologic symptoms or signs should be administered thiamin parenterally. Low magnesium, which is often present in alcoholics, may intensify withdrawal and seizures. Magnesium levels should be obtained and deficits replaced with oral or intramuscular magnesium sulfate.

Treatment of alcohol withdrawal syndrome. Physical dependence on alcohol and alcohol withdrawal syndrome are due to compensatory CNS changes in response to a chronically administered depressant substance (ethanol). Manifestations of withdrawal are primarily excitatory and consist of hyperarousal from central and sympathetic stimulation. Signs of alcohol withdrawal are hand and body tremors, diaphoresis, tachycardia and hypertension, dilated pupils, increase in temperature, seizures, restlessness, behavioral hyperactivity, mental hyperarousal, agitation, ataxia, and clouding of consciousness. Symptoms of alcohol withdrawal are anxiety, panic attacks, paranoid delusions or ideation, illusions, disorientation, visual hallucinations (often of animals), and auditory hallucinations.

Typically, symptoms of alcohol withdrawal peak from 1 to 3 days after withdrawal and last for 5 to 7 days. Approximately 5% of alcohol-dependent individuals undergoing detoxification develop severe withdrawal delirium (delirium tremens); of these, approximately 5% die. However, alcohol withdrawal is mild and requires minimal medical intervention for most alcoholics. The single best predictor of severe alcohol withdrawal is a previous history of seizures or delirium tremens. An underlying illness can contribute to the signs and symptoms of withdrawal. For example, an infection during withdrawal can predispose to a change in mental status.

Treatment of the alcohol withdrawal syndrome includes correction of physiological abnormalities, hydration, nutritional support, and pharmacological therapy for the increased activity of the nervous system. Administration of depressant substances markedly attenuates the signs and symptoms of withdrawal and may decrease medical morbidity and mortality.

Benzodiazepines are the most widely used medications to treat alcohol and sedative withdrawal because of their low toxicity and anticonvulsant activity. Their safety and effectiveness have been well established by double-blind, controlled studies. The benzodiazepine loading method matches dose of medication to a patient's tolerance and symptoms and avoids overmedication. Patients receive an initial oral or intravenous dose of a long half-life benzodiazepine (10 to 20 mg diazepam or 50 to 100 mg chlordiazepoxide hydrochloride), repeated every hour until the patient is sedated or has a significant decrease in withdrawal signs and symptoms. Most patients show marked reduction in withdrawal after several doses and usually require little or no additional medication, although patients with heavy sedative dependence or polysubstance dependence often require additional doses. Elderly patients and those with respiratory, cardiovascular, or hepatic disease require close observation to prevent overmedication. A short-acting benzodiazepine such as lorazepam is indicated when elimination time for benzodiazepines is prolonged, eg, when there is significant liver disease or in the elderly. In patients receiving calcium channel blockers and adrenergic blockers, some signs of withdrawal such as hypertension, tachycardia, and tremor may be obscured.

Other pharmacological agents, such as beta-adrenergic blocking drugs, anticonvulsants, and antipsychotics, are often administered to control symptoms. Antiepileptic medications, such as carbamazepine and valproic acid, effectively reduce most signs and symptoms of alcohol withdrawal and are widely used in some European countries. In using antiepileptics, patients are rapidly titrated to blood levels that are therapeutic for seizures. Additional benzodiazepines are administered for breakthrough symptoms. Beta-adrenergic blocking drugs are particularly useful as secondary agents for controlling tachycardia and hypertension in patients with coronary disease. Medications such as propranolol hydrochloride and atenolol have been used as primary agents in treating alcohol withdrawal. However, beta-blockers are most effective in reducing peripheral autonomic signs of withdrawal and are less effective for CNS signs such as delirium. Antipsychotics, such as haloperidol, are useful for treating hallucinosis and paranoid symptoms sometimes associated with withdrawal.

Many patients do not require pharmacological intervention. Nonmedically oriented treatment facilities use a nondrug method known as social-setting detoxification, which relies on peer and group support for patients. This behavioral method reduces withdrawal signs and symptoms without an increased incidence of medical complications. However, some patients do require careful monitoring and pharmacological treatment during the withdrawal process. In particular, a history of delirium tremens or seizures or the presence of medical or psychiatric comorbidities increases the need for inpatient detoxification. Some experts have expressed concern that repeated, untreated alcohol withdrawal might worsen subsequent withdrawal episodes due to kindling effects; they have suggested that any symptomatic withdrawing patient receive pharmacological treatment.

During and after detoxification, many alcoholic patients will appear to suffer from psychiatric symptoms, including major depression. Depression is often a substance-induced mood disorder related to alcohol and will resolve within several weeks of detoxification. Major depressive symptoms that persist beyond this time should be considered for treatment with antidepressants. Patients previously known to have recurrent mood disorders may be treated immediately after detoxification if mood symptoms are severe.

Rehabilitation and aftercare treatment. The goals of long-term treatment include maintaining a state of abstinence from alcohol and forming psychological, family, and social interventions to maintain this recovery. These goals are best achieved if the patient participates in a comprehensive treatment program, beginning after discharge from the acute care setting. Self-help programs such as AA are helpful for many patients and their families. Local AA groups often use hospitals and clinics as meeting sites, and patients may easily attend these meetings. Nevertheless, some aspects of long-term treatment may be initiated during an acute hospital stay.

Medications to reduce alcohol consumption. Several pharmacological agents have shown efficacy as adjuncts in treating alcohol dependence, decreasing drinking, and reducing relapse in patients who are in treatment. Of course, these agents should always be used as adjuncts to treatment, ie, as part of a comprehensive treatment program that addresses the patient's psychological, social, and spiritual needs.

Although benzodiazepines (chlordiazepoxide hydrochloride, diazepam, etc) have been shown to be efficacious in treating alcohol withdrawal, the use of maintenance benzodiazepines to reduce drinking and prevent relapse is strongly discouraged by most addiction professionals. In the past, some alcoholics were maintained on daily doses of benzodiazepines, barbiturates, or other sedatives in a poorly monitored and uncontrolled fashion. This uncontrolled use sometimes led to benzodiazepine dependence or combined alcohol and benzodiazepine dependence.

Disulfiram (Antabuse), an irreversible inhibitor of the enzyme acetaldehyde dehydrogenase, is used as an adjunctive treatment for selected alcoholics. If alcohol is consumed in the presence of disulfiram, the toxic metabolite acetaldehyde accumulates in the body, producing tachycardia, skin flushing, diaphoresis, dyspnea, nausea, and vomiting. Hypotension and death may occur if large amounts of alcohol are consumed. This unpleasant reaction is a strong deterrent to the consumption of alcohol. Monitoring patients for compliance with medication improves success with disulfiram.

The typical dose of disulfiram is 250 mg once daily. Daily doses of 125 to 500 mg are sometimes used, depending on side effects and patient response. The optimal duration of treatment is unknown—most patients use the medication for brief periods when the risk of relapse is high. However, some patients use the medication continuously for years. Some clinicians administer a small dose of alcohol to patients receiving disulfiram in order for them to experience a disulfiram-alcohol reaction. This is thought to provide a stronger deterrent to future alcohol use.

Patients who use disulfiram must understand its benefits and risks. Alcohol present in foods, shaving lotion, mouthwashes, and over-the-counter medications may produce a disulfiram reaction. In addition, disulfiram may interact with other medications. It is a potent inhibitor of the CYP2E1 oxidase and can interact with anticoagulants (warfarin sodium [Coumadin]), antiepileptics (phenytoin sodium), benzodiazepines (diazepam, chlordiazepoxide hydrochloride), and antidepressants (desipramine hydrochloride, fluoxetine hydrochloride). Disulfiram is contraindicated in patients receiving these medications. Patients with liver disease require close monitoring. A complete blood count and liver function tests should be monitored prior to starting disulfiram therapy and periodically during treatment.

Medications to reduce alcohol craving. The opioid neurotransmitter system has been strongly implicated in mediating alcohol consumption. In clinical trials with recently abstinent human alcoholics, naltrexone-treated subjects had reduced rates of relapse to heavy drinking, consumed fewer drinks per drinking day, and had lower dropout rates than did the placebo group. Subjects receiving naltrexone also report decreased craving and decreased "high" from alcohol.

The usual dose of naltrexone (Revia) is 50 mg per day, with a range of 25 to 150 mg per day. The most common side effects include anxiety, sedation, and nausea in approximately 10% of patients. Hepatic toxicity is an issue with this drug. Although high doses of naltrexone (300 mg per day) have been associated with hepatotoxicity, few deleterious hepatic effects have been observed with a 50-mg daily dose. However, naltrexone should probably be avoided in patients with hepatitis or severe liver disease. It is recommended that liver functions be monitored prior to naltrexone treatment, at 1 month, and periodically thereafter. Naltrexone should only be used in the context of a comprehensive alcoholism treatment program that includes counseling and other psychosocial therapies.

Certain medications that modify central serotonergic function appear to reduce ethanol consumption in animals and humans. Ondansetron hydrochloride, a serotonin-3 receptor antagonist used as an antiemetic, has been shown to reduce alcohol consumption, particularly in patients with early-onset alcoholism. Selective serotonin reuptake inhibitors (SSRIs) also appear to modestly reduce alcohol consumption in some patients. Several human studies on heavy drinkers found SSRIs to reduce overall alcohol consumption by approximately 15% to 20%. The effective daily doses were somewhat higher than those typically used in depression (eg, 60 mg fluoxetine, 200 mg sertraline). The effects appear to be most pronounced in late-onset, non-antisocial alcoholics.

Acamprosate (calcium acetylhomotaurine) is a structural analogue of γ-aminobutyric acid (GABA) and has agonist effects at GABA receptors and inhibitory effects at n-methyl-d-aspartate (NMDA) receptors. In clinical trials with alcoholics, acamprosate reduced relapse drinking and craving for alcohol and had minimal side effects. This medication has been approved in several European countries for preventing alcoholic relapse and is currently under clinical testing in the United States.

Sedatives and Hypnotics

Intoxication. Sedatives and hypnotics (benzodiazepines, barbiturates, ethchlorvynol, glutethimide, meprobamate, gamma-hydroxybutyrate, etc) are depressants that suppress brain function. Sedative medications are a major source of drug emergencies, including overdose, yet they are among the most prescribed drugs and are routinely used for their anxiolytic and hypnotic effects. Patients may obtain these medications illicitly from the street or from physicians who unwittingly (or purposely) are contributing to abuse or dependence. The medications in this group derive their pharmacological activity by affecting the chloride channel-GABA receptor complex in the brain. Specific binding sites exist for benzodiazepines, barbiturates, and other drugs, which increase hyperpolarization (inhibition) of neurons.

Manifestations of intoxication from sedatives include sedation, slowed mentation and coordination, confusion, loss of consciousness, and coma. Depressants can cause hypotension, bradycardia, and slowed respiratory rate. Prolonged slowing of respiratory rate can lead to respiratory acidosis, arrhythmias, arrest, and death. In emergency settings, flumazenil, a benzodiazepine antagonist, may be given intravenously to counter the respiratory depressant effects.

Gamma-hydroxybutyrate (GHB) is an easily manufactured, widely available sedative agent that is abused for its sedative and euphorigenic properties. Medically, it is used to treat narcolepsy and as an anesthetic and sedative. GHB use is popular in clubs and raves. Because the drug has been shown to release growth hormone from the pituitary, athletes and body builders use it to increase muscle mass. However, GHB causes overdoses and deaths due to respiratory suppression and has been used as a date rape drug. As with most sedatives, tolerance develops with continued use; heavy GHB users show withdrawal.

Withdrawal features. Typically, the peak period of withdrawal for short-acting benzodiazepines (eg, alprazolam) is 2 to 4 days, and duration of withdrawal is 4 to 7 days; the peak period of withdrawal for long-acting benzodiazepines (diazepam) is 4 to 7 days, with a duration of 7 to 14 days. Signs of withdrawal are agitation; increased psychomotor activity; tremulousness; fever; sweating; delirium; convulsions; tachycardia; hypertension; coarse tremor of tongue, eyelids, and hands; and status epilepticus. Symptoms of withdrawal are anxiety; euphoria; depression; incoherent thoughts; hostility; grandiosity; disorientation; and tactile, auditory, and visual hallucinations. The signs, symptoms, and treatment of withdrawal for other sedatives and hypnotics are similar to those for benzodiazepines.

As with alcohol, withdrawal from benzodiazepines and other sedatives is not usually marked by significant elevations in blood pressure and pulse. The anxiety of withdrawal is usually controlled with a prescribed taper that has a long-acting preparation, unless objectively it appears that the doses are too low. Caution in prescribing medication is urged because drug-seeking behavior must be differentiated from anxiety of withdrawal and anxiety from underlying psychiatric disorders, such as panic disorder. Nonbenzodiazepines, such as antidepressants, should be used to treat anxiety from other disorders whenever possible. The prescriber must be in control of dispensing medications. By definition, the addict is out of control regarding drug use and cannot reliably negotiate the schedule for medication administration.

Withdrawal treatment. Treatment of withdrawal is aimed at gradually tapering off the depressant drugs or substituting another depressant drug that shares pharmacologic cross-tolerance and dependence to suppress withdrawal symptoms. Benzodiazepines have cross-tolerance and dependence with each other, other sedative and hypnotic drugs, GHB, and alcohol. Consequently, benzodiazepines can be substituted for other sedatives and vice versa. The conversion for equivalent doses can be calculated if doses are known prior to taper (see Table 19-10 in Chapter 19). A long-acting benzodiazepine is more effective than short-acting preparations in suppressing withdrawal symptoms and producing a gradual and smooth transition to the abstinent state. In general, greater patient compliance and less morbidity can be expected when longer-acting benzodiazepines are used.

Duration of the tapering schedule is determined by the half-life of the sedative that is being withdrawn. For short-acting benzodiazepines such as alprazolam, a 7- to 10-day gradual taper with a long-acting benzodiazepine or barbiturate is often sufficient: 7 days for low-dose and short duration of use and 10 days for high-dose and long duration of use. Because of the higher rates of withdrawal seizures with alprazolam, phenobarbital substitution is recommended for the taper. For the long-acting benzodiazepines, 10 to 14 days of a gradual taper with a long-acting benzodiazepine or barbiturate is often sufficient: 10 days for low-dose and short duration of use and 14 days for high-dose and long duration of use. The doses can be given in a qid or tid interval. The long-acting preparations accumulate during the taper, resulting in a self-leveling effect of benzodiazepine or barbiturates in blood levels over time.

Anticonvulsants, such as carbamazepine or valproic acid, have been used to treat sedative benzodiazepine and GHB withdrawal. Patients are loaded with the anticonvulsant to produce therapeutic blood levels. The levels are maintained for 7 to 14 days and then tapered.

Following detoxification, the patient should take part in long-term treatment. Treatment should be individualized to the patient but may include residential drug-free programs, outpatient counseling, and self-help groups such as AA or NA.

Nicotine

Nicotine is an alkaloid drug present in the leaves of the tobacco plant, *Nicotiana tabacum*, which was used for centuries by Native Americans in rituals and folk medicine. Today, tobacco use has spread worldwide, and nicotine has become one of the most common psychoactive drugs used. More than 50 million persons in the United States use cigarettes daily, with another 10 million using another form of tobacco. Since publication of the first surgeon general's report, *Smoking and Health,* in 1964, the percentage of Americans who smoke, primarily in males, has gradually declined. However, the number of young women who smoke and the use of other tobacco products such as smokeless tobacco have increased. Tobacco use has also increased greatly in developing countries.

Pharmacology. To maximize the absorption of nicotine, tobacco products are usually smoked in pipes, cigars, or cigarettes or instilled intranasally or orally as snuff or smokeless tobacco. Two basic methods of using smokeless tobacco are dipping and chewing. Dipping involves placing moist or dry tobacco between the cheek and gum. Following absorption from the lungs or buccal mucosa, nicotine levels peak rapidly and then decline with a half-life of 30 to 60 minutes.

Nicotine affects the peripheral autonomic and central nervous systems in several ways. It is an agonist at nicotinic cholinergic receptor sites in autonomic ganglia of the parasympathetic and sympathetic nervous systems. Nicotine produces salivation, increases gastric motility and acid secretion, and releases catecholamine. The release of catecholamines produces cardiac stimulation and peripheral vasoconstriction. In the CNS, nicotine acts as a stimulant, producing increased alertness, attention, and concentration and suppressing appetite. The fact that tobacco use can prevent weight gain makes the drug attractive, especially to young women.

Repeated use of nicotine produces tolerance and dependence. The degree of dependence is considerable—more than 70% of dependent individuals relapse within 1 year of stopping use. Cessation of nicotine use in dependent individuals is followed by a withdrawal syndrome characterized by increased irritability, decreased attention and concentration, and an intense craving for and preoccupation with nicotine. Withdrawal symptoms, which may begin within several hours of ending use or reducing dosage, typically last about a week. Often, an increase in appetite and food consumption with weight gain occurs in the weeks and months following cessation of chronic nicotine use.

Medical consequences. The medical consequences of nicotine use are extensive and include coronary artery disease, vascular disease, respiratory disease, and cancers, particularly of the lung and oropharynx. Many deleterious effects of tobacco are not due to nicotine but are due to other toxic and carcinogenic compounds present in tobacco extract or smoke. There is a strong association between cigarette smoking and alcohol use. Although the overall prevalence rate of alcoholism is approximately 15% in the general population, 85% of alcoholics smoke cigarettes. Moreover, combined alcohol and tobacco use may increase the risk of several of types of cancer, including lung, oropharyngeal, and gastrointestinal cancers. Because 30% of smokers have comorbid alcoholism, smokers should be assessed for alcohol use.

Treatment. Treatment of nicotine dependence should follow the principles of treatment for other common addictions. Brief education and advice on smoking cessation provided by physicians has been shown to be effective in helping patients stop smoking. The most successful treatment programs use cognitive-behavioral techniques to educate patients about the health hazards of tobacco and provide patients with behavioral methods for coping with urges. Although some programs use gradual reduction in tobacco use over days to weeks (nicotine fading) for detoxification, others suggest abrupt discontinuation (going "cold turkey").

Pharmacologic therapy with nicotine replacement is increasingly popular in the treatment of nicotine dependence. The principle of nicotine replacement therapy is to provide the nicotine-dependent patient with nicotine in a form not associated with the carcinogenic and irritant elements in tobacco products. Five methods of nicotine administration have been approved: nicotine gum, nicotine lozenge, transdermal nicotine patch, intranasal nicotine, and nicotine inhaler. Nicotine gum, lozenge, and transdermal patch are now available to patients over the counter. Although nicotine replacement has been used primarily for detoxification and relief of withdrawal symptoms during smoking cessation, some patients use nicotine replacement in a maintenance fashion. The most successful treatment of nicotine dependence occurs with interventions that combine pharmacological and behavioral therapies.

Nicotine gum consists of a sweet, flavored resin containing 2 mg or 4 mg of nicotine that is released slowly when chewed. Its alkaline pH permits nicotine absorption across the buccal mucosa. The individual chews the gum whenever he or she feels the need for tobacco. When the mouth or tongue starts to tingle, chewing is ceased for a short period of time while the gum is held in the mouth. Chewing too rapidly may cause nausea. The gum is chewed for 20 to 30 minutes and then discarded. This method produces nicotine blood levels that rise and fall, partially mimicking smoking, thereby reducing the craving for tobacco and reducing withdrawal discomfort. After a daily maintenance dose is established, the frequency of chewing gum is gradually tapered. For example, a patient who uses 15 pieces of 2-mg or 4-mg gum each day during the first week of treatment may gradually reduce the number of pieces to 10 per day by the end of the first month and 5 per day by the end of the second month. Patients typically discontinue use of nicotine gum after 3 to 6 months of treatment.

Nicotine lozenges, which are used similarly to nicotine gum, contain 2 mg or 4 mg of nicotine that is released when the sweetened lozenge dissolves in the mouth. The nicotine inhaler and nicotine nasal spray mimic smoking by delivering small, measured doses of nicotine to the mucosa.

Nicotine transdermal patches contain various doses of nicotine (7 mg, 14 mg, or 21 mg) impregnated into an adhesive patch for transdermal administration. Nicotine patches deliver a steady, predictable, and measurable amount of nicotine. After the patient stops use of nicotine, one patch is applied to uncovered skin for a 24-hour period and the previous patch is discarded. Some individuals wear the patch during the daytime only and remove it while asleep. Nicotine withdrawal is treated by applying a high-dose patch to skin (hairless, dry, clean) for 1 to 2 weeks, an intermediate-dose patch for 1 to 2 weeks, and then the small-dose patch for 1 to 2 weeks. Side effects include irritation from the patch and nicotine effects (nausea, cardiac effects, etc). Patients must not use tobacco products while using the patch because toxic nicotine blood levels may occur.

Several clinical studies have shown a high incidence of major depression occurring within days to weeks following smoking cessation and nicotine withdrawal. Patients with a personal or family history of affective illness appear to be at greatest risk for depression. The antidepressant bupropion hydrochloride (Zyban) has been shown to improve the chances of remaining abstinent from nicotine, even in nondepressed smokers. The drug should be started several days prior to smoking cessation at a dose similar to that used for depression and should be continued for at least several weeks. Sleep disturbance is a common side effect.

Clonidine hydrochloride, an alpha-2-receptor agonist, has also been reported as efficacious in reducing nicotine withdrawal symptoms. The doses used are similar to those for treating mild hypertension. Clonidine hydrochloride is available in oral and transdermal preparations. Side effects include hypotension and sedation. It is usually prescribed for a period of 3 to 4 weeks, with the dose gradually reduced over the detoxification period. As with other forms of nicotine addiction treatment, clonidine hydrochloride should be used in conjunction with a behavioral recovery program.

Opioids

Opioid abuse and dependence are significant social and medical problems in the United States, with an estimated opioid addict population of more than 500,000. These patients frequently use medical and surgical services because of the multiple medical sequelae of intravenous drug use and the crime and violence associated with the addict lifestyle. The past decade has seen an increase in nonintravenous use of heroin and in the abuse of pill opiates, such as oxycodone hydrochloride.

Opioid drugs affect many organ systems. Their action is due to stimulation of receptors for endogenous hormones, enkephalins, endorphins, and dynorphins. Recent evidence suggests that there are at least three distinct opioid receptors, which are designated by the Greek letters mu, kappa, and delta. Drugs that act primarily through mu-receptor effects include heroin, morphine, and methadone; such drugs produce analgesia, euphoria, and respiratory depression. Drugs that are mediated through the kappa-receptor include the so-called mixed agonist-antagonists, buprenorphine hydrochloride, butorphanol tartrate, and pentazocine hydrochloride, which produce analgesia, but less respiratory depression. The delta-receptor appears to bind endogenous opioid peptides.

Opioid intoxication. During intoxication, opioid drugs cause a suppression of central and peripheral noradrenergic release. Mood and affect are depressed and inhibited. Important clinically, pupils are constricted and poorly reactive. Peripherally, hypotension and constipation from activation of opioid receptors and noradrenergic alpha and beta receptors are common. Other effects of severe intoxication include seizures and pulmonary edema. The acute effects of large amounts of opioids include respiratory suppression and cardiovascular arrest.

Opioid overdose is a life-threatening emergency and should be suspected in any patient presenting with obtundation or coma and respiratory suppression. Treatment of a suspected overdose includes emergency support of respiration and cardiovascular functions. Opioid suppression can be reversed with naloxone hydrochloride (Narcan), an opioid antagonist. Naloxone hydrochloride is given intravenously in doses of 0.4 mg to 0.8 mg every 20 minutes, as required. Although naloxone hydrochloride rapidly reverses the effects of opioids, including coma and respiratory suppression, it does not reverse CNS depression caused by other drugs, such as alcohol or sedative hypnotics. Naloxone hydrochloride will precipitate withdrawal in any patient who is dependent on opioids, causing the patient whose life was just saved to be most ungrateful.

Withdrawal. Opioid withdrawal, although by itself (ie, without substantial medical comorbidity) medically benign and rarely life threatening, is subjectively distressing and marked by an intense drive to use more opioids. The peak period of acute withdrawal depends on the opioid used. For short-acting opioids, such as morphine, heroin, or meperidine hydrochloride, the peak withdrawal is 1 to 3 days and duration is 5 to 7 days. For longer-acting opioids, such as methadone, the peak is 3 to 5 days and the duration 10 to 14 days.

Symptoms of opioid withdrawal are intense muscular cramps, anxiety, arthralgias, nausea, malaise, and a compelling desire for more opioids. Signs of opioid withdrawal include:

- pulse rate of 10 beats per minute or more over baseline or over 90 if there is no history of tachycardia and the baseline is unknown; systolic blood pressure 10 mm Hg or more above baseline or above 160/90 mm Hg in nonhypertensive patients;
- dilated pupils;
- gooseflesh, diaphoresis, rhinorrhea, lacrimation, diarrhea;
- agitation, insomnia, mood lability; and
- drug-seeking behavior.

Opioid withdrawal can be treated using an opiate taper; using an opiate agonist, such as methadone with clonidine hydrochloride; or with a partial agonist, such as buprenorphine hydrochloride.

Opiate taper detoxifications are performed by substituting the abused opioid with the same or another opiate, then gradually decreasing the dose approximately 10% daily over a period of days. Although any opioid agonist can be used for detoxifications, in practice, methadone is commonly used due to its long half-life and once-daily oral administration. Initially, patients should be given 10 mg to 20 mg methadone orally every 2 to 4 hours until withdrawal symptoms are suppressed. The total daily dose received is typically 20 mg to 40 mg for heroin addicts. This dose is then decreased daily. For those patients who are unable to receive oral medications, the same dose of intramuscular methadone may be administered twice daily in divided doses. Federal law allows methadone detoxifications for periods up to 21 days.

The alpha-2-adrenergic agonist, clonidine hydrochloride, suppresses many autonomic signs and symptoms of opioid withdrawal. Clonidine hydrochloride acts at presynaptic noradrenergic nerve endings in the locus coeruleus of the brain and blocks the adrenergic discharge produced by opioid withdrawal. Clonidine hydrochloride has been reported as clinically effective for suppressing opioid withdrawal following opioid discontinuation in dependent inpatients and outpatients.

Clonidine hydrochloride detoxification is performed as follows: On day 1, the opioid is stopped completely and, instead, clonidine hydrochloride is given at a dose of 0.1 mg each 8 hours. From days 2 through 4 the clonidine hydrochloride dose is gradually increased to suppress withdrawal signs and symptoms but without allowing blood pressure to decrease below 80 mm systolic and 60 mm diastolic. For most patients, a dose of 0.6 mg to 1.2 mg clonidine hydrochloride is required by day 4, but the dose will depend on the quantity of opioid used. This dose continues until day 7 for patients using short-acting opioids, such as heroin, morphine, or meperidine hydrochloride, and until day 10 to day 12 for those using longer-acting methadone. The dose of clonidine hydrochloride is then reduced by 0.2 mg to 0.3 mg per day until discontinued. Clonidine hydrochloride is less effective in attenuating drug craving, insomnia, and arthralgias and myalgias. Insomnia is best treated with a hypnotic, such as chloral hydrate, or a benzodiazepine. Muscle and joint pains may respond to acetaminophen or ibuprofen. Clonidine hydrochloride side effects include orthostatic hypotension, sedation, and dry mouth. If clonidine hydrochloride detoxification is conducted in the outpatient setting, patients must be closely monitored with daily blood pressure determinations.

The partial agonist buprenorphine hydrochloride, available as a parenteral preparation (Buprenex) or as recently approved sublingual tablets (Subutex), has been shown to be effective for detoxifying opioid-dependent persons. Buprenorphine hydrochloride is initially administered at low doses, which are gradually increased until withdrawal signs and symptoms diminish. The medication is maintained for 7 to 14 days and then tapered and discontinued. Patients treated with buprenorphine hydrochloride for detoxification report less intense and shortened withdrawal. In addition, the analgesic properties of buprenorphine hydrochloride make it ideal for detoxifying patients with pain.

Ultra rapid opiate detoxification. Recently, a number of clinicians have combined opioid antagonists and clonidine hydrochloride with conscious sedation or general anesthesia in a technique called *ultra rapid opioid detoxification (UROD)*. Using this technique, opioid-dependent patients may be detoxified in less than 24 hours. Proponents of the technique claim that the detoxification is safe and results in long-term abstinence. However, there have also been deaths reported from the procedure. Controlled studies comparing the efficacy and safety of UROD with more traditional detoxification methods have yet to be conducted.

Maintenance treatment of opioid dependence. The most widely used pharmacological treatments for opioid-dependent individuals include pharmacological maintenance treatments with the opioid agonists methadone and l-alpha-acetylmethodol (LAAM); maintenance with the partial opioid agonist buprenorphine hydrochloride; and opioid antagonist therapy with naltrexone. All of these medications are best used in a structured maintenance treatment program that includes monitored medication administration; periodic, random urine toxicological screening to assess compliance; and intensive psychological, medical, and vocational services. Maintenance treatments increase opioid tolerance, thereby decreasing the subjective effects of illicitly administered opioids, and provide an incentive for involvement in counseling and therapies.

Methadone, a synthetic orally active opioid, possesses a long duration of action, produces minimal sedation or "high," and has few side effects at therapeutic doses. Since its introduction in 1965, methadone maintenance has become a major modality of long-term treatment of opioid abuse and dependence. Currently, more than 100,000 individuals are maintained on methadone in the United States. Although some programs have waiting lists for treatment, patients who are pregnant or who have significant medical problems, such as renal failure, heart disease, or acquired immune deficiency syndrome (AIDS), are usually accepted immediately without a waiting period. Individual patients can receive methadone maintenance in an office setting with approval from the federal government.

Many studies have shown the efficacy of methadone maintenance in treating opiate addicts. Methadone-treated patients show increased treatment retention, improved physical health, decreased criminal activity, increased employment, and decreased chance of becoming HIV-positive. Methadone is most effective in the context of a program that provides intensive psychosocial and medical services and adequate methadone dosing. Methadone is dissolved in a flavored liquid and administered to patients daily, under observation. Methadone doses usually range from 20 mg per day to more than 100 mg per day. Higher doses are shown to be generally associated with better retention in treatment. Long-standing patients are allowed take-home doses of methadone, which they self-administer. Urine toxicological screening is performed randomly and periodically to assess compliance with treatment. Counseling and other rehabilitative services are regularly provided to patients.

If patients receiving methadone maintenance are hospitalized, their usual daily dose of methadone should be continued in the hospital. Frequent communication must be maintained with the methadone program, particularly to confirm the patient's actual daily dose and to communicate any changes in methadone dosage. If pain medication is necessary, patients should receive additional short- to intermediate-acting opioids, such as meperidine hydrochloride or oxycodone hydrochloride, in addition to their usual dose of methadone, rather than increasing the methadone dose (see below). Certain mixed agonist-antagonist medications, such as pentazocine hydrochloride and butorphanol tartrate, should be avoided because they may precipitate opioid withdrawal.

LAAM is a long-acting, orally active opioid with pharmacological properties that are similar to methadone. Studies on LAAM have shown it to be equal or superior to methadone maintenance in reducing IV drug use when used in the context of a structured maintenance treatment program. The advantages of LAAM include a slower onset of effects and a longer duration of action than methadone. This allows LAAM to be administered only three times per week and potentially reduces the use of take-home medications, which may be diverted to illegal uses. Patients treated with LAAM should be started on 20 mg administered three times weekly, with the dose increased weekly in 10-mg increments as necessary. Doses up to 80 mg three times weekly are safe and effective.

Buprenorphine hydrochloride is a partial agonist opioid medication (mixed agonist-antagonist), originally used medically as an analgesic: The agonist properties predominate at lower doses, and antagonist properties predominate at higher doses. Buprenorphine hydrochloride tablets containing naloxone hydrochloride (Suboxone, 2 mg and 8 mg) were approved for maintenance treatment of opioid dependence in 2002. Daily dosing of buprenorphine hydrochloride is effective in the maintenance treatment of narcotics addicts and may also reduce cocaine use. Physicians who receive specialized training and register with the Center for Substance Abuse Treatment may prescribe buprenorphine hydrochloride to individual patients without being part of a specialized program. This enables physicians to treat opioid dependence in an office-based setting, like any other chronic illness.

Buprenorphine hydrochloride doses usually range from 2 mg per day to up to 16 mg per day, administered sublingually because the medication is not effective orally. Advantages of buprenorphine hydrochloride include a milder withdrawal syndrome on discontinuation and less potential for abuse because agonist effects diminish at higher doses. Opioid-dependent patients may be started on 2 mg to 4 mg buprenorphine hydrochloride immediately after opioids are discontinued, with the buprenorphine hydrochloride dose titrated to 8 mg to 16 mg over several days.

Opioid antagonist therapy reduces the use of illicit drugs by blocking the drugs' effect at neurotransmitter receptors, leading to decreased use. There is some evidence that opioid antagonists block the craving for drugs other than opioids as well. Naltrexone is an orally active opioid antagonist, approved for the treatment of opioid dependence and narcotic addiction. Naltrexone blocks the intoxicating effects of opioids and has few side effects in individuals not dependent on opioids. The usual dose of naltrexone is 50 mg per day, administered orally, although three times weekly dosing with 100 mg, 100 mg, and 150 mg has been shown to be effective. High doses of naltrexone have been associated with hepatotoxicity; however, few deleterious hepatic effects are observed using a dose of 50 mg per day. Other possible side effects include anxiety, sedation, and nausea. Naltrexone therapy has been shown to be most effective in motivated individuals who have good social supports and less effective for street heroin addicts. Although any physician may prescribe naltrexone, it is most effective when part of a comprehensive rehabilitation program.

Nonpharmacological and behavioral treatment modalities are quite efficacious in treating the opioid abuser. Programs may differ in their lengths of stay, intensity, and theoretical orientation. Long-term residential treatment and therapeutic communities may be helpful for the chronic opioid abuser who requires a change in lifestyle, with vocational and psychological rehabilitation. Attending NA is helpful for many patients.

Pain and addiction. A particularly difficult clinical problem is the treatment of pain in patients with addiction. Patients with addictive disorders are prone to conditions that produce pain and require analgesic treatment. Drug and alcohol use are major causes of injuries due to accidents and violence. The medical consequences of drug and alcohol use include painful conditions such as pancreatitis, cancers, infections, and HIV-related illnesses. Important issues in treating patients with combined addictive disorders and pain include the type of drug producing dependence (eg, alcohol, opioids), whether the patient is in addiction treatment, and the type of addiction treatment (drug-free, substitution, or antagonist therapy).

These patients should be entered into an addiction treatment program that can work in a coordinated fashion with the clinicians providing the pain treatment. When analgesic medications are required, nonnarcotic substances should be used, if possible. If narcotic analgesics are required, the type of addiction treatment the patient is receiving has important implications for analgesic therapy. Patients receiving drug-free, abstinence-oriented therapy will respond to opioids but require careful monitoring to reduce the chances of abuse and dependence. Those receiving substitution therapies with methadone, LAAM, or buprenorphine hydrochloride may require higher doses of narcotic analgesics because of their increased tolerance.

If narcotics are needed for analgesia, patients should receive a different opioid medication, such as meperidine hydrochloride or oxycodone hydrochloride. This differentiates the concept of opioids for analgesia from the concept of opioids for maintenance and does not change the dose of the agent used for substitution therapy. In those patients receiving antagonist therapy with naltrexone, the effect of opioids will be blocked for 24 to 72 hours after dosing. Stopping the antagonist 1 to 3 days prior to scheduled surgery or dental procedures will remove the opioid blockade. If opioids are needed emergently, higher doses can acutely overcome the blockade because naltrexone is a competitive antagonist. However, administration of high opioid doses must be carefully monitored.

Case Vignette

Ms Lynn is a 54-year-old woman with breast cancer diagnosed 2 years earlier who comes to her primary care physician for low back pain. She had been dependent on heroin during most of her 30s and 40s, but she has been enrolled in a methadone maintenance program for the past 3 years. She has been working regularly. Ms Lynn's mother has looked after her two children for the past 2 years. The physical examination reveals several points of tenderness in the lumbosacral area, and x-rays of her spine reveal several lytic lesions that are eventually determined to be metastatic from a recurrence of her breast cancer. She is treated with nonsteroidal antiinflammatory drugs (NSAIDs) for pain with fair relief and referred to an oncologist. Chemotherapy proves unhelpful over the next 6 months, and she develops new bony lesions in her ribs and liver and lung metastases; the NSAIDs are no longer controlling her pain adequately. Her physician contacts the physician at her methadone program and her oncologist to discuss the situation. They decide to continue methadone at the same dose and add an oral codeine preparation for pain control. Over the next 2 months she has worsened pain; eventually an oral morphine preparation is added to her ongoing methadone regimen.

Cocaine and Other Stimulants

The use of CNS stimulants, such as cocaine and amphetamines, is extremely common. Government surveys of drug use find that more than 20 million Americans have tried cocaine at least once and more than 10 million used it during the preceding year. Cocaine and amphetamines are administered by intranasal snorting of powder, smoking, or intravenous injection. Amphetamines may also be used orally. Freebase cocaine is now widely available as crack, which is potent, inexpensive, and easily distributed. Crack is self-administered by smoking, usually by adding a small piece to a burning cigarette and inhaling the vapor.

Pharmacology. Cocaine has major physiological and behavioral effects because it acts as a:

- highly potent local anesthetic that blocks the initiation and propagation of nerve impulses by affecting the sodium conductance of nerve cell membranes;
- potent sympathomimetic agent that potentiates the actions of catecholamines in the autonomic nervous system, producing tachycardia and hypertension; it is a potent vasoconstrictor; and
- potent stimulant of the CNS, potentiating the action of central catecholamine neurotransmitters, norepinephrine, and dopamine.

Amphetamines have actions similar to those of cocaine, although they are not local anesthetics. The short-term effect of stimulants is to block the reuptake and increase the release of dopamine and other catecholamines to act on postsynaptic receptors. However, after prolonged use, stimulants deplete the presynaptic supplies of these neurotransmitters.

Signs and symptoms of cocaine and amphetamine intoxication are sympathomimetic: dilated and reactive pupils, tachycardia, elevated temperature, elevated blood pressure, dry mouth, perspiration or chills, nausea and vomiting, tremulousness, hyperactive reflexes, repetitive compulsive behavior, stereotypic biting or self-mutilation, cardiac arrhythmias, and flushed skin. Particularly common and serious psychiatric symptoms during intoxication are depression and suicidal and homicidal ideation. Chronic users have poor self-care, weight loss, and wasting. Cocaine overdose produces hyperpyrexia, hyperreflexia, and seizures, which may progress to coma and respiratory arrest.

The plasma half-life of cocaine following oral-nasal or intravenous administration is approximately 1 to 2 hours, which correlates with its behavioral effects. As plasma levels decline, most users experience a period of dysphoria or crash, which often leads to additional cocaine use within a short period of time. The dysphoria is intensified and prolonged following repeated use.

Treatment. The treatment of acute stimulant intoxication is essentially supportive. Propranolol and haloperidol administration has been reported as useful in acute cocaine intoxication to reduce the tachycardia, anxiety, and psychosis. Stimulant use is not followed by a physiological withdrawal syndrome of the magnitude seen with opioids or alcohol. The dysphoria, depression, and drug craving that follow chronic cocaine use are, however, often intense and make abstinence difficult. Psychotherapy, group therapy, and behavior modification are useful in maintaining abstinence. Recently, a variety of pharmacological agents have shown promise as adjunctive treatments. Several reports have shown the efficacy of antidepressant agents, such as desipramine hydrochloride, in reducing cocaine craving and usage. The doses of medication used were similar to those used for antidepressant therapy. Although there have been reports that carbamazepine, amantadine hydrochloride, and bromocriptine mesylate may partially block cocaine craving, controlled clinical trials have not shown them to be effective in treatment.

Many psychiatric and drug hospitals now offer short-term inpatient cocaine treatment, providing intensive psychological treatment and drug education in a drug-free environment. For recidivists, long-term residential drug-free programs, including therapeutic communities, may be helpful. Self-help groups such as NA may be useful both as a primary treatment modality for cocaine dependence and as an adjunct to other treatment.

Certain psychiatric disorders such as depression and attention deficit disorder may be common in stimulant users. Recognition and treatment of these underlying disorders may be necessary to stop cocaine use. In addition, many stimulant users also use alcohol or other drugs, particularly sedatives and heroin, and may require treatment for these substances as well.

Caffeine

Caffeine and the related methylxanthines—theophylline and theobromine—are consumed by more than 80% of the US population. These agents are found in coffee, tea, cola and other carbonated drinks, chocolate, and many prescribed and over-the-counter medications, including stimulants (NoDoze), appetite suppressants (Dexatrim), analgesics (Anacin, acetylsalicylic acid [APC] tablets), and cold and sinus preparations (Dristan, Contac).

Effects of caffeine use. CNS effects of caffeine include psychomotor stimulation, increased attention and concentration, and suppression of the need for sleep. Even at low or moderate doses, caffeine can exacerbate symptoms of anxiety disorders and may increase requirements for neuroleptic or sedative medications. At high doses and in sensitive individuals, methylxanthines may produce tolerance and behavioral symptoms of tremor, insomnia, jitteriness, and agitation. In moderate to heavy users, a withdrawal syndrome, characterized by lethargy, hypersomnia, irritability, and severe headache, follows cessation of use. Clinically significant caffeine-withdrawal symptoms are commonly observed in even low to moderate users and may occur with reduced caffeine intake during a medical or psychiatric hospitalization. The duration of withdrawal is usually 24 to 72 hours. The signs and symptoms of caffeine intoxication or caffeine withdrawal may complicate medical or psychiatric treatment by increasing patient distress, leading to an unnecessary workup for other disorders.

Methylxanthines produce physiological effects through actions at the cellular level. They produce cardiac stimulation, diuresis, bronchodilation, and CNS stimulation through several mechanisms. They have a direct inhibitory effect on adenosine receptors in the brain. Methylxanthines also inhibit the enzyme cyclic AMP phosphodiesterase and increase intracellular cyclic AMP levels, thereby augmenting the action of many hormones and neurotransmitters, such as norepinephrine.

Treatment. Treatment of caffeine dependence limits consumption of caffeine-containing foods, medications, and beverages. Beverages such as coffee or cola may be substituted with decaffeinated forms. Many patients are unaware of the extent of their caffeine consumption and of the caffeine content of their diet. They require education about the caffeine content of these substances. Withdrawal symptoms such as headache and lethargy are best treated with slow caffeine taper, analgesics, and rest.

Cannabis

Cannabis, which includes marijuana and hashish, is the most frequently used illicit drug in the United States. Although perhaps 60% or more of the adult population have tried the drug, probably no more than 2% report daily use. The main psychoactive compound, Δ^9-tetrahydrocannabinol (THC), produces effects within minutes of being smoked that last for up to several hours. THC-related compounds exert their behavioral effects by binding to cannabinoid receptors on brain cells.

Effects of cannabis use. Adverse effects from cannabis use alone are seldom identified in medical settings. However, cannabis use may complicate other substance use disorders, and the number of injuries (particularly automobile crashes) associated with cannabis use is probably not insignificant. An unresolved question is whether cannabis may serve as a gateway to the use of other, even more problematic drugs. In addition, the pulmonary effects from combustion products in smoked cannabis may be as detrimental as tobacco smoke. There is considerable anecdotal evidence that cannabis may be useful for managing chemotherapy-induced nausea and vomiting or for appetite stimulation in the AIDS wasting syndrome, but confirmatory empirical research has not been done.

Intoxication. Acute use of cannabis is characterized by an altered sense of time (time seems to pass more slowly), lassitude, somnolence, increased appetite, diminished short-term memory, and decreased psychomotor performance. Dysphoric reactions, including anxiety, panic, and depression, may be seen, especially in naive users or those taking it in an unfamiliar setting. Paranoia or delirium may develop in very rare cases. A calm environment with low stimulation and interpersonal reassurance is generally sufficient to manage most reactions. Anxiolytics (eg, diazepam 10 mg to 20 mg) may be administered for severe anxiety, and antipsychotics (eg, haloperidol 2 mg to 5 mg) are sometimes used for psychosis.

Abuse and dependence. Regular use of cannabis can cause tolerance and dependence; cannabis abuse and dependence are disorders defined in the DSM-IV. Chronic use of cannabis is associated with the so-called amotivational syndrome, characterized by apathy, diminished initiative, and impaired learning. The abstinence syndrome can be subtle, probably due to the long half-life of the drug in the body. However, irritability, insomnia, dysphoria, myalgias, and nausea may follow abrupt cessation of cannabis after heavy use. Pharmacologic approaches are generally not used in detoxification or relapse prevention. Structured programs, including self-help groups and, at times, psychotherapy are used to maintain drug abstinence.

Hallucinogens, Ketamine and Phencyclidine, and Ecstasy

Many drugs are used for their hallucinogenic or psychotomimetic effects. These include the psychedelics lysergic acid diethylamide (LSD), mescaline, psilocybin, and dimethyl-tryptamine; phencyclidine (PCP), ketamine, and similar-acting arylcyclohexylamines; and anticholinergics, such as scopolamine. All cause a state of intoxication characterized by hallucinosis, affective changes, and delusional states. The mechanism of action of hallucinogens is not well understood and varies according to the drug. Hallucinogens of the LSD and amphetamine class are thought to act on dopaminergic and/or serotonergic brain systems, especially the 5HT-2 receptor. Hallucinogens related to ketamine and PCP act at NMDA-glutamate receptors. Anticholinergics act at muscarinic cholinergic receptors.

Effects of hallucinogens use. Cognitive or memory impairment, disorientation, and confusion often occur in intoxication from psychedelic use. Psychedelic agents produce electroencephalogram (EEG) changes similar to those seen during REM sleep, which may account for the dreamlike quality of the high reported by those using this class of drugs. The duration of the intoxication effects may last days to weeks following last use. Users may report persistent visual trails and flashbacks of the hallucinogen experience. Hallucinogens can precipitate mania or psychosis in susceptible individuals with a previous history or a strong family history of these disorders.

PCP and the related dissociative anesthetic ketamine can induce a state of intoxication characterized by hyperactivity, insensitivity to pain, hallucinations, paranoid delusions, and memory loss. Physical manifestations include hypertension, tachycardia, eyelid retraction (producing a wide-eyed stare), dry flushed skin, dilated pupils, nystagmus, and an excitable, angry affect. Because the perception of pain (analgesic and anesthetic action) is reduced, the user is capable of great feats of strength, eg, breaking out of restraints or overpowering staff. Insensitivity to pain, disturbed thinking, and increased motor activity make PCP-intoxicated patients threatening to themselves and others.

Ecstasy (methylenedioxymethamphetamine, MDMA), methylenedioxyamphetamine (MDA), and other hallucinogenic amphetamines produce a state of euphoria, heightened sensory awareness, and empathy and positive feelings toward others. Since introduction in the 1970s, their use has steadily increased. Ecstasy has become popular among adolescents and young adults who use it as a club drug and rave drug. Ecstasy can cause hyperthermia, the effect of which may have led to deaths from its use, particularly in overheated dance clubs. Also of concern is the observation that methoxylated amphetamines like ecstasy can cause long-term reductions of neurotransmitters (serotonin and dopamine) in the brains of rodents and monkeys who receive the drug. Similar neurotransmitter depletions probably occur in humans; however, the consequences of such depletions are unknown.

The differential diagnosis of hallucinogen- or PCP-induced psychosis includes schizophrenia, bipolar affective disorder, delusional disorder, and organic mental disorders such as encephalitis, brain tumors, and toxic encephalopathies.

Treatment of hallucinogen intoxication. The most effective treatment of acute hallucinogen intoxication is supportive care in a quiet environment until the effects of the intoxication subside. Treatment of the psychotic state includes supportive measures to prevent patients from harming themselves or others, maintaining cardiovascular and respiratory functions, and ameliorating agitation and psychotic symptoms. Psychedelic agents commonly require combined pharmacological and psychosocial treatments for the management of intoxication and withdrawal. Lorazepam 1 mg to 2 mg PO or IV q1h to q2h prn or diazepam 5 mg to 10 mg PO q2h to q4h prn can be given to calm and sedate. For PCP, the acute symptoms of intoxication and withdrawal are diminished or reversed by haloperidol 5 mg to 10 mg intramuscularly or orally every 1 to 6 hours as needed for behavioral control. Lorazepam 1 mg to 2 mg IV or diazepam 5 mg to 10 mg PO q1h to q6h can also be given as needed. Following detoxification, the patient should be engaged in long-term treatment, which may include residential drug-free programs, outpatient counseling, and self-help groups such as NA.

Inhalants

Inhalants are volatile organic compounds that are inhaled for their psychotropic effects. Substances in this class include organic solvents (gasoline, toluene, ethyl ether, fluorocarbons) and volatile nitrates (nitrous oxide, amyl and butyl nitrate). Inhalants are readily available in households and at work sites, or users may easily purchase them. At low doses, inhalants produce mood changes (especially euphoria), hallucinosis, and ataxia; at high doses they may produce dissociative states and sedation. A primary danger of inhalants is suffocation because sufficient oxygen may not be available and many inhalants also reduce respiratory drive. Consequences of organic solvent use include bone marrow suppression, hepatotoxicity, and both central and peripheral neuropathies. Cardiac arrhythmias may occur, leading to sudden death. Inhaled nitrates may produce hypotension and methemoglobinemia.

The typical inhalant user is a male adolescent. According to the National Household Survey on Drug Abuse, 9.1% of 12- to 17-year-olds and 12.8% of 18- to 25-year-olds have tried an inhalant at least once.

The optimal treatment of the inhalant user is similar to that for any substance dependence. Patients need comprehensive medical and psychiatric assessments as well as addiction treatment. Because inhalant users are usually adolescents, treatment should involve the family. Long-term residential treatment may be helpful in treating heavy users.

SUMMARY

Addictive disorders, which cause substantial medical morbidity and mortality, are extremely common in the general population and in medical settings. Primary care physicians can play an important role in screening for, recognizing, and diagnosing addictive disorders. Treatment generally requires an initial phase of drug withdrawal followed by a long-term plan to encourage and maintain abstinence. Pharmacologic strategies may be used to block the effects of the addicting drug, reduce drug craving, offer a less harmful substitute, or create aversion to drug use. Self-help groups, structured psychosocial programs, and some forms of psychotherapy may be important components of overall management.

ADDITIONAL READINGS

American Psychiatric Association. *Diagnostic and Statistical Manual of Mental Disorders*. 4th ed, Primary Care Version. Washington, DC: American Psychiatric Association; 1995.

Brewer C. Recent developments in disulfiram treatment. *Alcohol Alcohol*. 1993;28(4):383-395.

Compton PA, Wesson DR, Charuvastra VC, Ling W. Buprenorphine as a pharmacotherapy for opiate addiction. *Am J Addict*. 1996;5:220-230.

Ewing JA. Detecting alcoholism: the CAGE questionnaire. *JAMA*. 1984;252:1905-1907.

Galanter M, Kleber HD. *Textbook of Substance Abuse Treatment*. Washington, DC: American Psychiatric Press Inc; 1994.

Hester R, Miller W, eds. *Handbook of Alcoholism Treatment Approaches: Effective Alternatives*. 3rd ed. Boston, Mass: Allyn & Bacon; 2002.

Hoffmann NG, Miller NS. Perspectives of effective treatment for alcohol and drug disorders. *Psychiatr Clin North Am*. 1993;16(1):127-140.

Koob GF, LeMoal M. Drug addiction, dysregulation of reward and allostasis. *Neuropsychopharmacol*. 2000;24(2):98-129.

Liskow BI, Goodwin DW. Pharmacological treatment of alcohol intoxication, withdrawal and dependence: a critical review. *J Stud Alcohol*. 1987;48:356-370.

McLellan AT, Lewis DC, O'Brien CP, Kleber HD. Drug dependence—a chronic medical illness. Implications for treatment, insurance and outcomes evaluation. *JAMA*. 2000;284(13):1689-1695.

Mee-Lee D, ed. *ASAM Patient Placement Criteria for the Treatment of Substance-Related Disorders*. 2nd ed. Chevy Chase, Md: American Society of Addiction Medicine; 2001.

Miller NS, ed. *Principles and Practices for Addictions in Psychiatry*. Philadelphia, Pa: WB Saunders Co; 1996.

Miller NS, Gold MS, Smith DE, eds. *Manual of Therapeutics for Addictions*. New York, NY: John Wiley & Sons; 1997.

National Institute on Alcohol Abuse and Alcoholism. *The Physician's Guide to Helping Patients With Alcohol Problems*. Washington, DC: NIH Publication (No. 95-3769); 1995.

O'Brien CP. Range of research-based pharmacotherapies for addiction. *Science*. 1997;278(5335):66-70.

Prochaska JO, DiClemente CC, Norcross JC. In search of how people change: applications to the addictive behaviors. *Am Psychol*. 1992;47:1102-1114.

Samet JH, Rollnick S, Barnes H. Beyond CAGE. A brief clinical approach after detection of substance abuse. *Arch Intern Med*. 1996;156:2287-2293.

Senay E. Methadone maintenance treatment. *Int J Addict*. 1985;20:803-821.

Stein M. Medical consequences of intravenous drug abuse. *J Gen Intern Med*. 1990;5:249-257.

Swift RM, Griffiths W, Camara P. Special technical considerations in laboratory testing for illicit drugs. In: Stoudemire A, Fogel BS, eds. *Medical Psychiatric Practice*. Vol 1. Washington, DC: American Psychiatric Association Inc; 1991.

Swift RM. Drug therapy of alcohol dependence. *N Engl J Med*. 1999;340(19):1483-1489.

Volpicelli JR, Alterman AI, Hayashida M, et al. Naltrexone in the treatment of alcohol dependence. *Arch Gen Psychiatry*. 1992;49:876-880.

Chapter **7**

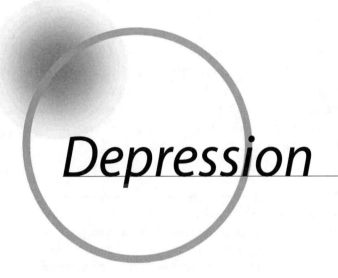

Depression

Michael J. Roy, MD, MPH
Roger G. Kathol, MD
Kurt Kroenke, MD

In the general US population, 5% to 12% of men and 10% to 25% of women experience at least one episode of major depression during their lifetime. As many as 5% to 10% of primary care patients suffer from major depression at any one time, and an additional 10% to 15% will experience lesser degrees of depression. Overall, at least one in every four patients treated in the primary care setting has some sort of mental disorder, and there is significant associated morbidity and functional impairment with such conditions. It is therefore imperative that primary care physicians be comfortable in evaluating and managing patients with depressive disorders.

A CASE OF DEPRESSION

Depression in the primary care setting presents special problems that are frequently overlooked in psychiatric texts about depression. It is for this reason that this chapter emphasizes major depression in the primary care setting. Special strategies that can be used in primary care to facilitate diagnosis and ensure timely treatment are discussed. The following case highlights numerous problems that the primary care physician may encounter when diagnosing and treating a patient with depression.

Case Vignette

Mrs Manning, 39, is a successful businesswoman who runs a flower shop. She is married to a family physician and has two children, Monica age 14 and Jesse age 17, who are good students and well respected by their peers. Mrs Manning grew up in a middle-class family, married at age 20, and struggled to complete college. She helped her husband through medical school and raised their family. She started her own business when her youngest entered grade school, receiving emotional and financial support from her husband.

Dr Crane has been Mrs Manning's doctor for nearly 15 years. Through the years, she has seen Dr Crane on several occasions for nonspecific complaints, sometimes fatigue, sometimes headache. Sometimes she just wanted to talk. Each time nothing serious was found. Months and occasionally years would pass before Mrs Manning would return. She always seemed to have a positive attitude, though it occasionally seemed contrived. Nonetheless, she had been stronger than other members of her family during times of trial. This is why Dr Crane was so surprised when Dr John Manning called one Saturday afternoon to ask if he could see Mrs Manning. She had threatened to kill herself. Dr Crane arranged to see her immediately.

During her conversation with Dr Crane that afternoon, Mrs Manning was clearly distraught. She had been feeling run-down for several weeks and admitted that she wasn't coping well. She reported that she had been experiencing frequent and severe headaches. Initially she said that everyone would be better off if she wasn't around. Later, she admitted she had no plan to kill herself and eventually settled down after 30 minutes of ventilating her feelings. She did not appear so much depressed as excessively upset about an impending visit from her in-laws as well as about turning 40 soon. She had been worrying about these and other issues more than usual, and her worrying was making it difficult for her to get to

Acknowledgment: The authors acknowledge Henry Chung, MD, for the concept of the PHQ-9 as a "blood pressure" for depression and the potential actions corresponding to the PHQ-9 score.

sleep at night. Dr Crane ordered a CT (computed tomography) scan of her head, which was normal. She was sent home with instructions to call if things didn't get better and encouraged to see a counselor. She demurred.

When she was seen 2 weeks later, it was as though the previous Saturday counseling session had never occurred. The usual as-needed schedule was resumed. For the next 2 years, Mrs Manning continued to visit her physician intermittently; however, no significant disease was uncovered. Again, Dr Manning made an urgent phone call to Dr Crane. Mrs Manning was talking about killing herself again. Dr Manning noted that this had happened several times in the past couple of years, but that Mrs Manning had convinced him that she was just tired and upset. This time it was somehow different, and Dr Manning was afraid something was going to happen. He said that Mrs Manning refused to see a psychiatrist or counselor, saying, "think of how it would look," but she agreed to see Dr Crane.

While Dr Manning was on the phone, he revealed that Mrs Manning had always had periods during which she became despondent, even times when she talked of killing herself. However, she never missed work, even when she was at her worst. She always had a good appetite, although occasionally she would have trouble sleeping. Mrs Manning never refused to participate in an active sex life but lost her spontaneity and interest when she felt overwhelmed.

When Dr Crane saw Mrs Manning this time, she was clearly depressed and suicidal. She spontaneously cried during their conversation and described a dismal future with suicidal thoughts, even though she knew how hard it would be on John, Jesse, and Monica. She stated that she hadn't slept well for weeks and had been forcing herself to eat to keep her strength up. It had become harder for her to keep up at the flower shop, although she didn't think that anyone had noticed. Mid-afternoon crying spells, when she would sneak home to be alone, helped her to cope. It was during these times that she had the most difficulty resisting the aspirin she had stockpiled in the medicine cabinet.

Dr Crane was now very uncomfortable with a patient he recognized to be seriously depressed and suicidal. He tried to persuade her to see a psychiatrist, but she refused. Dr Crane advised admission to the hospital. Again, she said no. However, she was willing to take medication because she felt so bad.

Dr Crane left the examining room and called a psychiatrist colleague to ask her advice. She suggested encouraging referral to a psychiatrist or using involuntary commitment if needed. Dr Crane noted that a referral had been suggested and that Mrs Manning didn't feel comfortable with involuntary commitment. The psychiatrist advised making sure that the patient did not have any organic or psychiatric conditions that could be contributing to her symptoms, such as thyroid disease, diabetes mellitus, or substance abuse, and that she was not on any medications that could contribute to depression. If nothing was found, she suggested that Mrs Manning be given a 2- to 3-week course of zolpidem tartrate (Ambien) to help with her sleep disturbance, and that she be started on sertraline hydrochloride (Zoloft). In addition to the medication, the psychiatrist strongly advised that Dr Manning take time off, starting immediately, and stay continuously with Mrs Manning until her suicidal ideation subsided.

Dr Crane told Dr Manning in front of Mrs Manning that he was to stay with her until she no longer felt she wished to harm herself. Dr Manning agreed. Dr Crane gave a pamphlet on depression to Mrs Manning and also gave one to Dr Manning so that he and the children could read about the trouble their mom was having and could help out. Because Mrs Manning had little motivation, Dr Crane encouraged Dr Manning to read the pamphlet to her. This would remind both of them that depression is treatable and that Mrs Manning would get back to her usual self. An appointment to see Mrs Manning in a week was made, and Dr Manning was encouraged to keep Dr Crane informed by phone of how things were going.

It was about 3 weeks before Mrs Manning showed signs of real progress. At that point, she was continued at the same dose of sertraline hydrochloride but the zolpidem tartrate was stopped. By week 4, Mrs Manning agreed to see a psychiatrist; however, there was a 4-week wait. Mrs Manning did not wish to enter psychotherapy, so she canceled the upcoming appointment. Within 6 weeks, Mrs Manning returned to euthymia. She was back to work and enjoying life once again.

In looking back, it became apparent to Dr Crane that a number of Mrs Manning's clinic visits prior to the crisis were very likely related to depression, but symptoms of depression were not elicited. After she had been successfully treated for depression, Mrs Manning admitted that her father was an alcoholic, her mother had committed suicide at age 40, and a sister had had periods of depression. She indicated that the pamphlets on depression had been very helpful, not particularly at the time for her but for her family. However, later she was able to concentrate on the information enough to see its importance and had talked to others who had similar problems.

Dr Crane discussed the advisability of long-term medication with Mrs Manning during the next several office visits because she had experienced several episodes of depression.

The preceding case illustrates a number of problems that primary care physicians encounter when they try to diagnose and treat depression. These problems may be divided into three categories: those related to patients, those related to the physician, and those related to the health care delivery system.

Patient-related problems have these characteristics:

- Many patients present with depression by complaining of physical symptoms that do not have readily identifiable causes. In fact, depressed patients report significantly more somatic symptoms than nondepressed patients.
- Most patients are reluctant to seek help from the mental health sector.
- Symptoms of depression in the primary care setting sometimes improve with limited counseling as part of a simple office visit.
- Even when symptoms of depression are blatant, patient resistance to mental health intervention remains high.

Physician-related problems have these characteristics:

- Information from collateral sources (eg, family members) is seldom obtained.
- Family history of psychiatric problems is seldom obtained.
- There is great discomfort with using interventions such as involuntary commitment.
- For patients with persistent depression, treatment is often delayed because the physician's index of suspicion is low or comfort with making the diagnosis is low.
- Physicians often want to rule out organic causes first, ordering studies such as head CTs, and then considering depression as a diagnosis of exclusion after other potential etiologies have been ruled out.
- Medication is the most likely treatment to be used in depressed patients.
- Formal psychotherapy, other than short-term, nonspecific counseling, is uncommonly used.
- Medical causes for depression are often overlooked before treatment is started.
- Education about depression is often undervalued.
- The duration of treatment is as important as the initiation of treatment.

System-related problems have these characteristics:

- Although assistance through psychiatric consultation may be desired by the primary care physician and accepted by the patient, timely appointments may be difficult to arrange.
- In some managed care or other reimbursement systems, psychiatric care may be difficult to obtain or is not covered adequately under the patient's insurance plan.
- Diagnosing and/or treating depression in primary care may not be reimbursed commensurately, or at all, by some third-party payers.

EVALUATION

Many primary care physicians balk at initiating evaluation for depression, perceiving it as a relatively nebulous and time-consuming condition that is both more difficult and less amenable to diagnosis and treatment than other medical conditions. However, there are tools that can facilitate the diagnosis, and therapy is about as effective as that for other common conditions such as diabetes mellitus and hypertension. Moreover, depression is associated with significant morbidity and mortality, both directly and indirectly through a negative impact on such comorbid medical conditions as cardiovascular disease.

Risk Factors

Some primary care patients are at particularly high risk for depression, as outlined in Table 7-1. The presence of one or more factors should serve as flags prompting expedient evaluation for depression.

Presentation

Although it has been estimated that 88% of individuals who are worried about having a psychological disturbance first seek help from a general medical practitioner, it has been widely reported that primary care physicians miss the diagnosis of depression at least

---

TABLE 7-1 Risk Factors for Primary Major Depressive Disorder

- Female gender
- Postpartum
- History of depression, alcoholism, or other psychiatric illness in first-degree relatives
- Prior episodes of major depression
- Greater risk with first occurrence between ages 20 and 40 years
- Lack of social support
- Frequent use of medical resources in the absence of serious illness
- Several unexplained somatic complaints
- Nicotine dependence or multiple failed attempts at smoking cessation
- Persistent failure to adhere to management recommendations
- Failure to improve as expected

half the time. This is the case in part because depressed patients typically present with somatic symptoms such as insomnia, fatigue, or weight change rather than depressed mood. Such symptoms have many potential etiologies, and primary care physicians may be more attuned to seeking organic rather than psychological causes.

Rarely do depressed primary care patients spontaneously volunteer emotional distress as a chief complaint. In fact, depressed patients often report primary physical symptoms that are not even diagnostic criteria for depression, such as dyspepsia, joint or muscle pain, or headaches. In general, depressed patients tend to have more physical symptoms, and more medical and psychological comorbidity, than other primary care patients. The primary care physician must think about depression when patients present with physical complaints and must routinely ask about depressed mood and loss of interest in activities. Depression should be considered up front rather than as a diagnosis of exclusion after performing numerous costly and time-consuming diagnostic tests for symptoms that have no clear organic basis. Not only does extensive testing delay treatment, incurring the potential for interim morbidity and mortality, it may also undermine satisfaction in patients who desire dialogue on psychosocial issues.

The stigma surrounding mental illness may lead patients and physicians to avoid direct discussions of mood disorders. Patients either mention their symptoms at the end of an appointment (not infrequently while getting up to leave) or fail to verbalize them at all; physicians may avoid the subject so as not to embarrass patients. Ironically, and perhaps contrary to many physicians' beliefs, patients seem to derive greater satisfaction from discussing psychosocial issues than from discussing biomedical subjects. In addition, as physicians face progressively more onerous time constraints, they may feel there is not enough time to discuss depression with their patients. On the rare occasions when patients are up-front about their feelings of depression, primary care physicians usually handle them well. However, it usually takes several visits for the physician to recognize that the somatic complaints or conditions that fail to improve, eg, diabetes and hypertension, in fact have depression embedded in their foundation.

Diagnosis

Major depression. Researchers have found that formal DSM-IV (*Diagnostic and Statistical Manual of Mental Disorders,* fourth edition) diagnoses are often not made in the primary care setting. Instead, patients are treated without clarifying the exact diagnosis. As long as significant variables such as suicidality, psychosis, and bipolar features are ruled out, this approach may not necessarily be inappropriate. It is likely that third-party payers, which frequently do not reimburse primary care physicians for managing mental disorders but do reimburse them for treating symptoms, have a role in propagating this practice. Nevertheless, there are many ways to clarify a diagnosis, including implementing appropriate treatment plans, following up on the patient over time, and utilizing referral when indicated.

When diagnosing depression, the physician must ask about nine symptoms:

- Depressed mood
- **S**leep disturbance
- Loss of **I**nterest or pleasure, ie, anhedonia
- Feelings of **G**uilt or worthlessness

- Low **E**nergy
- Poor **C**oncentration or memory
- **A**ppetite disturbance
- **P**sychomotor agitation or retardation
- **S**uicidal ideation

At least five of these symptoms must be persistently present for at least 2 weeks for a diagnosis of major depression. A popular mnemonic, **SIG = E CAPS** ("the prescription for depressed patients is energy capsules") applies to eight criteria in addition to depressed mood. Numerous randomized controlled trials have shown that major depression can be improved by medication, psychotherapy, and electroconvulsive therapy.

Although the *Diagnostic and Statistical Manual of Mental Disorders,* fourth edition, for Primary Care (DSM-IV-PC) [MJR1]suggests that symptoms of depression that are related to an underlying medical condition or medication should not count toward a depressive diagnosis, this is subject to considerable clinician judgment and potential bias. Several studies have shown that it is the number of symptoms, regardless of their relationship to an underlying illness, that is the key to identifying patients who might benefit from depression treatment. Patients whose depression-like symptoms are related to an underlying medical condition, such as fatigue in an anemic patient, will typically have only one or two such symptoms and not even come close to the syndrome of depression. On the other hand, medical patients with the syndrome of major depression, in whom some of the symptoms could potentially be attributed to an underlying medical condition, typically have other psychological symptoms that could replace the physiologic symptoms. In the diagnostic process, all symptoms should be taken at face value. If five of nine criteria are present, the diagnosis should be made. In fact, comorbid depression contributes to morbidity from common medical conditions such as diabetes mellitus and coronary artery disease.

Nevertheless, it can be helpful to determine whether identifiable causes or contributing factors are present when diagnosing depression. As with all syndromes, depression can occur in association with a variety of conditions and with varied presentations. Thus, not only must the syndrome be identified, it is also necessary to determine whether the symptoms are caused or aggravated by an underlying medical or psychiatric illness or a medication, ie, secondary major depression. If these factors are absent, the depression is said to be primary.

When depression is identified, how carefully should a physician look for an occult medical explanation? A complete history and physical examination, with attention to new medications and to the conditions noted above, is sufficient in most cases, with additional studies as directed by this initial approach. Even thyroid tests, which are commonly used in depression evaluations, are unnecessary if nondepression-related thyroid signs, such as tachycardia, bradycardia, eye signs, or skin changes, are not present. Thyroid disease is no more common in depressed patients than in the general population.

MOOD DISORDERS OTHER THAN MAJOR DEPRESSION

Common mood disorders other than major depression are discussed below. Figure 7-1 offers a diagnostic approach to identifying these disorders. Diagnostic criteria for other mood disorders can be found in the Appendix at the end of this chapter.

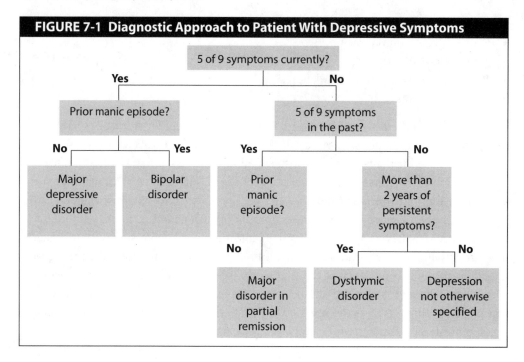

FIGURE 7-1 Diagnostic Approach to Patient With Depressive Symptoms

Bipolar Disorders

Bipolar disorders are characterized by the presence of mania (bipolar I) or hypomania (bipolar II) in addition to depression. A manic episode is a period of 1 week or more that is marked by an abnormally and persistently elevated, expansive, or irritable mood. During this period, three or more of the following symptoms should be present: inflated self-esteem or grandiosity; decreased need for sleep; unusually pressured, rapid, and/or prolonged speech; racing thoughts or flight of ideas; distractibility; increased goal-directed behavior (eg, sexual, political, religious); and excessive involvement in activities that have the potential for significant adverse consequences (eg, spending sprees and sexual indiscretions), often characteristic of impaired judgment. Hypomanic episodes may be as brief as 4 days, featuring a clear change in functioning that is less than marked impairment, in addition to having three or more of the accompanying manic symptoms. Psychotic features may occur in bipolar disorders even more commonly than in unipolar depression. The need for mood stabilizers rather than commonly used antidepressants for bipolar disorders often leads primary care physicians to refer such patients to psychiatrists. In fact, the potential for precipitation of mania by treatment with anti-depressants alone indicates a need to ask about a personal or family history of manic symptoms before starting an antidepressant.

Initial screening question: Have you had a period of several days or more where you have had a lot of energy, required little or no sleep, or had difficulty keeping up with thoughts racing through your head?

Dysthymia

Dysthymia represents a milder but chronic depressed mood present over the better part of at least 2 years. Two or more of the following symptoms should accompany the depressed mood: poor appetite or overeating, insomnia or hypersomnia, low energy or fatigue, low self-esteem, poor concentration or difficulty making decisions, and feelings of hopelessness. In order to diagnosis dysthymia, symptoms should be absent for no more than 2 consecutive months, and criteria for major depressive episode should not be met during the first 2 years of the disturbance. In fact, if the patient has a history of major depression, it should be in full remission for at least 6 months in order to make a diagnosis of dysthymia (otherwise, the diagnosis of major depression in partial remission should be considered). However, after the initial 2 years, major depression may be superimposed, yielding a diagnosis of "double depression." Comorbidity with other psychiatric conditions is frequent enough that the presence of dysthymia should lead physicians to look for associated conditions, including alcohol and substance abuse. Patients with dysthymia may have a poorer response to therapy and worse prognosis than those with major depression, highlighting the importance of identifying such patients.

Initial screening question: Have you felt down or depressed for more days than not for at least 2 years?

Minor or Subthreshold Depression

Some patients will have symptoms of depression that do not meet the above criteria, generally because they have fewer symptoms and/or symptoms of shorter duration. This can be characterized in a variety of ways, including "depression not otherwise specified" or "subthreshold," "subsyndromal," or "minor" depression. Although disagreement on the most appropriate terminology and classification remains, it appears that this type of depressive disorder is more common than major depression and dysthymia combined. In addition, patients who fit this category have significant associated disability and have more in common with depressed patients than with nondepressed patients. Compared to major depression, the lifetime prevalence of clinically significant depressive symptoms is fourfold greater, thereby accounting for greater use of medical services and social morbidity on a population basis. Some patients with several features of depression that are accompanied by excessive worrying or other symptoms of anxiety disorders do not meet the criteria for major depression, generalized anxiety disorder, or panic disorder. Researchers disagree as to how such patients should be categorized, but it is clear that many primary care patients fall into this category. Studies of intervention have not consistently demonstrated improved outcomes with treatment. However, as newer antidepressants become easier for physicians to use and better tolerated by patients, primary care physicians should consider treating such patients, particularly those with more functional impairment or who fail to improve with watchful waiting.

Bereavement

The reaction to the death of a loved one may have several features of major depression, including depressed mood, sleep disturbance, and altered appetite. If depressive symptoms do not improve within 2 months, the diagnosis of major depression should be considered. In addition, presence of the following features should lead the physician to consider depression as the more likely diagnosis: guilt about things other than what the individual did or did not do at the time their loved one died; excessive preoccupation with worthlessness; thoughts of death beyond wishing that they had died with, or instead of, the deceased; striking psychomotor retardation; prolonged, marked functional impairment; hallucinations other than transiently hearing the voice of, or seeing images of, the deceased. In one study of widows and widowers, about half had no depressive symptoms 2 months after loss of their spouse and they tended to remain symptom-free. Of the 21% with major depression after 2 months, many improved by 13 months—36% no longer had depressive symptoms and an equal percentage had subsyndromal depression—but 28% still had major depression. Those with subsyndromal depression at 2 months fared significantly better: 63% were asymptomatic at 13 months, 28% stayed the same, and 9% developed major depression.

Seasonal Affective Disorder

Seasonal affective disorder (SAD) is a depressive disorder characterized by a regular temporal relationship between the onset of the episodes at a particular time of the year, full remission at a particular time of the year, and at least two major depressive episodes within the past 2 years with this temporal seasonal relationship. Although mild seasonal changes in mood and behavior are common in the general population, groups at higher risk for SAD include women between the ages of 20 and 40 and those living in northern latitudes (presumably due to the lack of sun exposure during winter months). Typically, depressive symptoms develop in the fall or winter and remit in the spring. However, a summer SAD, exacerbated in sunny summer months and ameliorated in the winter, has also been reported. Interestingly, most patients in the case series that comprised the first report of SAD in the medical literature also met criteria for a bipolar disorder. Also, a subsyndromal form of SAD appears to be two to three times more common than the full disorder. Primary care physicians should consider seasonal patterns in depressed patients because this influences options for therapy.

Initial screening question: Do your symptoms seem to recur at the same time each year?

Premenstrual Dysphoric Disorder (PMDD)

This diagnosis should be considered in women with mood symptoms that are temporally related to their menstrual cycle. Symptom onset should be in the week prior to menses with complete remission within a week after menses. Five or more of the following symptoms should be reported, including at least one of the first four:

- Markedly depressed mood, feelings of hopelessness, or self-deprecating thoughts
- Marked anxiety, tension, feelings of being keyed up or on edge
- Marked affective lability
- Persistent and marked anger or irritability or increased interpersonal conflicts
- Decreased interest in usual activities
- Subjective sense of difficulty concentrating
- Lethargy, easy fatigability, or marked lack of energy
- Marked change in appetite, overeating, or specific food craving
- Hypersomnia or insomnia
- Subjective feeling of being overwhelmed or out of control
- Other physical symptoms such as breast tenderness or swelling, headaches, joint or muscle pain, a sense of bloating, weight gain

In addition, the symptoms should impair functional status at work, at school, or in social settings; should persist for at least two consecutive cycles; and should not merely represent an exacerbation of another mental disorder. PMDD has been identified in 3% to 5% of menstruating women; like other disorders, subthreshold symptoms seem to be much more common than the disorder itself. There are additional parallels with mood disorders, including evidence of disturbances in serotonin metabolism. The diagnosis should be considered in women who develop symptoms of recurring dysphoria, irritability, and tension in association with menstrual periods. Effective responses have been demonstrated with both cyclical and continuous treatment with selective serotonin reuptake inhibitors (SSRIs). See Chapter 18 for further information.

Initial screening question: Do your symptoms seem to be related to your menstrual cycle?

Postpartum Depression

Postpartum blues, characterized by 1 to 4 days of labile mood and tearfulness, has been reported by 50% to 80% of women within 5 days after delivery. Postpartum depression is seen in 10% to 15% of women at 3 to 6 months postpartum, more frequently in those with a psychiatric history. Life stressors related to delivery and childcare are additional risk factors. Psychosis is far less common than depression and may occur with or without depressive symptoms. Typically beginning within 3 days after delivery, psychosis has a good prognosis but often recurs with subsequent pregnancy. As might be expected, the risk of depression after perinatal death has been found to be even higher (relative risk, 2.4) than after a live birth. Miscarriage is also associated with depression, with a relative risk of 2.5 compared to women who had not been pregnant in the previous year. Factors that particularly raise risk after miscarriage include being childless and having a previous history of major depression.

Perimenopausal Symptoms

Although initial studies indicated an increased prevalence of depression in women at the time of menopause, these studies had methodologic flaws. Today it is felt that there is no significant increase in risk for depression associated with menopause. However, mild mood and anxiety symptoms are common perimenopausally, particularly for women with prolonged physical symptoms of menopause (eg, hot flashes). For women with menopausal symptoms, it has been shown that depressive symptoms and emotional measures of quality of life are improved with hormone replacement therapy. However, hormone replacement therapy is most effective for menopause-specific symptoms such as hot flashes. Thus, for the perimenopausal woman with major depression, antidepressants or psychotherapy may be indicated either initially or in the absence of substantial improvement in the first month of hormone replacement. In women who do develop depression at menopause, a prior history of depression again seems to be the strongest predictor.

SCREENING

There are a number of good reasons to consider screening for depression in some high-risk populations. These include the facts that depression:

- is a major health problem from an epidemiologic point of view;
- contributes substantially to the cost of nonpsychiatric health care;
- causes personal, social, and economic hardships for patients and families;

- is missed half the time without screening;
- is treatable;
- can be screened for using a brief, simple, validated instrument developed to identify depression in the primary care setting;
- is as cost effective as other accepted preventive measures when used for one-time screening or screening at 5-year intervals.

Screening Instruments

Various instruments to facilitate screening for depression in the primary care setting have been developed. Although several have been validated and proved useful to researchers, most have been ignored by primary care providers who find them too cumbersome and time-consuming to use in their busy, short-visit-dominated practices. The PRIME-MD® (Primary Care Evaluation of Mental Disorders) has been the most successful and widely used instrument, effectively screening DSM-IV criteria–based diagnoses of depression, alcoholism, anxiety, and somatoform disorders. The PRIME-MD® has been validated in urban primary care and academic centers, as well as in rural medical practices.

The first iteration of the PRIME-MD® used two screening phases. First, a one-page questionnaire (PQ), to be completed by the patient, featured a series of screening questions, including the following two pertaining to depression: (1) During the past month, have you often been bothered by feeling down, depressed, or hopeless? and (2) During the past month, have you had little interest or pleasure in doing things? The second phase, the Clinician Evaluation Guide (CEG), provides questions for the physician to ask in the event of positive responses on the PQ. For example, a positive response to either of the two screening questions for depression would lead the clinician to ask a series of nine questions based on the DSM criteria for depression. Physicians who used the CEG were able to identify twice as many mental disorders as they had detected without the tool, with high specificity as well. The initial version has largely been replaced by a self-administered version known as PRIME-MD Today™. This new version has comparable validity and takes no more than 1 to 2 minutes of a clinician's time, compared to a mean of 8.4 minutes for the original version. The depression module asks nine simple questions based on the DSM-IV criteria for major depression. This module can also be used independently as the PHQ-9 (see Appendices 1 and 2 in Chapter 3).

The PHQ-9 is ideal for screening for depression, uniquely combining the following features:

- Brief and compatible with time constraints
- Easy and inexpensive to administer
- Makes accurate, validated diagnoses
- Educates patient and provider
- Provides a score to connote severity and to facilitate longitudinal monitoring
- Use has been associated with improved outcomes (in conjunction with provider education and mental health consultation)

In thousands of primary care and obstetrics/gynecology patients, PHQ-9 scores were strongly correlated with self-reported quality of life; interference of symptoms with usual activities; number of physician visits; and difficulty at work and at home and with others. Using a cutoff score of 10 for the diagnosis of major depression, the PHQ-9 has a sensitivity of 88% and specificity of 88%. Most valuable of all, the PHQ-9 score can be used as blood pressure or blood sugar are used to follow hypertension and diabetes mellitus, respectively, enabling a primary care provider to follow a patient's depression. The initial score can be used to guide management as follows (at this time, use of the scores in this manner is empirical and awaits validation):

PHQ-9 Score	Action
1–4	None
5–9	Watchful waiting with periodic screening
10–14	Treatment plan, considering counseling, follow-up, and pharmacotherapy
15–19	Immediate implementation of therapy
≥ 20	Pharmacotherapy and, if severe impairment or poor response to therapy, expedited referral to a mental health specialist

Although one can make a cogent argument for administering the full PRIME-MD Today™, based in particular on the high rates of psychiatric comorbidity seen with depression, busy primary care physicians have found the PHQ-9 to be much more appealing and practical. An even briefer approach is to use two screening questions for depression from the CEG, following up positive responses with the PHQ-9. Williams, Mulrow et al found that even a single question, "Have you felt sad or depressed much of the time in the past year?" was nearly as sensitive (85%) and specific (66%) as more comprehensive questionnaires. The characteristics of this "diagnostic test" compare favorably with many tests commonly used by primary care providers to screen for cancer or heart disease.

Overdiagnosis

Although the literature is replete with studies documenting that depression is missed in up to half of patients presenting with its symptoms in the primary care setting, some patients may be diagnosed with depression prematurely or inappropriately. Unfortunately, the frequency of this phenomenon is not known. As with any clinical disorder, the diagnosis of depression should be based on the presence of characteristic symptoms. Although the presence of unexplained symptoms warrants screening for mood and anxiety disorders, careful evaluation for subtle medical conditions such as sleep apnea is also warranted.

Additional Considerations

Medical conditions and medications. Many medical conditions are associated with higher rates of depression, and although causality is often ambiguous, it is nevertheless important to recognize the greater likelihood of depression in patients with such problems (see Table 7-2).

Depressive symptoms are also seen as a side effect of some medications (Table 7-3), although it should be noted that virtually any medication may cause an idiosyncratic reaction. Consequently, a history of new medications temporally related to the onset of symptoms should be taken. Careful consideration should be given to stopping a potential offending medication and observing the patient for improvement of the depressive symptoms.

TABLE 7-2 Prevalence of Depression in Selected Populations

Condition	Prevalence (%)
Hemodialysis	6.5
Coronary artery disease	16–19
Cancer	20–38
Chronic pain	21–32
Neurological disorders	
• Stroke	27–32
• Parkinson disease	28–51
• Multiple sclerosis	6–57
• Epilepsy	55
• Huntington disease	41
• Dementia	30–40
Endocrine conditions	
• Hyperthyroidism	31
• Diabetes mellitus	24–32.5
• Cushing syndrome	66.6
Other	
• HIV disease	30.3
• Chronic fatigue syndrome	17.2–46.4

Source: Rouchell et al. In: Rundell JR, Wise MG, eds. *Textbook of Consultation-Liaison Psychiatry.* Washington, DC: American Psychiatric Press Inc; 1996.

TABLE 7-3 Medications Associated With Depressive Symptoms

• Alcohol	• Metoclopramide
• Benzodiazepines	• Methyldopa
• Corticosteroids	• Opiates
• Levodopa	• Propranolol
• Neuroleptics	• Reserpine
• Marijuana	• Isotretinoin
• Stimulant, cocaine withdrawal	

Two thirds of primary care patients with a depressive disorder will have at least one other mental disorder. Perhaps the most common association that primary care physicians think about is anxiety: At least 30% of patients with an anxiety disorder also have depression. A number of other psychiatric illnesses have an increased prevalence of depression:

- Substance abuse, 15% to 25%
- Eating disorder, 25% to 50%
- Schizophrenia, 28%
- Dementia, 30% to 40%
- Obsessive-compulsive disorder (OCD), 75%

Another group of psychiatric disorders, the somatoform disorders, are frequently seen in primary care but not often formally diagnosed. These conditions have one of the highest levels of comorbidity with depression, 50% to 80%. Some physicians call patients with unexplained somatic complaints "complainers" or "somatizers" or, when less charitable, "crocks" or "hysterics." Psychiatrists frequently diagnose these patients as having hypochondriasis, conversion disorder, (psychogenic) pain disorder, body dysmorphic disorder, or somatization disorder. Somatoform disorders are discussed more fully in Chapter 15.

Suicidal ideation. Suicidal ideation is a core symptom of depression, though depressed primary care patients have a lower rate of suicide than depressed patients seen in psychiatric practice. Part of the reason for this is that patients who present to primary care physicians with suicidal ideation are typically referred on to psychiatrists. Nonpsychiatrists are often uncomfortable with this symptom of depression. However, at least half of suicide victims are reported to have seen their physician within 1 month, and more than 70% within 2 months, preceding their death. Suicide is the ninth leading cause of death in the United States. It is imperative that primary care physicians know how to detect and evaluate suicidal ideation and to develop strategies for dealing with the patient who presents with suicidal thoughts—whether the physician chooses to help the patient or to refer the patient to a psychiatrist for continued care. See Chapter 4 for a full treatment of this issue.

OVERVIEW OF TREATMENT OF DEPRESSION

Pharmacotherapeutic options for depression have increased dramatically in number over the past 2 decades, and even more important, many of the newer agents are far better tolerated than the original tricyclic antidepressants. However, a variety of other methods also deserve careful consideration in the management of patients with depression, and it is important for the physician to be aware of the full range of alternatives.

Initial Management

The primary care physician has a wide range of options in approaching a patient with depressive symptoms, from watchful waiting to pharmacotherapy and urgent referral. Physicians are accustomed to advising a program of exercise and dietary modifications for conditions such as hypertension, impaired glucose tolerance, and hyperlipidemia, with appropriate follow-up and monitoring. Patients with mild depression may be handled in a similar manner. Three factors are helpful in determining the need for treatment of a depressive disorder:

- *Symptom count:* to qualify for major depression, a patient must meet at least five of nine criteria.
- *Impairment:* the degree that depression has interfered with a person's occupational, social, or physical functioning must be sufficient to warrant the costs and complications of treatment.

- *Duration of the symptoms:* for major depression, symptoms must be present nearly every day for a minimum of 2 weeks.

All three factors should be considered when deciding whether to initiate therapy immediately or to monitor via close follow-up. Although most patients meeting five or more criteria merit early treatment for major depression, there are some patients with recent onset of symptoms and only modest impairment for whom an initial discussion of depression coupled with an early follow-up visit may be warranted, particularly those who require a little time to accept the diagnosis and prepare for therapy. On the other hand, there are patients with fewer than five criteria (eg, depressed mood, fatigue, insomnia, and loss of appetite) whose symptoms are persistent and distressing. Common examples include the patient with prior depressive episodes who experiences a partial recurrence of major depression and the patient with mixed anxiety and depression. Immediate initiation of antidepressants in such patients is preferable to waiting until the patient has developed at least five criteria. In addition, a strong family history of depression or a personal history of prior depression or suicide attempt favors early treatment. Use of the PHQ-9 score in the algorithm described above provides a particularly facile way to determine the urgency of treatment, readily incorporating not only the number of symptoms but their severity. In addition, the PHQ-9 includes a separate question about impairment.

Serious suicidal ideation and/or psychotic depression, typified by severe retardation, delusions (of guilt, persecution, or nihilism), or hallucinations are relatively uncommon in primary care and are indications for urgent referral to a psychiatrist.

Education

The first step in treating any patient who has a depressive syndrome is to provide the patient with information about the condition. This alleviates some of the patient's anxiety about the implications of the diagnosis and improves the likelihood that the patient will adhere to syndrome-specific treatment recommendations. Patients should be told that depression is common and that it is treatable with a high rate of symptom resolution. They should be informed that although depression can occur in response to life events or stresses, it is more likely to occur in individuals who have a predisposition to its development, somewhat like hypertension or headaches. It can be helpful to emphasize that depression is a medical illness, with chemical changes in the brain, not an indication of poor psychological makeup or weak will. This is supported by the fact that depression tends to run in families and is associated with hormone and sleep changes not typically present in the general population. It may be helpful to note the high prevalence of depression in the general population and even to mention some celebrities and historical figures that have experienced depression.

This information helps the patient appreciate that it is not his or her fault that they are depressed. It can also provide an expectation of improvement and resolution, something that is difficult to see in the depths of the current emotional state. Patients often look back on this information and see it as one of the things that helped them make it through their worst period. In fact, there is some evidence that the educational process, through simple statements of support and empathy, can be therapeutic. At the same time, the physician legitimizes the patient's emotional response to his or her condition and offers to work with the patient for recovery.

Education regarding the cause and course of illness is also important for the family or significant others. Family members and friends often think that they did something to cause their loved one to sink into depression. This is particularly troublesome for patients' spouses or children, who may wonder if their relationship with the patient will ever return to normal.

Adherence to treatment has historically been problematic; patients often discontinue therapy as soon as they feel better, putting themselves at higher risk for relapse. Adherence can be improved by educating patients on the need for a satisfactory duration of therapy and the risk of relapse, as well as by recognizing patient preferences. Cognitive-behavioral and interpersonal psychotherapy are as effective as medication in the treatment of mild to moderate depression. If patients know that there is an option to use either with the same likelihood of success, they may choose one over medication as an initial treatment. Other patients will initially prefer medication. This improves the likelihood that patients will complete a treatment course because they are not forced to use the preferred recommendation of their physician.

Support

The second important component of management after education is patient support with nonspecific interventions and help with social adjustments until symptoms improve. Depression is certainly unpleasant for the patient, but it can be made worse by the effect that it has on the way the patient relates to others. This can show up at home in the form of irritability, social isolation, or misperception of others' motivations or interest, which can lead to strained family relationships, lost friendships, and altered expectations.

At work, similar problems can occur. Patients with depression often use their short-term disability, which can put an undue burden on their coworkers. When the patient is able to make it to work, the hostility of others who don't understand the reason for their less-than-optimal performance is taken out on the patient either directly or indirectly.

Recognizing the impact that depression can have on relationships with others, it is helpful to include questions about work and social life during a patient's clinic visits to see if there are areas to focus on as the patient's depression improves. Simple things such as avoiding high-stress situations, getting help with housework or meals, taking a weekend off, or attending couples or family therapy may be extremely beneficial. As the depression improves, so will the relationships; helping them along while the patient is still sick may lessen the time for this to occur.

SPECIFIC TREATMENTS FOR PRIMARY DEPRESSION

Patients with no preexisting cause for depressive symptoms are said to have *primary depression*. Although a variety of predisposing factors are likely to contribute to symptom onset, such as biologic vulnerability or stressful life circumstances, treatment of primary depression, regardless of cause, will lead to improvement in up to 60% to 90% of patients. This section focuses on treatment of unipolar patients, ie, those who have not experienced a manic episode and are not predisposed to one, using interventions with efficacy demonstrated in randomized controlled trials.

Before discussing unipolar major depression, it should be noted that individuals with bipolar affective disorder, typified by manic symptoms at some time during the course of illness, require mood stabilization with thymoleptics such as lithium, carbamazepine, or sodium valproate. Although standard antidepressants may be therapeutic adjuncts, their use alone without concomitant thymoleptics is ill advised because they may promote more rapid (and treatment-resistant) cycling between different mood states. Psychotherapy alone is not a reasonable treatment option. Because of the frequent incapacitating nature of this illness and the specialized therapies required, most patients with bipolar disorder are best referred to psychiatrists for treatment.

Medication

Unipolar major depression can be treated with medication, certain specific forms of psychotherapy, and electroconvulsive therapy. In primary care practice, the only realistic intervention that is usually readily available is medication. The time commitment and minimal amount of reimbursement for psychotherapy usually obviates its use by primary care physicians. General principles for using pharmacotherapy in major depression are shown in Table 7-4 and Figure 7-2.

All antidepressants are of comparable efficacy when subjected to meta-analysis of randomized controlled trials, although there is emerging evidence that venlafaxine, a serotonin-norepinephrine reuptake inhibitor, may be associated with more sustained remission. Consequently, decisions regarding their selection are based on ease of use, prior response, side-effect profile, contraindications, and cost. Each of these will receive differential weight depending on circumstances related to the patient. The initial antidepressant selected can be expected to be efficacious 50% to 70% of the time. SSRIs or other relatively new antidepressants should be the first choice for most patients. They are remarkably well tolerated, safe, and effective. SSRIs are also effective for many other psychiatric conditions (eg, OCD, anxiety, or eating disorders) that are often comorbid with depression. They are also the only agents with proven efficacy for women with PMDD.

TABLE 7-4 Principles of Medication Use for Major Depression in Primary Care

- Document symptoms and associated difficulties.

- Evaluate for preexisting or comorbid factors (bereavement, medical illness, medication, other psychiatric illness).

- Start single-agent antidepressant, starting at or titrating to therapeutic dose.

- Assess compliance and initial response at 1 to 2 weeks, followed by another assessment at 4 to 6 weeks to judge need for change to different medicine (no response), increased dose (partial response), or continuation (good response).

- Follow up in another 4 to 6 weeks to assess continuing compliance, increasing dose, adding second agent, or changing medication if incomplete response (more frequent visits may be necessary if compliance and/or nonresponse become apparent).

- For a single episode treat 4 to 9 months after symptom resolution; for two episodes, treat at least 4 to 9 months but consider prolonged treatment; for three or more episodes, treat for lifetime (greater than 90% chance of recurrence).

- Refer patient to psychiatrist if patient is treatment resistant (poor response to adequate course of two or more agents).

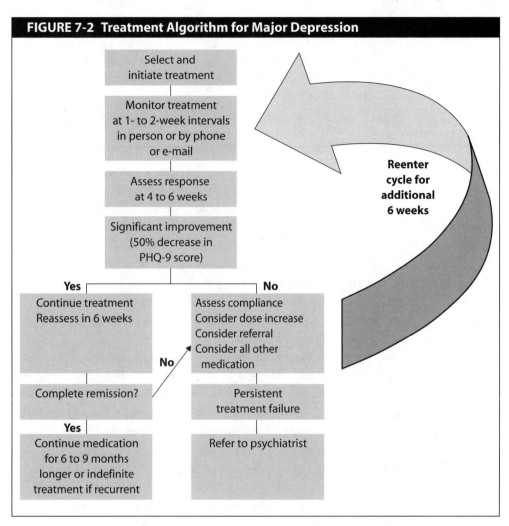

FIGURE 7-2 Treatment Algorithm for Major Depression

Tricyclic antidepressants (TCAs) or monoamine oxidase inhibitors (MAOIs) should rarely be the first choice for depression, especially in primary care. Their side effects are often intolerable or severe, they are more likely to interact with other medicines or exacerbate other medical conditions, they can be difficult to titrate to an effective dose, and they can be lethal in an overdose. However, previous treatment history is important: A patient who has responded to a particular antidepressant in the past is likely to respond to it again, so if a TCA had excellent results previously, it should be considered to treat a recurrence of symptoms.

The ARTIST (A Randomized Trial Investigating SSRI Treatment) trial demonstrated similar efficacy for the three SSRIs most widely prescribed in the United States—fluoxetine hydrochloride, paroxetine hydrochloride, and sertraline hydrochloride—and it is likely that others such as luvoxamine and citaloprim are equally effective. Selecting the appropriate medication may be done based on the cost for some patients, but differences between them may be of greater importance for other patients. For example, paroxetine hydrochloride is more likely to cause weight gain than other SSRIs, which could be beneficial or deleterious depending on the individual patient. Paroxetine hydrochloride has a shorter half-life than the others and consequently may cause serotonin-withdrawal symptoms (headache, tremulousness, nausea) in noncompliant patients. Fluoxetine hydrochloride and paroxetine hydrochloride have a greater effect on the liver's P450 system, making interactions with some other drugs a potential concern. Chapter 19 reviews the side-effect profiles, dosing, and drug-drug interactions of antidepressant medications in greater detail.

Although the SSRIs are far better tolerated than TCAs, they are not universally well tolerated (a variety of effects on sexual function are common to all SSRIs currently available), nor are they effective for everyone. Therefore, primary care physicians should also be comfortable prescribing at least a few other classes of antidepressants. The 5HT-2 antagonists include trazodone hydrochloride and nefazodone hydrochloride, which rarely cause sexual side effects, although trazodone hydrochloride causes priapism in about 1 in 6000 men. Trazodone hydrochloride, which is most often used as a hypnotic, can be useful in conjunction with an SSRI in patients with sleep difficulties. Nefazodone hydrochloride is also a valuable adjunctive antidepressant for patients with partial response to an SSRI or as the sole treatment in individuals for whom an SSRI was ineffective or contraindicated. Rare cases of severe liver toxicity have been reported, leading to a recent recommendation for periodic monitoring of liver function in patients treated with nefazodone hydrochloride.

Venlafaxine hydrochloride acts like an SSRI at lower dose ranges. However, when the dose is increased, it also has significant norepinephrine reuptake inhibition. It is generally effective and well tolerated, without significant interaction with other medicines, although the most significant side effect of hypertension needs to be taken into account and monitored for because this is already a prevalent problem in primary care. In addition, a recent meta-analysis of 8 randomized double-blind placebo-controlled trials suggests that venlafaxine results in higher remission rates than SSRIs.

Two useful antidepressants that do not fit neatly into another category are bupropion hydrochloride and mirtazapine. Bupropion hydrochloride, which is also approved for smoking cessation, might be a judicious choice for a depressed patient who also desires to quit smoking. It rarely causes sexual side effects, but insomnia can occur in some patients. It can also lower the seizure threshold, so it should not be used in patients with a history of seizures. Mirtazapine is sedating and causes weight gain, making it a consideration for patients with insomnia or who have had undesirable weight loss with their depression.

TCAs are as effective as any other class of antidepressants if patients actually continue to take them and should be considered for patients who did not respond to the first choice of medication. Nortriptyline hydrochloride, in particular, has less anticholinergic side effects than some others in its class and provides the physician with the advantage of being able to check blood levels, which can help in assessing compliance and confirming a therapeutic level.

Finally, some patients may ask about or even self-medicate with alternative medicines, most notably St John's wort (*Hypericum perforatum*). Although there were initial suggestions that St John's wort might be effective for mild to moderate depression, more rigorous recent trials have shown no benefit. In addition, there are concerns about quality control with products that are not under the jurisdiction of the US Food and Drug Administration.

Persuading Patients

Some patients are reluctant to begin antidepressant medication because of misconceptions and fears. Several suggestions may overcome this resistance:

- Describe depression as a neurotransmitter imbalance (of serotonin and catecholamine pathways) that can be restored by medical therapy, not unlike other medical conditions such as hypertension.
- Inform patients of the numerous medical conditions with certain symptoms in common with depression that are frequently treated with antidepressants, such as fibromyalgia, chronic insomnia, migraine headaches, peripheral neuropathies and other pain disorders, and chronic fatigue syndrome.
- Emphasize that antidepressants are not nerve pills or habit forming because many people mistakenly equate antidepressants with prescription medicines that can lead to abuse and to which the media have drawn attention, such as benzodiazepines and narcotic pain medications.

A second challenge is to decrease the likelihood that the patient will prematurely discontinue his or her medication. At least one third of patients stop antidepressant medication within the first several weeks, and half or more stop before completing the recommended 6 to 9 months of therapy. Patients should be informed that side effects, if they occur, typically diminish within the first several weeks and that benefits of the medicine are not immediate but unfold gradually over the first 2 to 4 weeks of therapy. Lin et al (1995) have reported that providing five specific educational messages can improve patient adherence to pharmacotherapy. Following are the most common messages:

- Take the medication daily.
- Antidepressants must be taken for 2 to 4 weeks for a noticeable effect.
- Continue to take medicine even if feeling better.
- Do not stop taking the antidepressant without checking with the physician.
- This is what to do if questions arise (eg, call the office).

When TCAs were the mainstay of antidepressant therapy, primary care physicians often provided subtherapeutic doses of antidepressant medication. In fact, studies found that although half of patients went undiagnosed, only one third of those who were diagnosed and treated received an effective course of treatment. This is far less of a problem with SSRIs, where the starting dose is often effective. However, if age or comorbidities lead to selection of a lower starting dose, the medication should be titrated to effect and continued for at least 6 months. Monitoring response to therapy, such as with the PHQ-9 score, is helpful. After a therapeutic dose is reached, if a 50% reduction in symptoms at 4 to 6 weeks or a near complete response at 10 to 12 weeks is not seen, consider giving a referral, dosage adjustment, or adjunctive therapy, such as psychotherapy.

Another problem facing primary care physicians when prescribing antidepressants is determining how long to keep the patient on medication. Based on several large follow-up studies of patients with depression, evidence suggests that patients who have a first episode of depression should be treated 4 to 9 months *after symptom resolution* because continuation therapy decreases the chance of relapse from 65% to 20%. Maintenance therapy beyond this time is usually not needed because 50% will remain symptom-free the rest of their lives. Clinical judgment may suggest, even in these patients, that a longer course of medication is necessary if a patient has a particularly severe episode, prior untreated episodes have been missed, there has been an incomplete response to medication, or there is a strong family history of depression.

Patients with two prior episodes have a 70% chance of recurrence. Although at least 6 to 9 months should elapse before medication is discontinued in these patients, greater consideration should be given to prolonged and/or lifetime therapy based on clinical circumstances. Many factors contribute to this decision, such as episode severity, time interval between episodes, and family history. Patients with three or more episodes or those with poor interepisode recovery should be considered for lifetime antidepressant therapy because they have a 90% chance of experiencing another episode.

Prophylaxis, ie, the goal of prolonged treatment, is most effectively achieved with medication rather than psychotherapy. Full, not subtherapeutic, doses should be used. If this is done in patients with recurrent depression, relapse is reduced from 90% to 20%.

Psychotherapy

Multiple forms of psychotherapy have demonstrated efficacy in randomized controlled trials, including interpersonal psychotherapy (IPT), cognitive-behavioral psychotherapy (CBT), problem-solving therapy (PST), and behavior therapy (BT). (These therapies are described more fully in Chapter 20.)

Psychotherapy is as effective as pharmacotherapy for mild to moderate depression, although it may take longer to produce improvement—up to 6 to 8 weeks, or perhaps 2 to 3 weeks longer than with medication. Psychotherapy requires the patient to become an active participant, ie, trying new behaviors and doing homework assignments in order for improvement to occur. This may be a significant hurdle, but it is often beneficial for the patient to take a more active role. Because the interpersonal relationship between therapist and patient plays a significant role in motivating the patient to be a participant, the therapist plays a potentially greater role in treatment outcome than a physician prescribing medication. However, any given antidepressant can be anticipated to be ineffective for up to 40% of patients. Consequently, the fact that a patient may not establish a productive relationship with his or her first therapist should not lead to avoidance of psychotherapy. However, it may be helpful to inform the patient that he or she may need to try more than one therapist before achieving success.

It is important to recognize that as many as half the patients referred for psychotherapy never follow through with seeing a therapist, although the percentage of patients who comply with antidepressant therapy is no better. The primary care physician has the opportunity to improve the likelihood of follow-through. First, concerns that the patient might have regarding seeing a therapist should be raised up front. In the course of diagnosing depression and then educating the patient about his or her condition, the effective physician demonstrates compassion, initiates a dialogue, and provides an opportunity to work together to achieve improvement. In advising the patient to see a therapist, the physician can note that the patient will be able to talk more frequently and at greater length with a therapist. In some instances, a primary care practice may be able to incorporate a therapist within the practice's walls, enabling the patient to see a therapist in a known, trusted environment, thus avoiding additional stigma.

Combining medication and psychotherapy, compared to medication alone, has been shown to be cost effective, saving money by lowering hospitalization rates and reducing lost workdays. It has also been associated with improved outcomes, especially in patients with more severe depression. Psychotherapy should be considered as an adjunctive therapy for seriously depressed patients, as well as for patients with comorbid panic disorder, posttraumatic stress disorder, obsessive-compulsive disorder, and eating disorders.

Electroconvulsive Therapy

Electroconvulsive therapy (ECT) has been shown to be effective in treating depression, although it is often reserved for severe or treatment-resistant depression. As such, even though a knowledgeable primary care physician can administer it, it is usually administered by psychiatrists. ECT is discussed further in Chapter 19.

Disorders With Specific Therapies or Considerations

Individuals with *seasonal affective disorder* have been shown to respond well to light therapy (use of artificial light to replace seasonally diminished sunlight). Light therapy is discussed further in Chapter 19.

Patients with *premenstrual dysphoric disorder* have been shown to respond to either cyclic or continuous therapy with SSRIs. In general, SSRIs are particularly effective for a wide spectrum of mood and anxiety disorders. In particular, one or more types of antidepressants have proved efficacious for panic disorder, generalized anxiety disorder, social anxiety disorder, and obsessive-compulsive disorder. The fact that many depressed patients have other comorbid mental disorders, coupled with their benign side-effect profile, makes antidepressants particularly appealing as first-line therapy for many patients with this type of mood disorder.

Bereavement does not require specific therapy; it can be treated symptomatically with support and/or medication if the clinical situation warrants. Generally, treatment can be stopped in 6 to 9 months. Patients whose symptoms persist longer than 2 to 3 months should be treated for depression. Similarly, patients with depressive symptoms atypical for uncomplicated bereavement (eg, suicidal ideation, marked guilt, or anhedonia) should be treated.

Alcoholism should be considered a distinct disorder separate from major depression. The prevalence of alcoholism in patients with primary depression is probably no greater than in nondepressed patients, and numerous studies have found that alcoholism is rarely a result of depression. Even when alcoholism is felt to be the primary disorder, diagnosing depression is important because it can modify the course of the alcoholism and appropriate treatment improves prognosis.

Cocaine and amphetamines can mimic mania, and they should be evaluated for in patients presenting with bipolar symptoms.

Medical Illness and Nonpsychiatric Medication

As with any medical condition, etiology of depressive symptoms influences initial management. The coexistence of a mood disorder and a medical condition may be coincidental or the relationship may be related biologically and/or psychologically. If the patient is on medication for a medical condition, first consider whether depressive symptoms could be induced by medication. If so, consider alternative treatment. If the medical condition is known to be a biological cause of depression (eg, hypothyroidism and Cushing disease), primary treatment of the underlying medical disorder should be the initial approach. If the relationship between the general medical condition and the mood disorder is not clear, it is prudent to screen for major depression and to treat it if it is identified. In addition, patients who are psychotically or suicidally depressed even though their symptoms are caused or exacerbated by medical illness or medication may require immediate depression-specific therapy in an effort to accomplish early improvement. This type of patient should in most cases be referred to a psychiatrist. However, when one is unavailable, depression-specific intervention should be considered along with treatment of the medical condition and/or medication adjustment. Patients with these serious depressive symptoms should also be admitted to the hospital for close observation except in unusual cases when family support and close follow-up can provide the care needed.

If the depression seems to be psychologically induced, such as a reaction to the prognosis of a malignancy or HIV infection, treatment of the depression should not be delayed. Many physicians do not initiate treatment in these patients because they consider the patient's clinical circumstances a plausible explanation for depression. Although it is possible, if not likely, that the negative life situation is contributing to the patient's depression, it is inhumane not to treat the depression just because it makes sense given the clinical circumstances. The wisest approach is to try to alleviate the depressive symptoms as quickly as possible. Not only does the patient have a better chance of emotional improvement or recovery, effective treatment is also likely to improve functional capacity and satisfaction with care and to decrease use of general medical health care services due to better compliance, all good reasons to treat even though a legitimate explanation for symptoms is available. Of course, this should be done while medical management of the chronic physical condition is optimized. Likewise, coincident depression that does not seem to be a consequence of the medical condition(s) deserves prompt treatment.

Somatization disorder deserves special consideration, given that more than half of patients who present in a primary care setting with affective disorders have significant somatic components to their illness. Somatic pain has been present in 60% to 100% of depressed patients in some studies, and chronic pain is particularly nettlesome. Most patients with somatization should be approached using the steps outlined for reassurance therapy (Table 7-5) at initial symptom presentation. This involves addressing a few more

TABLE 7-5 Reassurance Therapy

- Examine the patient.
- Assure the patient that serious medical illness is not present (educate).
- Suggest the symptom will resolve.
- Tell the patient to return to normal activity.
- Consider nonspecific treatment.
- Follow the patient.

issues than simply stating that nothing is wrong or that the physical examination and test results are normal. If reassurance therapy fails to alter the course of depressive symptoms, depression-specific treatment can be tried. A general rule of thumb in somatizing patients is to use as few medications as possible because somatizing patients tend to be more sensitive to side effects or to attribute new coincidental symptoms to the medicine. Cognitive-behavioral psychotherapy is useful for patients with symptom-based syndromes such as fibromyalgia, chronic fatigue syndrome, or other unexplained somatic symptoms. This can be an effective alternative to medication.

If a decision is made to use antidepressant medications in a somatizing patient, the target symptoms should be well documented and systematically followed. In these situations, it is useful to follow the patient's progress using an instrument such as the PHQ-9 to determine if the patient is benefiting from treatment.

It is noteworthy that antidepressants, often at low doses, have proved effective for various conditions manifested by chronic physical symptoms, such as fibromyalgia, migraine headache, tinnitus, premenstrual syndrome, atypical chest pain, and chronic pain disorders. Patients with these types of conditions should be informed that these medications, although well known as antidepressants, are also helpful in treating certain physical disorders, probably because of the broad effects neurotransmitters such as serotonin and catecholamines have throughout the body. A useful analogy, for clinicians as well as patients, is that of beta-blockers, which are effective for numerous disorders including hypertension, angina, cardiac arrhythmias, migraine headaches, essential tremor, and stage fright.

Referral

A common question that primary care physicians have about their involvement with depressed patients is when to make a referral. This is, of course, a function of the knowledge and skills of the physician considering the referral. Some physicians have had excellent training in the care of uncomplicated depression, while others feel uncomfortable with a patient's emotional distress in response to an acute crisis. Referral therefore depends on each physician's comfort with a particular patient and the patient's psychiatric problems.

Nonetheless, there is a point at which most clinicians should involve a psychiatrist (Table 7-6). This decision is based on treatment resistance, suicidal or psychotic behavior,

---

TABLE 7-6 Indications for Referral of the Depressed Patient to a Psychiatrist

- *Suicidal* ideation or plans
- *Bipolar* disorder, either currently or prior episodes
- *Psychotic* features (delusions, hallucination, catatonia)
- *Refractory* to the antidepressants with which primary care physician feels comfortable
- *Psychotherapy* needed for optimal response (eg, deep-seated family, interpersonal, or personality issues)
- *Diagnostic* uncertainty (eg, atypical features; psychiatric or medical comorbidity; personality disorder)

the need for combination or extraordinary medication, bipolar symptoms or history, or the need for hospitalization. Some primary care physicians are interested in early referral of patients, even though they technically could handle the clinical situation. This may be the case because their practice demands full attention to medical conditions with little time devoted to the emotional difficulties of their patients. Physicians in this situation should prepare their patients for referral and provide basic information about depression, as well as provide encouragement for follow-through. Of course, there are some patients for whom the primary care physician is comfortable treating pharmacologically but would refer for adjunctive psychotherapy; this includes patients who seem to have significant insight and seemingly can benefit from greater attention and/or expertise than the primary physician is able to provide. Regardless of the indication for referral, the primary care physician should schedule the patient for follow-up, demonstrating continued involvement and interest in their care and preventing feelings of abandonment.

National and Community Resources

The National Institute of Mental Health has a mood and anxiety disorders program (MAP, 866-627-6464). They offer free information, available in many languages, for patients, families, and employers. They also provide information about treatment trials, which may be useful for patients who have unusual complications or are not responding well to treatment.

The following organizations provide information and support for patients with depression: the Depression and Bipolar Support Alliance (DBSA, formerly the National Depressive and Manic Depressive Association, or NDMDA, www.ndmda.org) and the Depression and Related Disorders Association (DRADA, www.drada.org). Patients who have experienced mood disorders run both organizations. They provide informational resources through mail order bookstores and sponsor support groups for patients and family members coping with mood disorders. The organizations also encourage local hospital behavioral medicine programs or community mental health centers to develop support groups. Both have national and regional conventions at which patients can share ideas with patients with similar problems. DRADA also has a peer-counseling program. Referral to resources such as these assists patients and families who find it difficult to cope with the symptoms of depression before recovery has occurred with appropriate treatment. The physician should periodically review the material provided by such groups to ensure that their message is consistent.

Web sites also provide useful information for physicians, including the MacArthur Foundation Depression and Primary Care web site (www.depression-primarycare.org) and the web site of the American Psychiatric Association (www.psych.org).

SUMMARY

Depression is common in primary care and presents special challenges to physicians who diagnose and treat it. Numerous medical and psychiatric conditions often complicate depression. Fortunately, a tool exists (the PHQ-9) that rapidly and easily facilitates initial diagnosis and subsequent monitoring of patients with depression. The test can even serve as a guide for when to initiate treatment, modify or supplement initial therapy, and make a referral.

A number of effective, well-tolerated medications are also available for use in primary care, narrowing the need for referral to a psychiatrist to patients who do not respond to medication or who have complicating features such as psychosis, suicidal ideation, or bipolar depression. Ideally, care of less seriously ill depressed patients is coordinated by both psychiatrists and primary care physicians, with the help of other mental health professionals. Although most patients can be effectively treated for depression in the primary care setting, it is helpful to have psychiatric assistance when needed, particularly in light of demands in the primary care setting. Adequately addressing the needs of these patients is likely to reduce the amount of medical services required by these patients and to improve their ability to return to a more productive life.

ADDITIONAL READINGS

Ackerman RT, Williams JW. Rational treatment choices for non-major depressions in primary care. *J Gen Intern Med.* 2002;17:293-301.

Cassem EH. Depressive disorders in the medically ill: an overview. *Psychosom.* 1995;36:S2-S10.

Depression Guideline Panel. *Clinical Practice Guideline Number 5: Depression in Primary Care: Volume 1. Detection and Diagnosis.* Rockville, Md: US Department of Health and Human Services; 1993. Agency for Health Care Policy and Research. AHCPR Publication No 93-0550.

Depression Guideline Panel. *Clinical Practice Guideline Number 5: Depression in Primary Care: Volume 2. Detection and Diagnosis.* Rockville, Md: US Department of Health and Human Services, Agency for Health Care Policy and Research; 1993. AHCPR Publication No 93-0551.

Enssuah R, Gao B. Global benefit-risk evaluation of antidepressant action: comparison of pooled data for venlafaxine, SSRIs, and placebo. *CNS Spectr.* 2002;7:882-888.

Hall RCW, Wise MG. The clinical and financial burden of mood disorders: cost and outcome. *Psychosom.* 1995;36:S11-S18.

Hays RD, Wells KB, Sherbourne CD, et al. Functioning and well-being outcomes of patients with depression compared with chronic general medical illnesses. *Arch Gen Psychiatry.* 1995;52:11-19.

Kathol RG. Reassurance therapy: what to say to symptomatic patients with benign or non-existent medical disease. *Int J Psychol Med.* 1997;27:2, 173-180.

Katon W, Von Korff M, Lin E, et al. Collaborative management to achieve treatment guidelines: impact on depression in primary care. *JAMA.* 1995;273:1026-1031.

Kroenke K, Spitzer RL, Williams JBW, et al. Physical symptoms in primary care: predictors of psychiatric disorders and functional impairment. *Arch Fam Med.* 1994;3:774-779.

Kroenke K, Jackson JL, Chamberlin J. Depressive and anxiety disorders in patients presenting with physical complaints: clinical predictors and outcome. *Am J Med.* 1997;103:339-347.

Kroenke K, West SL, Swindle R, et al. Similar effectiveness of paroxetine, fluoxetine, and sertraline in primary care: a randomized controlled trial. *JAMA.* 2001;286:2947-2955.

Kroenke K, Spitzer RL, Williams JBW. The PHQ-9: validity of a brief depression severity measure. *J Gen Intern Med.* 2001;16:606-613.

Lin EHB, Von Korff M, Katon W, et al. The role of the primary care physician in patients' adherence to antidepressant therapy. *Med Care.* 1995;33:67-74.

Perez-Stable EJ, Miranda J, Munoz RF, et al. Depression in medical outpatients: underrecognition and misdiagnosis. *Arch Intern Med.* 1990;150:1083-1088.

Pignone MP, Gaynes BN, Rushton JL, et al. Screening for depression in adults: a summary of the evidence for the US Preventive Services Task Force. *Ann Intern Med.* 2002;136;765-776.

Roy-Burne PP. Generalized anxiety and mixed anxiety-depression: association with disability and health care utilization. *J Clin Psychiatry*. 1996;57(suppl 7):86-91.

Schulberg HC, Katon W, Simon GE, Rush JA. Treating major depression in primary care practice: an update of the Agency for Health Care Policy and Research Practice guidelines. *Arch Gen Psychiatry*. 1998;55:1121-1127.

Simon GE, Von Korff M. Recognition, management, and outcomes of depression in primary care. *Arch Fam Med*. 1995;4:99-105.

Spitzer RL, Kroenke K, Williams JBW, Patient Health Questionnaire Primary Care Study Group. Validation and utility of a self-report version of PRIME-MD. *JAMA*. 1999;282:1737-1744.

Whooley MA, Simon GE. Managing depression in medical outpatients. *N Engl J Med*. 2000;343:1942-1950.

Williams JW, Barrett J, Oxman T, et al. Treatment of dysthymia and minor depression in primary care: a randomized controlled trial in older adults. *JAMA*. 2000;284:1519-1526.

Williams JW, Mulrow CD, Chiquette E, Noel PH, Aguilar C, Cornell J. A systematic review of newer pharmacotherapies for depression in adults: evidence report summary: Clinical guidelines, part 2. *Ann Intern Med*. 2000;132:743-756.

Zajecka JM, Ross JS. Management of comorbid anxiety and depression. *J Clin Psychiatry*. 1995;56(suppl 2):10-13.

Appendix

Criteria for Mood Disorders Other Than Major Depression

Bipolar I Disorder

I. Current and/or previous history of a manic or mixed episode, defined as:

  A. Manic episode

    1. A 1-week or longer period of abnormally and persistently elevated, expansive, or irritable mood

    2. During this period, three or more of the following symptoms have been persistent and significant:

      a) Inflated self-esteem or grandiosity

      b) Decreased need for sleep

      c) More talkative than usual or pressure to keep talking

      d) Flight of ideas or feeling that thoughts are racing

      e) Distractibility

      f) Psychomotor agitation or increase in goal-directed activity

      g) Excessive involvement in pleasurable activities that have a high potential for painful consequences

    3. Symptoms do not meet criteria for a mixed episode

    4. Function is markedly impaired

    5. Symptoms cannot be attributed to substance abuse, medication, or medical condition

  B. Mixed episode

    1. Criteria are met for both a manic episode and a major depressive episode nearly every day for at least 1 week

    2. Function is markedly impaired

    3. Symptoms cannot be attributed to substance abuse, medication, or medical condition

II. The mood symptoms cause clinically significant distress or impairment in social, occupational, or other important areas of functioning

III. The mood symptoms are not better accounted for by, or superimposed on, another diagnosis such as schizoaffective disorder or schizophrenia

IV. The mood symptoms are not due to a substance, medication, or medical condition

Bipolar II Disorder

I. As opposed to bipolar I, this is characterized not by mania but by a history of one or more hypomanic episodes, defined as:

  A. A distinct period of persistently elevated, expansive, or irritable mood, lasting throughout at least 4 days, that is clearly different from the usual nondepressed mood

  B. During the period of disturbance, three or more of the following symptoms have been persistent and significant:

    1. Inflated self-esteem or grandiosity

    2. Decreased need for sleep

    3. More talkative than usual or pressure to keep talking

    4. Flight of ideas or feeling that thoughts are racing

    5. Distractibility

    6. Psychomotor agitation or increase in goal-directed activity

    7. Excessive involvement in pleasurable activities that have a high potential for painful consequences

C. There is an unequivocal change in functioning associated with the episode, but it is not so marked as to require hospitalization or to severely impact social or occupational function, and psychosis is absent

D. The change in mood and functional status is noticed by others

E. The mood symptoms are not due to a substance, medication, or medical condition

Dysthymia

  I. Depressed mood for most of the day, for more days than not, as indicated either by subjective account or observation by others, for at least 2 years

 II. Presence, while depressed, of two or more of the following:

    A. Poor appetite or overeating

    B. Insomnia or hypersomnia

    C. Low energy or fatigue

    D. Low self-esteem

    E. Poor concentration or difficulty making decisions

    F. Feelings of hopelessness

III. During the 2-year period the individual has never been without the symptoms in criteria A and B for more than 2 months at a time

IV. No major depressive episode has been present during the first 2 years of the disturbance

 V. There is no history of mania or hypomania

Chapter **8**

Anxiety Disorders

Phillip R. Reeves, MD
Kenneth N. Panitch, MD
Troy L. Thompson II, MD

Primary care physicians frequently diagnose and manage anxiety, which is the most common psychiatric complaint in the primary care setting, estimated to occur in 10% to 15% of the general population. Untreated anxiety disorders impact the general economy through lost wages and productivity, as well as the strain put on the health care system. Anxiety may be a symptom of an underlying medical condition, a response to medications, the result of idiosyncratic or metabolic drug interactions, a complication of withdrawal from a prescribed or abused substance, a feature of many psychiatric illnesses, one of several primary anxiety disorders, or a combination of the above.

The root of the word *anxiety* comes from the Latin verb *angere*, meaning to choke, strangle, and give pain or distress. Indeed, the anxiety sufferer often complains of chest pain and shortness of breath, irritability, and a feeling of apprehension and doom. This is often accompanied by a fear that one will start to scream, lose control, or go insane. Not all anxiety is bad, however. Any student, musician, actor, or athlete can tell you that a little anxiety heightens the senses and improves performance, but that beyond a certain threshold it is crippling and will impair the skillful execution of difficult tasks.

Primary care physicians are the clinicians who are most likely to make an anxiety diagnosis. It is the chief complaint for 10% to 15% of primary care outpatient visits; and for at least 2% to 5% of those afflicted, the result will be incapacitation. Given the high prevalence of anxiety in the general population and in primary care settings, primary care physicians must be knowledgeable about anxiety and its various manifestations. This chapter addresses how anxiety is recognized and managed in a primary care practice. A discussion of techniques the physician can use to increase the yield of detecting clinically significant anxiety is also provided. Specific disorders, as described in the *Diagnostic and Statistical Manual of Mental Disorders,* fourth edition (DSM-IV), that the primary care physician will encounter in practice are presented, as is a discussion of the neurobiology of anxiety and the case of anxiety in the medically ill patient.

ASSESSING THE PATIENT WITH ANXIETY

A common challenge faced by the primary care physician is identifying anxiety and anxiety disorders in patients who present with concern over a specific symptom or "medical" disorder. The manifestations of anxiety are so varied that they overlap with a broad array of physical disorders and medication effects, as shown in Tables 8-1 and 8-2.

Some physical clues to the diagnosis of anxiety may include fidgety and hyperactive behavior, facial expressions of fear or panic, tachycardia, palpitations and chest pains, shortness of breath, lightheadedness and dizziness, headache, diarrhea, heartburn and abdominal pains, urinary frequency, faintness, diaphoresis, dry mouth, and paresthesia. Some psychological clues may include complaints of worry and tension, a sense of doom and panic, difficulty with concentration, preoccupation with self, complaints of chronic fatigue, lack of energy, feeling like the world seems odd, observance that the patient feels he or she is not the same person he or she used to be, problems with sexual performance, abuse of medications and alcohol, and a tendency toward being accident-prone.

Physicians in training are often taught to rule out every possible underlying medical disorder before assigning a diagnosis of an anxiety disorder. Typically, a battery of

TABLE 8-1 Medical Conditions That Often Have Anxiety as a Symptom

Endocrine
- Hypothyroidism
- Hyperthyroidism
- Pheochromocytoma
- Hyperadrenalism

Cardiovascular
- Congestive heart failure
- Pulmonary embolism
- Arrhythmia

Respiratory
- Chronic obstructive pulmonary disease
- Pneumonia
- Hyperventilation

Metabolic
- Vitamin B_{12} deficiency
- Porphyria

Neurologic
- Neoplasms
- Vestibular dysfunction
- Encephalitis

Source: *Diagnostic and Statistical Manual of Mental Disorders*. 4th ed, Text Revision. Copyright 2000. American Psychiatric Association.

diagnostic tests is ordered, and when nothing is found, patients are given the diagnosis of anxiety. This process leaves the patient feeling frustrated that his or her physician feels the problem is "all in the head" and not real or serious. Because many patients distrust this process of assessment, they seek further medical or alternative health care opinions and are often subjected to additional testing. This approach, which is unsatisfying to physicians and patients alike, often results in poor care and waste of medical resources.

An alternative approach that may be helpful in evaluating patients with symptoms suggestive of anxiety is to first thoroughly evaluate the patient within the construct of the biopsychosocial model. Gather as much information as possible about the onset and progression of presenting symptoms, including exacerbating and alleviating factors. Both the medical and the psychological histories should be taken in parallel. Other useful strategies in obtaining the history and lessening anxiety in the patient-physician relationship include the following:

- Greet your patient in a friendly, genuine manner, offering a caring gesture such as a handshake or touch on the shoulder.
- Make a positive comment on something personal that your patients have with them, demonstrating interest.

TABLE 8-2 Medications and Other Substances That May Produce Anxiety

Intoxication	Withdrawal	Medications	Toxins
Alcohol	Alcohol	Anesthetics	Gasoline
Amphetamines	Cocaine	Analgesics	Paint
Caffeine	Sedatives	Sympathomimetics	Organophosphates
Cannabis	Hypnotics	Bronchodilators	Insecticides
Cocaine	Anxiolytics	Anticholinergics	Nerve gases
Hallucinogens		Insulin	Carbon monoxide
Inhalants		Thyroid preparations	Carbon dioxide
Phencyclidine		Oral contraceptives	
		Antihistamines	
		Antiparkinsonians	
		Corticosteroids	
		Antihypertensives	
		Cardiovascular	
		Antidepressants	

Source: *Diagnostic and Statistical Manual of Mental Disorders.* 4th ed, Text Revision. Copyright 2000. American Psychiatric Association.

- Sit down and don't appear rushed; this will put the patient at ease. Then say something like, "Let's take some time to talk. How have you been doing?"
- Be attentive: maintain good eye contact and body posture that does not lean away from the patient.
- Take a thorough, careful history.
- Ask the patient to tell you about the stresses in his or her life. This questioning often opens up areas that would otherwise be left untouched.
- Ask about subjects that may be sensitive, such as intimate relationships, family violence, sexual functioning, financial and legal stresses, etc.
- Try to get more detail when a patient seems uncomfortable with a question or takes a long time to answer, asking for clarification and more details to vague responses or unexpected answers.
- Look for the meaning of the illness to the patient, what he or she is most concerned about, and temporal connections between symptoms and life events.
- Avoid rushing.
- Normalize the patient's emotional reactions with destigmatizing comments, such as, "It is very common and understandable for patients to feel the type of distress you've been having when they experience the symptoms you have had. What are your specific worries?"
- Make a treatment alliance with the patient: "I will stick with you through this; we will get to the bottom of this."
- Agree to follow up regularly.

The mental status examination includes noting whether the patient seems tense or anxious as well as the range of emotions and mood expressed during the interview.

Another important aspect of the evaluation is the physical exam. Even when an anxiety disorder is likely, based on the history alone, the physical examination enables the clinician to determine if another condition is present that may be completely or partially responsible for the physical symptoms. It also serves as a screen for an underlying condition that may mimic anxiety and helps to tailor which, if any, diagnostic tests are necessary. Finally, the exam may have a therapeutic effect because the physician has direct contact with the patient (through the "laying on of hands") and can reassure the patient that everything checks out well. Table 8-3 summarizes the key points of this initial evaluation.

This type of evaluation for anxiety symptoms is time-consuming and can be carried out over a few appointments. However, the data gathered and insight gained are invaluable in subsequent care of the patient. In some instances, this evaluation may be all that is needed to confidently diagnose an anxiety disorder. The time invested in performing this initial evaluation and making an accurate diagnosis may be saved many times over by avoiding the pursuit of blind leads and unnecessary testing.

When it seems clear that a patient has an anxiety disorder and not some other medical illness, frankly and honestly discuss the illness with him or her. Patients appreciate a more medicalized approach and the time spent on patient education, which should explain that modern scientific research confirms that anxiety symptoms are the expression of an endocrine/neurotransmitter imbalance. Discussing normal physiologic reactions to abnormal life stressors helps to destigmatize the experience. Assure your patients that you do not think they are crazy. Patients will feel validated, and this reassurance will open the door to a more meaningful and stronger patient-physician relationship. When patients experience an alliance with their physician, they can begin to feel less stress and trust their physician's recommendations. Patients want and need to feel that their physicians care about them. This empathy is the crux of the therapeutic relationship and a core aspect of psychotherapy. The empathy that you demonstrate will build trust and improved compliance with medical treatments.

A goal of the initial assessment is to make as specific a diagnosis as possible within the spectrum of anxiety disorders delineated in the DSM-IV. There are significant differences in the course and prognosis of these conditions. At times, treatment may be initiated to control symptoms before a significant diagnosis can be made.

TABLE 8-3 Key Steps in Evaluating Anxiety Symptoms

- Gather initial specific information relative to presenting symptoms.
- Obtain a thorough past medical, psychiatric, and social history.
- Assess the likelihood of an underlying medical condition and substances causing or exacerbating anxiety.
- Assess patient's level of stress.
- Inquire about past trauma, violence, or abuse.
- Convey willingness to listen.

TABLE 8-4 DSM-IV Anxiety Disorders

- Panic disorder (with or without agoraphobia)
- Agoraphobia without a history of panic attacks
- Specific phobias, including social phobias
- Obsessive-compulsive disorder
- Posttraumatic stress disorder
- Acute stress disorder
- Generalized anxiety disorder
- Anxiety disorder due to a general medical condition or substance-induced
- Anxiety disorder not otherwise specified

Source: Reprinted with permission from *Diagnostic and Statistical Manual of Mental Disorders*. 4th ed, Text Revision. Copyright 2000. American Psychiatric Association.

Table 8-4 lists the current classification of anxiety disorders in DSM-IV. Five disorders are discussed here: panic disorder, specific and social phobias, obsessive-compulsive disorder (OCD), posttraumatic stress disorder (PTSD), and generalized anxiety disorder (GAD). DSM-IV diagnostic criteria, epidemiological data, treatment strategies available to primary care physicians, and indications for the involvement of a psychiatrist or other mental health professional are discussed in the following sections.

PANIC DISORDER

Case Vignette

Mrs Alison, a 26-year-old taxicab dispatcher, had sudden onset of chest tightness, palpitations, and dizziness for the first time as she walked around a large shopping mall near her home. She feared she was having a heart attack, even though she had no personal or family history of cardiac disease. She drove herself to the nearest emergency department. Her vital signs revealed mild tachypnea and tachycardia, and an electrocardiogram (ECG) showed sinus tachycardia. She was referred to a cardiologist, who obtained an echocardiogram, a 24-hour Holter monitor, and a thallium stress test, all of which were normal. Mrs Alison experienced four more episodes, each lasting about 10 minutes, over the next 2 weeks. She avoided the mall, where she had previously shopped regularly, as well as her local supermarket, where she had her third episode. The cardiologist sent her to a neurologist, who, suspecting demyelinating disease, performed a magnetic resonance imaging (MRI) of the head and visual evoked responses; both were normal. Mrs Alison then sought out her primary care physician, Dr Rhine, who reviewed her history and the workup previously performed (including basic chemistries and thyroid function tests). She told Mrs Alison that she believed she was suffering from panic disorder and recommended a trial of a selective serotonin reuptake inhibitor. After obtaining reassurances from her physician that this condition was neither life threatening nor "all in her head," she agreed to start the medication.

Panic attacks are discrete, time-limited events that have both emotional and physical features. They are the key feature of panic disorder (PD) but may occur in other anxiety disorders as well. Typically, they occur spontaneously, increasing in intensity over several minutes and then taking another several minutes to begin to resolve. The physical symptoms, particularly chest pain and shortness of breath, are the result of autonomic hyperarousal. Such attacks often lead to avoidance of the situations the individual associates with the attack or at least a desire to feel that there is a safe and rapid route for escape if the need should arise. Another feature of PD is the anticipatory fear of the consequences of a panic attack. As defined by DSM-IV criteria, a panic attack is accompanied by at least four of the following somatic or cognitive symptoms:

- Palpitations, pounding heart, or accelerated heart rate
- Sweating
- Trembling or shaking
- Sensations of shortness of breath or smothering
- Feeling of choking
- Chest pain or discomfort
- Nausea or abdominal distress
- Feeling dizzy, unsteady, light-headed, or faint
- Derealization (feeling of unreality) or depersonalization (being detached from one's self)
- Fear of losing control or going crazy
- Fear of dying
- Paresthesia
- Chills or hot flashes

Interestingly, there are models of chemical induction for this physiologic/psychologic event. Because the infusion of lactic acid may provoke panic attacks in individuals who previously had spontaneous episodes, some have proposed using a lactic acid challenge as a diagnostic tool. Because change in blood pH and hypersensitivity to carbon dioxide may be involved, inhalation of carbon dioxide and infusion of bicarbonate of soda also may initiate panic attacks. Other panicogenic substances include yohimbine hydrochloride, a noradrenergic stimulant; doxapram hydrochloride, a respiratory stimulant; and cholecystokinin (CCK).

Diagnosing Panic Disorder

The distinguishing feature of panic attacks in patients with PD is that the attacks are uncued or unexpected, differentiating PD patients from those with social phobia, specific phobia, PTSD, and OCD, for whom the panic attacks are often either situationally triggered or situationally predisposed. The specific DSM-IV criteria for PD are shown in Table 8-5.

The lifetime prevalence of PD is 1% to 5%, with a 2:1 female:male ratio. Typically, panic attacks begin in the third decade; the average age of onset is 25 with a 10-year standard deviation. One third to one half of individuals with panic attacks have agoraphobia, a complication that often limits activity outside the home. Patients who have panic attacks often have other symptoms of generalized anxiety and will deny psychiatric symptoms. This can cause them to become frustrated, thinking their physician feels it is "all in their head." These patients may make multiple visits to emergency rooms or urgent care outpatient centers in an attempt to find a source of their symptoms. There

TABLE 8-5 DSM-IV Criteria for Panic Disorder

A. Recurrent, unexplained, or unexpected panic attacks with at least one of the attacks followed by 1 month of:

   1. Persistent concern of additional attacks

   2. Worry about the implications of the attacks

   3. Change in behavior related to the attacks

B. The panic attacks cannot be due to direct physiologic effects of a substance or general medical condition.

C. The panic attacks are not better explained by the presence of another mental disorder.

Note: Panic disorder can be with or without agoraphobia, anxiety, and avoidance of situations or places from which escape might be difficult or embarrassing or in which help might not be available in the event of having a panic attack.
Source: Reprinted with permission from *Diagnostic and Statistical Manual of Mental Disorders*. 4th ed, Text Revision. Copyright 2000. American Psychiatric Association.

is often absenteeism from school and work, which can lead to social and financial hardships. Many patients who have panic attacks become depressed; this occurs comorbidly in 50% to 60% of patients with PD. In two thirds of the cases, the panic disorder appears first.

Pharmacologic Treatment of Panic Disorder

When choosing a psychiatric medication, comorbid conditions and prior response history for the patient and first-degree relatives (parents, siblings, and children) should be taken into account. Effective pharmacologic and nonpharmacologic therapies are available for treating PD. At 6 to 10 years posttreatment, 30% are asymptomatic, 40% to 50% have improved but are still symptomatic, and 20% to 30% are the same or worse.

The benzodiazepine alprazolam (Xanax) was the first US Food and Drug Administration (FDA)-approved medication to treat PD. Tricyclic antidepressants and monoamine oxidase inhibitors (MAOIs) have also been used with success. Formerly, these classes of medications were first-line agents. Today, however, medications that, at least in part, are serotonin reuptake inhibitors are the pharmacologic intervention of choice. Their efficacy is comparable to the older MAOIs without the risk of hypertensive crisis, due to the ingestion of tyramine-containing food products.

Common side effects of selective serotonin reuptake inhibitors (SSRIs) include anxiety, gastrointestinal (GI) distress, agitation, sexual dysfunction, and insomnia. They all raise synaptic levels of serotonin but differ with respect to structure, cytochrome P-450 interactions, half-life, and side-effect profile. When given to patients with PD at therapeutic doses for depression, they may be overly stimulating and therefore poorly tolerated. Care must be taken to start low and gradually increase the dosage, as tolerated by the patient. Sertraline hydrochloride, eg, should be started at 25 mg every other day and titrated to 50 to 100 mg per day, as tolerated. Paroxetine hydrochloride is usually started at 10 mg daily and titrated up to 20 to 40 mg. Citalopram hydrobromide is usually prescribed at an initial dose of 20 mg, and escitalopram oxalate at an initial daily dose of 10 mg, which may prove to be therapeutic.

High-potency benzodiazepines may have significant benefit during the initial phase of treatment with an antidepressant. The dose can often be titrated downward and sometimes discontinued as the dosage of antidepressant reaches therapeutic levels.

Nonpharmacologic Treatments

Supportive therapy. Supportive therapy is perhaps the type of nonpharmacologic therapy at which primary care physicians are most adept. Providing a supportive, educational, and caring environment for the patient may be particularly beneficial when used in concert with pharmacologic treatment. However, these nonpharmacologic approaches alone have not been shown to be effective in improving outcomes for patients with PD.

Cognitive-behavioral approaches. A full explanation of cognitive-behavioral therapy (CBT) can be found in Chapters 1 and 20. Several points about this approach may be useful to the primary care physician. Patients are often fearful about their panic attack symptoms. Literature that provides a good explanation of the prevalence and nature of panic disorder or a pamphlet listing signs and symptoms of panic can be used to validate what the patient is experiencing. The patient can share this information with his or her family to prove he or she has a bona fide medical disorder and is not crazy.

The physician may then explain that the body is misinterpreting internal and external signals as being more dangerous than they actually are. The physician should address the physical symptoms the patient is experiencing and try to allay his or her fears of more serious illness. Certain diagnostic tests can often be helpful in proving to the patient, and the physician, that another diagnosis is not being missed. If the physician is not concerned about other pathology, the tests may be used to demonstrate to the patient that nothing else is causing the symptomology. Helping patients gain an awareness and understanding of PD and relieving them of the fear of a life-threatening condition is often a useful first step in treatment.

Another helpful aspect of CBT that the primary care physician may use is applied relaxation and respiratory control techniques. These exercises, which are described later, teach patients to reduce arousal levels and instill a sense of control in the event of a panic attack.

An additional component of CBT involves exposure techniques. Gradual exposure and confrontation with feared stimuli while practicing relaxation and respiratory control techniques are often beneficial to patients with panic disorder and specific phobias as well. Exposure can take the form of actual or imaginary confrontation with the feared situation or object.

The type of therapy a patient receives depends in part on the person's willingness to take medication, comorbid psychological conditions, and acuity of the situation. A patient should be referred to a mental health professional if he or she does not want pharmacologic therapy and the physician is not knowledgeable or comfortable with CBT. Alternatively, if adequate response is not achieved after 6 to 8 weeks of pharmacotherapy, with or without informal cognitive-behavioral techniques, a change in medication or referral to a mental health professional is appropriate. Failure to respond to usual approaches should prompt the physician to consider a comorbid psychiatric condition.

SPECIFIC PHOBIA

A specific phobia is clinically significant anxiety provoked by exposure to a specific feared object or situation, leading to avoidant behavior. The DSM-IV diagnostic criteria are shown in Table 8-6.

Diagnosing Specific Phobia

Specific subtypes of phobias include, as examples, animal, natural, environmental (heights, storms, water), blood-injection-injury, and situational (airplanes, elevators, enclosed spaces). There is a 10% to 11% lifetime prevalence in the general population. Simple phobias predominantly occur in women: 75% to 90% of the animal, natural, environment, and situational and 50% to 70% of blood-injection-injury phobias occur in females. Onset is usually in childhood or early adulthood, with variation among the different types of specific phobias. The etiology of specific phobias is often felt to be either exposure to traumatic events (either personally or observing someone else undergoing a traumatic event) or via informational transmission from a parent, eg, being told repeatedly about the dangers involved in going in elevators. Many childhood phobias remit spontaneously; however, phobias that persist into adulthood remit spontaneously only approximately 20% of the time.

TABLE 8-6 Diagnostic Criteria for Simple (Specific) Phobia

A. Marked and persistent fear that is excessive or unreasonable, cued by the presence or anticipation of a specific object or situation.

B. Exposure to the phobic stimulus almost invariably provokes an immediate anxiety response, which may take the form of a situationally bound or situationally predisposed panic attack. Note: In children, the anxiety may be expressed by crying tantrums, freezing, or clinging.

C. The person recognizes that the fear is excessive or unreasonable. Note: In children, this feature may be absent.

D. The phobic situation(s) is either avoided or endured with intense anxiety or distress.

E. The avoidant anxious anticipation or distress in the feared situations interferes significantly with the person's normal routine, occupation, academic functioning, or social activities or there is marked distress about having the phobia.

F. In individuals under 18 years, the duration is at least 6 months.

G. The anxiety, panic attacks, or phobic avoidance associated with a specific phobia or situation is not better accounted for by another mental disorder such as obsessive-compulsive disorder (fear of dirt in someone with an obsession about contamination), posttraumatic stress disorder (avoidance of stimuli associated with a severe stressor), separation anxiety (avoidance of school), social phobia (avoidance of social situations because of fear of embarrassment), panic disorder with agoraphobia, or agoraphobia without history of panic disorder.

Source: Reprinted with permission from *Diagnostic and Statistical Manual of Mental Disorders*. 4th ed, Text Revision. Copyright 2000. American Psychiatric Association.

Treatment of Specific Phobia

Pharmacologic therapy is usually not used for specific phobias. The mainstay of treatment is behavioral (exposure) therapy, sometimes in conjunction with the cognitive techniques described earlier for PD. The primary care physician can first help patients learn anxiety-reducing techniques such as progressive muscle relaxation, diaphragmatic breathing, and mental imaging. These can be demonstrated in the office or given as homework assignments for patients to practice between appointments. (See the appendix at the end of this chapter for a brief description of each of these exercises.)

The primary care physician can also help patients identify automatic fearful thoughts that occur when thinking about or confronting the phobic situation or object. As patients learn which of their automatic thoughts result in heightened anxiety levels, they can try to block or counteract them with thought processes learned in therapy sessions. Ultimately, patients are instructed in gradual exposure to a hierarchy of increasingly fearful situations in which they use relaxation, breathing, and cognitive therapy techniques until they are able to encounter their most feared object or situation.

For some phobias, such as fear of flying, commercial courses are available. These classes use the same principles described here; they teach about the safety of planes, give arguments to dispute automatic thoughts, teach breathing and relaxation exercises, and then gradually increase exposure. One such course in the northeast celebrates the last day of class with a flight from New York to Boston for dinner and a return home the same night. Unless the primary care physician has a particular interest or expertise in these approaches, referral to a mental health professional or phobia clinic is appropriate.

SOCIAL PHOBIAS

Social phobias are phobias associated with certain types of social or performance situations. The DSM-IV criteria are shown in Table 8-7. The two main types of social phobia are classic and generalized. In the classic type there may be fear of spilling coffee or wine at a social gathering or talking to someone of the opposite sex. In most cases, people with classic phobias had normal personalities before onset of the phobia; there is an equal male-to-female representation. In generalized social phobia there are broad social skill deficits and social dysfunction. Many people with generalized social phobias were excruciatingly shy as children. There is a male predominance in this condition. Not surprisingly, substance abuse is a common comorbid condition.

Diagnosing Social Phobia

Common features seen in social phobia include blushing, acute fear of being looked at by others, fear of scrutiny, and fear of people (individuals, not crowds). Those affected experience concern about embarrassment, and they are afraid that others will judge them to be anxious, weak, crazy, or stupid. There is often a fear of being inarticulate and an avoidance of eating in public. Typically, patients have the usual anxiety symptoms, such as palpitations, tremor, sweating, GI distress, muscle tensing, blushing, confusion, or even panic attack, when they are in a feared situation. Common features of social phobia include difficulty being assertive, low self-esteem, feelings of inferiority, and hypersensitivity to criticism and negative evaluations. Social skills are generally poor. This condition

TABLE 8-7 Diagnostic Criteria for Social Phobia

A. The marked and persistent fear of one or more social or performance situations in which the person is exposed to unfamiliar people or to possible scrutiny by others. The individual fears that he or she will act in a way or will show anxiety symptoms that will be humiliating or embarrassing. Note: In children, there must be evidence of the capacity for age-appropriate social relationships with familiar people and the anxiety must occur in peer settings and not just in interactions with adults.

B. Exposure to the social situation almost invariably provokes anxiety, which may take the form of a situationally bound or situationally predisposed panic attack. Note: In children, the anxiety may be expressed by crying, tantrums, freezing, or shrinking from social situations with unfamiliar people.

C. The person realizes that the fear is obsessive or unreasonable. Note: In children, this feature may be absent.

D. The feared social or performance situations are either avoided or endured with intense anxiety or distress.

E. The avoidance, anxious anticipation, or distress in the feared social or performance situation interferes significantly with the person's normal routine, occupation/academic functioning, or social activities or relationships.

F. In individuals under 18 years, the duration is at least 6 months.

G. The fear or avoidance is not due to the direct physiologic effect of a substance or drug abuse, a medication, or a medical condition and it is not better accounted for by another mental disorder.

H. If a general medical condition or another mental disorder is present, the fear in the first criteria is unrelated to it. The fear is not of stuttering or trembling in Parkinson disease, or exhibiting abnormal eating behavior in anorexia nervosa or bulimia nervosa. Specify, if generalized, if the fears include most social situations.

Source: Reprinted with permission from *Diagnostic and Statistical Manual of Mental Disorders*. 4th ed, Text Revision. Copyright 2000. American Psychiatric Association.

can significantly interfere with work and social life. With generalized social phobia, there is 92% occupational impairment, 70% social impairment outside of work, and 50% have used alcohol at some point to allay their anxiety.

Nonpharmacologic Treatment of Social Phobia

CBT has been shown to be effective for social phobia. Patients with generalized social phobia who have significant interference with daily functioning should be referred for such therapy. Cognitive-behavioral group therapy gives patients the opportunity to review maladaptive automatic thoughts, to analyze and question these automatic assumptions in individual and role-play situations, and to have successful social experiences to counter their profound demoralization. This type of therapy is superior to placebo and supportive therapy.

Other nonpharmacologic methods include exposure therapy, cognitive restructuring techniques, and social skills training. Exposure therapy refers to any of the classic interventions that use confrontation with a feared stimulus by a patient, including play-acting or imagination. Cognitive restructuring attempts to change patient perceptions and interpretations of feared situations. Social skills training presumes that interpersonal anxiety is the result of deficient social skills. It incorporates modeling of appropriate behavior, behavior rehearsal, corrective feedback, social reinforcement, and homework assignments. CBT has been shown to have more lasting effects than treatments with MAOIs or benzodiazepines. It is, however, more labor and cost intensive for the patient. Pharmacologic intervention may be more suited to situations in which a more rapid response is needed.

Pharmacotherapy for Social Phobia

If CBT is used alone and is ineffective after 3 months, medication should be considered. Medications may be chosen from several different classes, such as SSRIs, benzodiazepines, buspirone hydrochloride, MAOIs, and beta-blockers. Prior to introduction of antidepressants that inhibit serotonin reuptake, the MAOI phenelzine sulfate was commonly used and was often quite effective. Today, SSRIs and venlafaxine have become the first choice in treating social phobia. Their relative safety, generally well-tolerated side-effect profile, and efficacy make them preferable. In addition, the risk of hypertensive crisis due to a tyramine response that complicates the use of MAOIs is eliminated. Benzodiazepines may have some benefit, particularly for short-term use, but the risk of relapse is high and caution must be used due to the potential for abuse. Buspirone hydrochloride has limited efficacy. Although ineffective for generalized social phobia, beta-blockers such as propranolol hydrochloride have been used successfully for performance anxiety. Typically, a dosage of 10 to 40 mg is administered a half hour prior to the performance; many musicians and actors who take this medication find they no longer suffer the distress of autonomic dyscontrol that typically interferes with their ability to perform.

OBSESSIVE-COMPULSIVE DISORDER

Obsessive-compulsive disorder (OCD) is characterized by repeated obsessions (or ruminations) that cause marked anxiety or distress and/or compulsions that serve to reduce or neutralize the anxiety. Even though patients realize that these activities are irrational, they nevertheless feel powerless to stop their repetitive acts, such as hand washing, counting their steps as they walk down the street, or checking and rechecking whether the front door has been locked. Diagnostic criteria for OCD and the definitions of these terms are shown in Table 8-8.

OCD is often chronic and may be disabling, and the lifetime prevalence is estimated at 2% to 3% of the general population. It usually has its onset in adolescence or early adulthood. The course of the disorder is generally one of waxing and waning, with exacerbations often temporally related to stressful life events. The onset is usually earlier in males (6 to 15 years) than females (20 to 29 years).

The presence of OCD has been highly correlated with tic disorders and Tourette syndrome. Formerly, it was assumed that these ritualistic behaviors had a wide spectrum of causes, from demonic possession to unresolved neurotic conflicts. It is now known that there is a consistently demonstrated biologic component to OCD, which can be visualized by neuroimaging of the brain. In addition, one etiologic hypothesis is that

TABLE 8-8 Diagnostic Criteria for Obsessive-Compulsive Disorder

A. Either obsessions or compulsions. Obsessions are:

- Recurrent and persistent thoughts, impulses, or images that are experienced, at some time during the disturbance, as intrusive and inappropriate and that cause marked anxiety or distress.

- The thoughts, impulses, or images are not simply excessive worries about real-life problems.

- The person attempts to ignore or suppress such thoughts, impulses, or images or to neutralize them with some other thought or action.

- The person recognizes that the obsessional thoughts, impulses, or images are the product of his or her own mind (not imposed from without, as in thought insertion).

Compulsions are:

- Compulsive behaviors (eg, hand washing, ordering, checking), or mental acts (eg, praying, counting, repeating words silently) that the person feels driven to perform in response to an obsession or according to rules that must be applied rigidly.

- The behaviors or mental acts are aimed at preventing or reducing distress or preventing some dreaded event or situation; however, these behaviors or mental acts are either not connected in a realistic way with what they are designed to neutralize or prevent or are clearly excessive.

B. At some point during the course of the disorder the person has recognized that the obsessions or compulsions are excessive or unreasonable. Note: This does not apply to children.

C. The obsessions or compulsions cause marked distress, are time-consuming, take 1 or more hours per day, or significantly interfere with the person's normal routine, academic or occupational functioning, or usual social activities or relationships.

D. If another axis I disorder is present, the content of the obsessions or compulsions is not restricted to it, eg, preoccupations with food in the presence of an eating disorder, hair pulling in the presence of trichotillomania, concern with appearance in the presence of body dysmorphic disorder, preoccupation with drugs in the presence of substance abuse disorder, preoccupation with having a serious illness in the presence of hypochondriasis, preoccupation with sexual urges or fantasies in the presence of paraphilia, or guilty ruminations in the presence of major depressive disorder.

E. The disturbance is not due to the direct physiologic effects of a substance (ie, drug abuse or a medication), or a general medical condition, behaviors, or mental acts are either not connected in a realistic way with what they are designed to neutralize or prevent or are clearly excessive. [Author note: The thoughts or behaviors won't or can't realistically prevent what is bothering the patient, eg, repeated hand washing does not protect the patient from being infected by refuse on the ground.]

Source: Reprinted with permission from *Diagnostic and Statistical Manual of Mental Disorders*. 4th ed, Text Revision. Copyright 2000. American Psychiatric Association.

there is a relationship between OCD and post-beta-streptococcal infection, much like rheumatic fever, or (more closely in the central nervous system) Sydenham chorea. Antibodies to these bacteria are consistently found in individuals with OCD and Tourette.

Treatment of OCD

It has been repeatedly demonstrated that OCD responds favorably to SSRIs, venlafaxine, and clomipramine hydrochloride, which suggests a strong underlying dysregulation of serotonergic neurotransmission. Generally, a combination of pharmacologic and nonpharmacologic intervention is necessary. Medications may be more useful when obsessions predominate, and behavioral therapy may be of more benefit when compulsions are the main problem. Behavioral therapy with exposure and response prevention is effective when performed by an experienced clinician. It is helpful to involve family members in the process because they can monitor changes in the frequency and disruptiveness of symptoms.

Clomipramine hydrochloride, fluoxetine hydrochloride, and fluvoxamine maleate are FDA approved for treating OCD. The entire class of SSRIs, however, has shown efficacy, and there is no reason to assume that one would be superior to another. If a medication is tolerated, the dosage should be increased until a significant clinical response is seen. A 10- to 12-week trial is generally recommended. A trial of medication is not considered adequate until the following daily doses of medications are reached: clomipramine hydrochloride, 250 mg; fluoxetine hydrochloride, 60 mg; fluvoxamine maleate, 300 mg; paroxetine hydrochloride, 60 mg; and sertraline hydrochloride, 200 mg. If one SSRI is not successful, it is often useful to try a second SSRI or venlafaxine before switching to clomipramine hydrochloride.

POSTTRAUMATIC STRESS DISORDER

Case Vignette

Mr Bradley is a 34-year-old man, previously in good health, whose car skidded on an icy road into oncoming traffic and who was then hit broadside by another car. He fractured a tibia and had diffuse soft-tissue injuries, but he had no head injury and experienced no loss of consciousness. Mr Bradley underwent open surgical repair of his leg fracture and remained off of work and on crutches for 6 weeks after the accident. During this recovery, he noted frequent intrusive thoughts about the automobile crash and he developed fragmented sleep, with frequent nightmares of life-threatening situations from which he would awaken, drenched in sweat. Mr Bradley found himself extremely uncomfortable driving again, and he avoided the road on which he had been injured, even though by doing so he doubled his commuting time. His wife complained that he was uncharacteristically yelling at her and his two children over the slightest provocation. She pressed him to see his primary care physician "for something to settle your nerves."

Posttraumatic stress disorder (PTSD) is relatively new as a discrete diagnostic entity, making its appearance just over 20 years ago. However, one form of the condition was previously referred to as "shell shock" and "war neurosis." It shares common features with acute stress disorder but differs in that there may be a time lag between the actual precipitating event and the onset of symptoms; there are also more dissociative symptoms in acute stress disorder. The specific DSM-IV criteria are listed in Table 8-9.

Flashbacks, ie, a vivid reliving and reexperiencing of an event, are the hallmark of this disorder. These flashbacks are often accompanied by physiologic symptoms of autonomic hyperarousal on exposure to events that are similar to or reminiscent of the traumatic

TABLE 8-9 Diagnostic Criteria for Posttraumatic Stress Disorder

A. The person has been exposed to a traumatic event in which both of the following were present:

- The person experienced, witnessed, or was confronted with an event or events that involved threatened death or actual or threatened serious injury or a threat to the physical integrity of self or others.

- The person's response involved intense fear, helplessness, or horror (in children, this may be expressed instead as disorganized or agitated behavior).

B. The traumatic event is persistently reexperienced in one or more of the following ways:

- Recurrent and intrusive distressing recollections of the event including images, thoughts, or perceptions (in children, repetitive play may occur in which themes or aspects of the trauma are expressed).

- Recurrent, distressing dreams of the event (in children, there may be frightening dreams without recognizable content).

- Acting or feeling as if the traumatic event were recurring (including a sense of reliving the experience, illusions, hallucinations, and dissociative feedback episodes that include those that occur on awakening or when intoxicated) (in children, trauma-specific reenactment may occur).

- Intense psychological distress at exposure to internal or external cues that symbolize or resemble an aspect of the traumatic event.

- Physiological reactivity on exposure to external or internal cues that symbolize or resemble an aspect of the traumatic event.

C. Persistent avoidance of stimuli associated with the trauma and numbing of general responsiveness (not present before the trauma) as indicated by three or more of the following:

- Efforts to avoid thoughts, feelings, or conversations associated with the trauma.

- Efforts to avoid activities, places, or people that arouse recollection of the trauma.

- Inability to recall an important aspect of the trauma.

- Markedly diminished interest or participation in significant activities.

- Feeling of detachment or estrangement from others.

- Restricted range of affect (eg, unable to have loving feelings).

- Sense of shortened future (eg, does not expect to have a career, marriage, children, or normal life span).

D. Persistent symptoms of increased arousal not present before the trauma and indicated by two or more of the following:

- Difficulty falling or staying asleep.

- Irritability or outbursts of anger.

- Difficulty concentrating.

- Hypervigilance.

- Exaggerated startle response.

(continued)

TABLE 8-9 (continued)

E. Duration of the disturbance is more than 1 month.

F. The disturbance caused significant clinical distress or impairment in social, occupational, or other important areas of function.

Source: Reprinted with permission from *Diagnostic and Statistical Manual of Mental Disorders*. 4th ed, Text Revision. Copyright 2000. American Psychiatric Association.

experience. Those with the disorder typically restructure their lives to avoid the people, places, and things that may evoke this response. Such avoidance can cause significant impairment in multiple spheres of functioning. Hyperarousal is characterized by sleep disturbances, irritability, agitation, poor concentration, hypervigilance, and an exaggerated startle response.

The lifetime prevalence of PTSD is estimated between 1% and 14% of the general population. Rates are significantly higher in specific populations, such as war veterans and sexual assault victims. PTSD can occur at any age, and symptoms typically begin within 3 months after the trauma and must persist more than 1 month for the diagnosis of PTSD to be made. One half of PTSD cases resolve within 3 months. More than 80% of patients also meet criteria for at least one other psychiatric diagnosis. OCD, PD, agoraphobia, and major depression are the most common comorbid psychiatric diagnoses. Treatment should be tailored to take these comorbid illnesses into account.

Treatment of PTSD

Initial therapy for PTSD should primarily be nonpharmacologic. Most forms of psychotherapy require that the patient discuss the traumatic event and its sequelae. Some elements of CBT and supportive therapy are suited to the primary care physician treating a patient with PTSD. Initial goals are to provide ample support and empathy, provide education about PTSD so that the patient understands the association of the symptoms to the trauma, and help destigmatize the condition, as being due to the traumatic event. Further goals are to help the patient repeatedly talk about his or her traumatic situation in the context of a safe, supportive environment; teach anxiety control exercises; explore hidden fears or concerns; and help the patient overcome avoidances both in and out of therapy. Even when the primary care physician is not the primary therapist, these principles should be kept in mind.

The role of pharmacotherapy in PTSD is mainly adjunctive. It can be used to treat anxious or depressive symptoms that accompany the PTSD. Medication also has a role in controlling aggressiveness or impulsivity as well as treating severe symptoms that occur as a result of trauma-focused therapy. Pharmacotherapy is felt to be most useful in patients who have symptoms of hyperarousal, numbing, and reexperiencing. Mixed results have been demonstrated with respect to the efficacy of the various classes of medications. At the time of this writing, SSRIs and venlafaxine are considered to be the first-line treatment for PTSD, with use of tricyclics and MAOIs reserved for treatment-refractory cases, typically by a psychiatrist. Drugs such as clonidine hydrochloride, propranolol hydrochloride, buspirone hydrochloride, clonazepam, carbamazepine, and valproic acid may also be useful in a secondary adjunctive role.

GENERALIZED ANXIETY DISORDER

Generalized anxiety disorder is a condition quite frequently seen in primary care settings. Patients suffering from this condition often have high baseline levels of anxiety (ie, they tend to feel tense and worry a lot), and they almost always react strongly to stressors with further increases in tension or negative thinking. While they may present complaining specifically about their stressors or worrying, more commonly they present with somatic complaints caused by the anxiety, such as insomnia, low energy, increased sweating, shakiness, palpitations, or trouble concentrating.

Diagnosing Generalized Anxiety Disorder

Generalized anxiety disorder (GAD) is the most common anxiety disorder and is characterized by at least 6 months of persistent and excessive anxiety and worry. The DSM-IV criteria are listed in Table 8-10.

Primary care physicians are certain to encounter many patients with GAD, because they comprise 4% to 5% of general medical outpatients. Lifetime prevalence estimates

---

TABLE 8-10 Diagnostic Criteria for Generalized Anxiety Disorder

A. Excessive anxiety and worry (apprehensive expectation) occurring more days than not for at least 6 months about a number of events or activities such as work or school performance.

B. The person finds it difficult to control the worry.

C. The anxiety or worry is associated with three or more of the following six symptoms, with at least some symptoms present for more days than not for the past 6 months (only one item is required in children):

- Restlessness or feeling keyed up or on edge
- Being easily fatigued
- Difficulty concentrating or mind going blank
- Irritability
- Muscle tension
- Sleep disturbance (difficulty falling or staying asleep or restless, unsatisfying sleep)

D. The focus of anxiety and worry are not confined to features of an axis I disorder, ie, the anxiety or worry is not about having a panic attack, being embarrassed in public, being contaminated, being away from home or close relatives, gaining weight, or having multiple physical complaints or serious illness, and the anxiety or worry do not occur exclusively during posttraumatic stress disorder.

E. Anxiety, worry, or physical symptoms cause clinically significant distress or impair social, occupational, or other areas of functioning.

F. The disturbance is not due to the direct physiological effects of a substance or general medical condition and does not occur exclusively during a mood disorder, psychotic disorder, or pervasive developmental disorder.

Source: Reprinted with permission from *Diagnostic and Statistical Manual of Mental Disorders*. 4th ed, Text Revision. Copyright 2000. American Psychiatric Association.

have varied widely from 2% to 31%. Patients with this disorder often undergo extensive laboratory testing and use extensive medical resources secondary to their excessive worries, which prompt them to seek medical attention. The diagnosis of GAD is missed in many individuals.

Estimates suggest that only 25% of patients with GAD actually receive appropriate treatment. GAD often has a chronic course and is associated with significant impairment in the quality of life. The mean duration of the illness is 6 to 10 years, and 40% of patients have the illness longer than 5 years before seeking treatment. Most patients have a comorbid psychiatric diagnosis. One fourth have PD or major depression; another one third have another axis I diagnosis. Successful treatment of GAD therefore depends on the clinician's awareness and treatment of comorbid conditions.

Treating Generalized Anxiety Disorder

Treatment for GAD often requires both pharmacologic and nonpharmacologic therapy. Unlike many of the other disorders that require specific psychotherapeutic techniques, GAD often responds to simple supportive therapy. Regularly scheduled appointments in which the patient can discuss environmental stressors and receive support and empathy from the primary care physician can often lead to a substantial decrease in anxiety. Techniques to evoke the relaxation response are also helpful in reducing overall anxiety levels (see the appendix at end of this chapter). CBT, which helps patients recognize and alter patterns of distorted thinking and dysfunctional behavior, is also often beneficial.

GAD is a chronic condition that requires long-term treatment. A full two thirds of patients will relapse within 1 year when taken off medication. Today, SSRIs and venlafaxine are the most frequently used medications for patients with GAD. All benzodiazepines are very effective for symptomatic relief of GAD, but none has been clearly shown to be superior. However, concerns about tolerance and misuse make some clinicians cautious about using this class of medications for GAD.

Buspirone hydrochloride is another antianxiety medication that may be effective in patients with GAD. An agonist of 5-HT1A receptors, it has the benefit of little tolerance (ie, patients do not need progressively higher doses to achieve the same beneficial effect), no abuse potential, no withdrawal symptoms, no alteration of cognitive or psychomotor functioning, and no interaction with alcohol. In contrast to the rapid onset of benzodiazepines, buspirone hydrochloride has a 2- to 4-week lag in onset of clinical efficacy. The usual daily dose requirement is 30 to 60 mg, divided into three daily doses. Patients who are benzodiazepine naïve are more likely to respond to buspirone hydrochloride. How well the patient responds to pharmacologic and supportive therapy will determine whether consultation and treatment by a mental health professional is necessary.

Many anxious patients use or ask their physicians about using alternative or complementary treatments to help manage their anxiety symptoms. All anxious patients should routinely be asked about their use of such treatments in a nonjudgmental way. Patients can be directed (if interested) to therapies that seem to help and have few adverse effects, such as aerobic exercise, yoga, and tai chi. Therapies with limited documented value for anxiety, such as homeopathy, aromatherapy, and acupuncture, should be approached with caution, as should therapies that may pose health risks, such as kava (hepatotoxicity) or St John's wort (potential drug interactions).

THE NEUROBIOLOGY OF ANXIETY

Over the last decade, great advances have been made in the understanding of the neurobiologic processes that are part of the stress response. It is now known that there are pathways for neuroendocrine pathology that are common to both anxiety disorders and major depression. Several neurotransmitter systems have been implicated, and the interplay of the endocrine system with the central nervous system is the focus of intense research at the molecular level. The dysregulation of the autonomic nervous system is intrinsically linked with cortisolic suppression of the function of the hippocampus and subsequent neuroplastic changes. The important point to remember is that antidepressants may mediate the transcription of genes at the nuclear level and the expression of their protein products. This is why there may be a lag time of weeks to months between initiating treatment and the full response to antidepressant therapy.

ANXIETY IN THE MEDICALLY ILL PATIENT

Serious medical illness frequently provokes anxiety, especially for those who require hospitalization. In addition to immediate concerns for their health, patients typically experience several other psychological stressors, including the following:

- Fear of loss of or injury to body parts
- Fear of loss of physiological function
- Pain, the fear of pain, disability, and death
- Threat to individual integrity and self-esteem
- Guilt and fear of retaliation for "sins" of omission and commission
- Loss of control and placing one's well-being and life in the hands of others
- Separation anxiety from home, family, and friends
- Fear of loss of love, approval, and acceptance

A diagnosis of a physical illness, particularly a serious one, can turn a patient's world upside down. To varying degrees, the fears and worries listed above go through the patient's mind, and the initial reaction may range from numbness and silence to hysteria and grief. Additionally, a particular illness often has a specific meaning to a patient. For example, patients tend to associate a diagnosis of cancer with all the people they have known who have had the illness and perhaps died. The desire to run, yell, and deny the diagnosis may be intense, and some struggle to hold such feelings totally in check, often attempting to stay strong for the sake of loved ones. Fear of death and dying may leave patients feeling as if they are being pulled under. Usually, there is a sense of grief over the loss, either real or imagined, of future health, functioning, and relationships. Such distress often manifests as depression, anxiety, and emotional regression. Typically, a patient's innate personality traits will become magnified to defend and cope with these stressors.

The amount of distress experienced by a patient who becomes ill is highly dependent on these factors:

- Their beliefs about the nature and severity of illness and its meaning to them
- The patient's premorbid personality characteristics
- The presence of comorbid psychiatric illness
- Personal and social supports

Medically ill patients are at risk for depression and anxiety; likewise, having a psychiatric illness increases the likelihood of developing many other biomedical illnesses. Depression occurs two to three times more often in primary care patients than in the general population, and rates of anxiety conditions, including panic disorder, are 10 times higher in primary care patients than in the general community. In addition, a medical illness may exacerbate underlying psychiatric conditions; the reverse is also true.

Because some medically ill patients fear abandonment by family, friends, and even their physician, it is critical that the primary care physician lets the patient know that he or she will be with the patient through an illness. Patients seldom openly say, and may not be actively aware, that they are afraid of being abandoned. The physician must assume that this is the case and bring up the topic. Note that a possible emotional issue will not become a prominent issue if the issue is not already present (eg, asking patients if they are suicidal will not cause nonsuicidal individuals to suddenly decide to kill themselves).

Remember that medically ill patients with secondary anxiety respond to the same antianxiety treatments as those with primary psychiatric anxiety disorders. However, before initiating pharmacologic therapies in medically ill patients, consider the following: First, will the side effects of a given psychopharmaceutical exacerbate symptoms of the medical illness? Second, what is the risk of creating an adverse metabolic drug reaction? For example, a patient with Crohn disease may not be able to tolerate the GI hypermotility associated with some SSRI agents. The patient may instead benefit from an antidepressant that may slow GI activity, such as bupropion hydrochloride. Another example relates to patients with an exacerbation of COPD who need an anxiolytic. Benzodiazepines are generally contraindicated in COPD patients due to the risk of respiratory depression. However, use of low-dose atypical neuroleptics, such as quetiapine fumarate or olanzapine, may be effective without producing side effects.

SUMMARY

Anxiety is a condition that is commonly encountered by primary care physicians. Because the etiology of anxiety may be complex and multifactorial, discerning the source requires excellent skills in listening and taking histories and the ability to perform an appropriate physical examination and laboratory testing. The alliance the primary care physician makes with his or her patients is inherently psychotherapeutic in nature and can be, in itself, healing. In addition to correct diagnosis and medication use, optimally treating anxiety requires caring, compassion, and empathy. By normalizing the experience, patients may communicate more freely, which in turn increases treatment compliance. Most patients who are significantly medically ill suffer from some degree of anxiety, and addressing this issue will improve their ability to cope with their primary illnesses. Finally, having professional psychiatric relationships within the medical community will help primary care providers to refer patients for definitive treatment, when necessary.

ADDITIONAL READINGS

Coplan JD, Mathew SJ, et al. Effects of LY354740, a novel glutamatergic metabotropic agonist, on nonhuman primate hypothalamic-pituitary-adrenal axis and noradrenergic function. *CNS Spectrums.* 2001;7:607-617.

Ely EW, Inouye SK, et al. Delirium in mechanically ventilated patients. *JAMA.* 2001;286:2703-2710.

Fallon BA, Mathew SJ. *Biological Therapies for Obsessive-Compulsive Disorder.* Mahwah, NJ: Lawrence Erlbaum Associates; 2000:113-128.

Fresco DM, Heimberg RG. Empirically supported psychological treatments for social phobia. *Psychiatr Ann.* 2001;8:489-496.

Gorman JM. Environmental stress and the brain's reaction. *CNS Spectrums.* 2001;7:551.

Kendler KS, Myers J, Prescott CA. The etiology of phobias. *Arch Gen Psychiatry.* 2002;3:242-248.

Kent JM, Sullivan GM, Rauch SL. The neurobiology of fear: relevance to panic disorder and posttraumatic stress disorder. *Psychiatr Ann.* 2000;12:733-742.

Levitt JT, et al. Empirically supported treatments for panic disorder. *Psychiatr Ann.* 2001;8:478-487.

Mathew SJ, Coplan JD, et al. Glutamate-hypothalamic-pituitary-adrenal axis interactions: implications for mood and anxiety disorders. *CNS Spectrums.* 2001;7:555-564.

Mathew SJ, Simpson HB, Fallon BA. Treatment strategies for obsessive-compulsive disorder. *Psychiatr Ann.* 2000;11:699-708.

Mikhail AG, Kent JM, Pine DS. Childhood obsessive-compulsive disorder: a review. *J Psychiatr Pract.* 2000;177-189.

Monti DA, Thompson TL. Key counseling/psychotherapy issues in primary care. *Primary Psychiatry.* 1999;6:34-37.

Persons JB. Understanding the exposure principle and using it to treat anxiety. *Psychiatr Ann.* 2001;8:472-476.

Persons JB, et al. Common misconceptions about the nature and treatment of generalized anxiety disorder. *Psychiatrc Ann.* 2001;8:501-507.

Scott EL, Heimberg RG. Social phobia: an update on treatment. *Psychiatr Ann.* 2000;11:678-685.

Simon NM, Pollack MH. The current status of the treatment of panic disorder: pharmacotherapy and cognitive-behavioral therapy. *Psychiatr Ann.* 2000;11:689-696.

Simpson HB, Fallon BA. Obsessive-compulsive disorder: an overview. *J Psychiatr Pract.* 2000;6:3-17.

Simpson HB, Kozak M. Cognitive-behavioral therapy for obsessive-compulsive disorder. *J Psychiatr Pract.* 2000;59-68.

Appendix

Relaxation Exercises

The following are simple relaxation exercises that are often useful alone or as an adjunct to therapy and medication for patients who feel a significant amount of stress. They are easy to teach in the office, or they can be shown on a handout to be given to patients as a homework assignment prior to the next visit. Patients may find certain exercises more effective than others; they can also be encouraged to find other techniques for inducing a relaxation response. Many books and tapes on relaxation are available at most bookstores. Each exercise should be performed in a quiet, peaceful environment where the patient will not be disturbed for at least 10 to 15 minutes.

Focused Breathing

- Sit in a quiet, comfortable position in a chair or lie on the floor with a pillow under the small of the back. The eyes may be left open or closed. If left open, focus on a blank wall or soothing object or image. If eyes are closed, make certain not to fall asleep.
- Breathe in slowly through the nose (or mouth if this is more comfortable), letting the air fill the chest and expand the stomach.
- Hold the breath momentarily, then let the air out slowly, listening to the sound of the breath as it courses the lips, and letting the stomach come in.
- Let the tension out with each exhalation and allow the body to feel the quietness and physiologic relaxation response that comes with deep breathing.
- Continue this breathing for 5 to 15 minutes.
- Repeat the entire exercise twice daily or at times of increased stress or tension.

Progressive Muscle Relaxation

Progressive muscle relaxation (PMR) is another way to release tension from the body. The process of tensing and relaxing sequential muscle groups teaches us how to physically relax. Because this exercise couples the mind with concrete instructions, it is particularly good for people with racing thoughts who otherwise have a hard time focusing on relaxation techniques.

- Begin by sitting in a comfortable chair with the back straight and head in line with the spine, feet on the ground, and hands resting in the lap or on arm rests. Close the eyes or focus on an object or wall. Breathe deeply and slowly, letting the stomach rise with each breath in and fall with each breath out.
- Now concentrate on the forehead. Consciously tighten the muscles of the forehead while counting slowly from one to five. Slowly relax the muscles of the forehead, letting go of the tension while taking a nice deep breath. Allow the stomach to rise with each breath in and fall with each exhalation. Notice the difference between the tense and relaxed state.

- Now move down to the eyes and repeat the same process. Tighten the muscles around the eyes while counting slowly from one to five. Slowly relax the muscles, letting go of the tension while breathing slowly and deeply.
- Continue this relaxation technique, moving downward through the following muscle groups: forehead and scalp, eyes, jaw, neck, back, upper extremity (one side at a time), shoulders, forearms, hands (fists), chest, abdomen, pelvis/buttocks, upper legs, calves, feet.
- As the exercise progresses, notice differences in tension between different parts or sides of the body. Return to areas that remain tense.
- This exercise should take 10 to 15 minutes. It can be done twice daily or on an as-needed basis, depending on stress levels and the use of other techniques.

Mental Imaging/Body Scan

Like progressive muscle relaxation, these mental imaging techniques also relax specific muscle groups of the body. This relaxation is done through visualization of each group of muscles to identify where the tension lies. While concentrating on an area of muscle tension, focused breathing allows release of specific areas of tension.

- Begin by sitting comfortably in a chair or lying on the floor. Focus on your breathing. Allow the stomach to rise with each breath in and fall with each breath out. Close the eyes and focus on a muscle group. Note the tension in the muscle group. As you exhale, let go of any tension in that muscle group. (One might wish to say to oneself, "My head feels heavy, limp, loose, and relaxed.")
- Begin at the head and scan all muscle groups listed above under PMR.
- Some individuals prefer to start at the feet.
- Alternatively, individuals can visualize stress and anxiety as a brightly colored liquid that drains slowly from various parts of the body.
- When finished, do a mental scan of the entire body. If there is any muscle group with tension, focus again on those body areas.
- This exercise should take 5 to 15 minutes and can be repeated as often as needed throughout the day.

Chapter 9

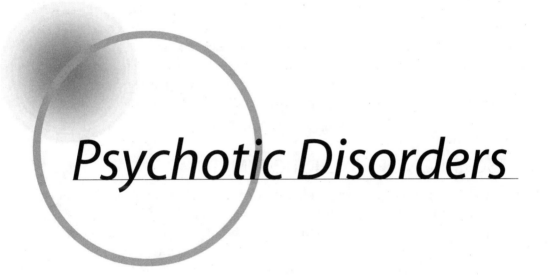

Psychotic Disorders

William R. Yates, MD
George R. Bergus, MD

Psychotic symptoms, which are among the most serious of psychiatric problems, are typical of severe and chronic illness such as schizophrenia. Primary care physicians may be the first to uncover psychotic symptoms. More commonly, primary care physicians provide medical care for patients who have already been diagnosed with a chronic psychotic disorder. Medical personnel may try to avoid contact with such patients because they misunderstand the real cause of these illnesses. However, an understanding of these disorders enables the primary care physician to bring high-quality care to suffering patients in what is often a challenging clinical situation.

Patients with psychotic disorders often have poor medical health. Medical illness is often the presenting problem for patients with schizophrenia or other psychotic disorders. For example, psychotic disorders may influence eating behavior and result in poor nutrition, including obesity. Schizophrenia and bipolar affective disorder are associated with high rates of nicotine dependence, resulting in increased risk for cardiovascular and pulmonary diseases. These relationships increase the risk for chronic medical conditions and medical utilization.

DESCRIPTION OF PSYCHOTIC SYMPTOMS

Precisely defining the term *psychosis* can be an elusive task. The term is roughly equivalent to the archaic term *insanity*. In general, the term refers to a patient's inability to appropriately assess reality. This assessment may be hampered by perceptual disturbances or marked dysfunctions in thinking. Some authors define psychosis as the presence of unusual mental experiences. This definition includes marked disturbances in cognitive functioning, whether arising primarily (as in dementia) or secondarily (as when depression impairs memory or concentration).

Psychotic symptoms may be quite obvious or they may be hidden and elicited only by careful probing in a nonthreatening manner. Typically, the most dramatic psychotic symptoms are delusions and hallucinations. Delusions are beliefs that are fixed (unchangeable) and false. Beliefs that a patient has in common with his religious or subcultural group are not considered delusional. The boundary between a delusion and an overvalued idea (eg, an emaciated patient with anorexia nervosa insisting she is fat) is not always clear. Delusions may be classified as follows:

- *Paranoid (persecutory) delusions* are a common type of delusion characterized by a belief that one is being persecuted (eg, a belief that the FBI is transmitting obscenities through a receiver implanted in the patient's body), followed, or harmed (such as by surreptitious poisoning).
- *Grandiose delusions* include the belief that one is unique or has special powers, gifts, talents, or abilities.
- *Somatic delusions* are the erroneous beliefs that something is wrong with one's body, eg, the patient is convinced he has cancer when he does not.
- *Nihilistic delusions* are the beliefs that one has died or that the world will be coming to an end.

- *Ideas of reference* are a set of beliefs that the actions of others are directed at the patient when they are not (eg, that the radio is broadcasting songs or shows to send a particular message to the patient).
- *Control delusions* include beliefs that others can read the patient's mind, steal his or her thoughts, or control his or her thinking or body.

The other common psychotic symptom, hallucination, is a perception experienced in the absence of an external stimulus. Hallucinations can be auditory, visual, olfactory, gustatory, or tactile. The most common type of hallucination seen in schizophrenia and other chronic psychotic disorders is an auditory hallucination, which is described as a sensation of hearing one or more people talking about the patient, arguing about the patient, or repeating aloud the patient's own thoughts. Visual hallucinations, which may be found in schizophrenia, are more often associated with delirium due to a general medical condition. Visual hallucinations are also associated with Lewy body dementia.

Although delusions and hallucinations form the key symptoms of psychosis, additional symptoms and signs suggest psychosis. Bizarre and unusual behavior can at times reflect a psychotic process. Patients with schizophrenia may have deterioration in social behaviors and in personal hygiene. Affect regulation can go awry and result in diminished affect, poverty of expression (limited verbal output in the absence of a speech or communication disorder), poor eye contact, and limited spontaneous and responsive speech. Psychotic signs and symptoms are summarized in Table 9-1.

The symptoms of psychosis can be grouped into positive and negative symptom classes. Positive symptoms include delusions, hallucinations, incoherent speech, and bizarre, agitated, or disorganized behavior. Negative symptoms reflect a deficiency in a mental function that is normally present. Negative symptoms include poverty of speech, flattening of affect, inability to experience pleasure (anhedonia), few friends (asociality), lack of initiative or sustained performance (avolition), and deficits in attention.

After discovery of psychotic symptoms, the next step is to determine the duration of the symptoms. If the symptoms have been long-standing, it is likely the patient has been previously hospitalized or has been in contact with mental health professionals. A review of medical records will be helpful in this presentation. If the symptoms have not been previously noted, differential diagnosis using a diagnostic algorithm can ensure a systematic review of potential causes for new-onset psychotic symptoms. Alternately, psychiatric consultation can be considered because new-onset psychotic symptoms are almost always clinically significant and require close monitoring and management.

DIAGNOSING PSYCHOTIC DISORDERS

Diagnosing mental disorders, including psychotic disorders, follows a pattern similar to that for diagnosing medical disorders. The patient's key symptoms are elicited with exploration of more detailed information for positive responses. For psychiatric disorders, a longitudinal history is very important. Many psychotic disorders are chronic with high rates of psychiatric hospitalization. Because of the chronic nature of psychotic symptoms, new-onset cases are relatively rare in primary care settings. Once key psychotic symptoms are elicited, clinicians can utilize an algorithmic approach to arrive at a specific diagnosis.

TABLE 9-1 Common Signs and Symptoms in Psychotic Disorders

Disturbances of Perception and Cognition

- Hallucinations: auditory, visual, tactile, olfactory, gustatory

- Delusions: paranoid, somatic, grandiose, religious, nihilistic

- First-rank delusions: thought broadcasting, thought withdrawal, thought insertion, delusions of passivity (ie, one is controlled by others)

- Thought disorder: derailment, poverty of speech or content of speech, tangentiality, perseveration, clanging (words strung together to produce sounds rather than actual meaning, ie, words that create a meaningless rhyme), neologisms (meaning "new words," idiosyncratic words a psychotic individual speaks that may not have meaning for others), echolalia (senseless repetition, echoing, of a word or phrase someone else has just spoken), blocking

Disturbances of Behavior and Motor Function

- Psychomotor agitation or retardation

- Aggressive verbal and motor behavior

- Catatonia: immobility, mutism, waxy flexibility, posturing, negativism (ie, refusing to carry out commands), stereotypy (repetitive nongoal-directed movements like rocking), mannerisms (repetitive goal-directed movements that are odd in appearance or context)

- Deterioration in social behavior or bizarre behavior

- Avolition (lack of goal-directed activity)

Disturbances of Affect

- Flat or inappropriate affect

- Anhedonia (loss of ability to experience pleasure)

Differential Diagnosis of Psychotic Symptoms

Figure 9-1 shows an algorithm for the differential diagnosis of psychotic symptoms. This algorithm has been adapted from the American Psychiatric Association's *Diagnostic and Statistical Manual for Mental Disorders*, fourth edition (DSM-IV).

The first step in evaluating psychotic signs or symptoms is to consider psychosis due to a general medical condition. Delirium is a common cause of new-onset psychotic features, especially in hospitalized patients with severe medical or surgical illness. Congestive heart failure, pneumonia, pyelonephritis, and uremia are just a few of the common disease states that can cause delirium in hospitalized patients. Psychotic symptoms are also common in dementia. Patients with Alzheimer dementia may develop delusions, typically voiced as beliefs that someone is entering the home and stealing or that family members may be trying to hurt them. A variety of central nervous system disorders, including tumors, temporal lobe seizures, HIV/AIDS, and cerebrovascular disease, can produce psychotic symptoms. Metabolic disturbances, such as hyponatremia or hypercalcemia, can also cause psychotic symptoms.

Drug-induced psychotic symptoms are common. Primary care physicians should search for a history of alcohol abuse or dependence or illicit drug use, especially cocaine,

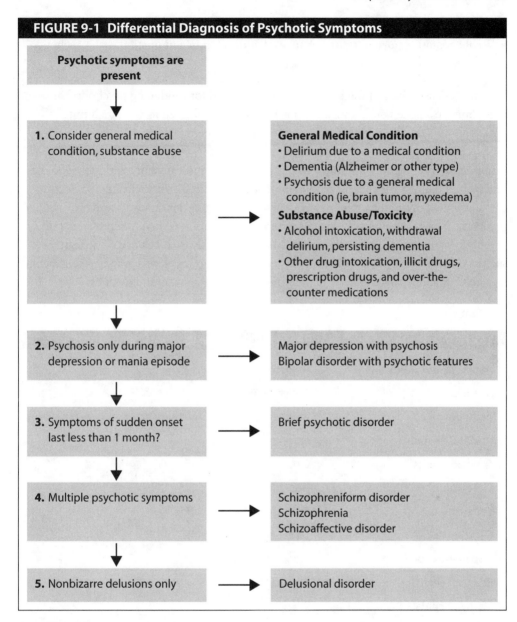

FIGURE 9-1 Differential Diagnosis of Psychotic Symptoms

Psychotic symptoms are present

1. Consider general medical condition, substance abuse

General Medical Condition
• Delirium due to a medical condition
• Dementia (Alzheimer or other type)
• Psychosis due to a general medical condition (ie, brain tumor, myxedema)

Substance Abuse/Toxicity
• Alcohol intoxication, withdrawal delirium, persisting dementia
• Other drug intoxication, illicit drugs, prescription drugs, and over-the-counter medications

2. Psychosis only during major depression or mania episode

Major depression with psychosis
Bipolar disorder with psychotic features

3. Symptoms of sudden onset last less than 1 month?

Brief psychotic disorder

4. Multiple psychotic symptoms

Schizophreniform disorder
Schizophrenia
Schizoaffective disorder

5. Nonbizarre delusions only

Delusional disorder

Source: Adapted with permission from the *Diagnostic and Statistical Manual of Mental Disorders, Fourth Edition, Text Revision.* Copyright 2000 American Psychiatric Association.

amphetamine, marijuana, phencyclidine, and hallucinogens. Urine drug screens can confirm historical information or be used when information is not available. Prescription drugs can produce psychotic symptoms in the context of intoxication, underlying brain disease, or idiosyncratic responses to a drug. It is important to note that a high percentage of patients with chronic psychotic disorders abuse alcohol and illicit medications.

Psychotic symptoms due to a medical condition or substances are more likely to be present in the following clinical situations:

• Age greater than 35 years
• Acute onset
• No family history of substance abuse

- Past history of substance use
- Acute cognitive (mental status) changes that develop in conjunction with psychotic symptoms

Table 9-2 lists some of the prescription drugs noted for producing psychotic symptoms. Some over-the-counter medications have been implicated as well, including sympathomimetic decongestants and anticholinergic hypnotics.

Psychotic symptoms can be present in mood disorders (step 2 in the algorithm). Major depressive disorder accompanied by psychosis is indicative of a serious mood disorder, often requiring treatment with combination psychopharmacotherapy or electroconvulsive therapy. Only a minority of patients with major depressive disorder display psychosis. Nevertheless, for undiagnosed psychotic symptoms, major depression with psychotic features should be considered. Mania frequently includes psychotic features such as delusions or hallucinations. Delusions in mania often have a grandiose character, ie, a belief that one is god or a belief that one has special powers and abilities.

TABLE 9-2 Prescription Drugs Reported to Cause Psychotic Symptoms

Paranoia and Delusions	Hallucinations
Acyclovir	Anticholinergic drugs
Amphetamines	Baclofen (on discontinuation)
Anabolic steroids	Calcium channel blockers
Cephalosporins	Cimetidine
Cimetidine	Dopamine agonists
Corticosteroids	Ethambutol hydrochloride
Cycloserine	5-Flucytosine
Dopamine agonists	Indomethacin
Ethosuximide	Isoniazid
Methylphenidate	Phenytoin
Theophylline	Vincristine sulfate

Other Unspecified Psychotic Symptoms	
Aminoglycosides	Procaine penicillin
Beta-blockers	Sympathomimetics
Bumetanide	Tocainide hydrochloride
Cyclobenzaprine hydrochloride	Trimethoprim
Ganciclovir sodium	Vinblastine sulfate
Hydralazine hydrochloride	Zidovudine (AZT)
Lidocaine	

Following step 2, a brief psychotic disorder should be considered (step 3 in the algorithm). Psychotic symptoms that are of sudden onset and have lasted less than 1 month are required for this diagnosis.

Step 4 focuses on the major psychotic disorders of schizophrenia, schizophreniform disorder, and schizoaffective disorder. These psychotic disorders often display multiple psychotic symptoms, producing severe impairment in daily function. A diagnosis of schizophrenia requires an illness lasting 6 months or longer with at least 1 month of active psychotic symptoms. Patients demonstrating symptoms of schizophrenia lasting less than 6 months can be diagnosed with schizophreniform disorder. Patients with schizoaffective disorder display both mood and psychotic symptoms. At some point in the illness, psychotic symptoms must be present in the absence of a mood disorder.

Step 5 in the algorithm focuses on the category of delusional disorder. This diagnosis differs from schizophrenia in that the patient has only a delusion that is not bizarre and that the global impairment characteristic of schizophrenia is not present. Delusions characteristic of this condition include infestation with parasites or paranoia concerning infidelity in a spouse.

Frequently, psychotic symptoms do not present with a clinical picture that allows assignment of a psychiatric diagnosis despite the steps outlined in the algorithm. In this situation, assigning the diagnosis of psychotic disorder as NOS (not otherwise specified) is appropriate. With clinical monitoring and the passage of time, a more specific diagnosis may emerge.

Case Vignette

Mr Ball is a 32-year-old man who presents to the emergency department with fever, abdominal pain, and bloody diarrhea. Being healthy and new to the community, he has no regular physician. Mr Ball is single, lives alone, and works intermittently as a carpenter doing new construction. A lower gastrointestinal endoscopy reveals that Mr Ball has inflammatory bowel disease. He is admitted to the hospital under the care of a newly assigned primary care physician and started on IV antibiotics (triple therapy with an aminoglycoside, cephalosporin, and ampicillin) and high-dose corticosteroids. Mr Ball's condition improves over the following 24 hours as his diarrhea stops and he becomes afebrile. On the second night in the hospital, he becomes very agitated and tells the nurses that god was talking to him. Mr Ball reports god told him that it is his life's mission to construct hundreds of small, model wooden houses so that "god would have a house all over the world." When Mr Ball is told no one else can hear the voice, he accuses the nursing staff of being evil and trying to disrupt god's work.

Mr Ball's case is an example of acute onset of psychotic symptoms, manifested as auditory hallucination, and the many possible etiologies of these symptoms. He had a serious medical condition that could provoke the change in mental status. The onset of psychotic symptoms could represent a serious deterioration of his condition, possibly as a result of intestinal perforation with resulting peritonitis and sepsis. Acute psychosis accompanied by cognitive impairment is consistent with a diagnosis of delirium. Another cause could be his medications: corticosteroids and some antibiotics are known to cause delirium. A third possibility is that Mr Ball had a chronic psychotic illness that became symptomatic when his medical condition improved. His episodic work history and lack of immediate friends and family also support this possibility.

Case Vignette

Mr Carl is a 40-year-old man seen by his physician, Dr Gladd, for evaluation of abdominal pain. He arrives from a nursing home where his primary diagnosis is chronic schizophrenia. Mr Carl has lost 20 pounds and is experiencing left lower-quadrant pain. After initial cooperation, he refuses testing, including blood work and diagnostic procedures. Mr Carl states he is refusing because he is frightened and worried the doctor is trying to poison him. Because the patient's delusional thinking places him at medical risk, arrangements are made for a guardian to authorize testing and treatment. Following review by the guardian *ad litem* and a judge, a guardian is appointed; Mr Carl undergoes the necessary tests and consultations and surgery is deemed necessary. Surgical exploration reveals perforated diverticula with abscess formation. Mr Carl improves with concurrent medical, surgical, and psychiatric treatment and is transferred back to his chronic care facility.

Key Clinical Features

Table 9-3 summarizes key clinical features of the psychiatric disorders characterized by the presence of psychotic features. Schizophrenia, with a lifetime prevalence of just below 1%, is not an extremely common psychiatric disorder. The risk is fairly stable across geographic, cultural, and socioeconomic groups. It contributes significantly to disability and decreased productivity because of an early age of onset and severe impairment in work

TABLE 9-3 Clinical Features of Psychotic and Related Disorders

Disorder	Key Features	Prevalence	Familial Risk	Course
Schizophrenia	Chronic symptoms lasting at least 6 months	0.5–1.0%	Increased tenfold	Variable, often and disabling
Schizophreniform disorder	Like schizophrenia but < 6 months	0.1–0.2%	Unknown	Brief
Schizoaffective disorder	Major mood disorder plus psychosis without mood symptoms	< 1.0%	Increased	Intermediate between schizophrenia and mood disorders
Delusional disorder	Nonbizarre delusions last >1 month	0.03%	Unknown	Variable, often chronic
Brief psychotic disorder	Acute psychosis of < 1 month duration	Rare	Unknown	Acute, self-limiting
Paranoid personality disorder	Lifelong, pervasive suspiciousness of others	0.5–2.5%	Increased	Chronic

and social function. Growing evidence suggests that schizophrenia is a biological brain disorder. Functional and structural brain imaging studies in groups of patients with schizophrenia are providing clues to the pathophysiology of the disorder.

Schizophrenia is classified into five subtypes in DSM-IV. These subtypes include paranoid, disorganized, catatonic, undifferentiated, and residual. The reliability and validity of these subtypes is unknown. The subtype classifications continue to be evaluated for their value in research and practice. There appears to be a significant genetic contribution to the risk for schizophrenia; for a first-degree relative the risk is 10%; for an offspring if both parents are schizophrenic the risk is 40% to 50%. Although recovery from schizophrenia has been described, a chronic course is more common. The chronic course may be punctuated by acute exacerbations. Additionally, progressive deterioration can occur, resulting in the eventual need for custodial care.

Schizophreniform disorder is diagnosed when features of schizophrenia are present for fewer than 6 months. Because a duration of illness of 6 months is required for schizophrenia, some patients will meet criteria for schizophreniform disorder prior to meeting criteria for schizophrenia. Schizophreniform disorder is less commonly diagnosed than schizophrenia. There is a higher rate of remission of schizophreniform disorders: The longer psychotic symptoms persist, the more likely the patient is to suffer from a chronic psychotic disorder. The familial risk associated with schizophreniform disorder is unknown.

Schizoaffective disorder is characterized by both psychotic symptoms and mood symptoms. Although unipolar depression and bipolar affective disorder can occur with psychotic features, psychotic features in mood disorders typically occur during exacerbation of the mood symptoms. In schizoaffective disorder, psychotic symptoms must occur in the absence of mood symptoms at least once in the course of the illness. Schizoaffective disorder appears less commonly than schizophrenia, with an increased familial risk. The prognosis for schizoaffective disorder is better than that for schizophrenia but not as good as that for mood disorders.

Delusional disorder is a relatively rare disorder characterized by delusions that are not considered bizarre. Bizarre delusions are fixed and false beliefs that are impossible and would be judged by most people to be unbelievable and irrational. Delusions typical of delusional disorder can be thought of as strange beliefs that are possible but highly unlikely. The familial risk in this disorder is unknown. The prognosis can be quite variable: Some delusional disorders remit spontaneously or with treatment, while others may persist for many years.

Brief psychotic disorder also appears quite rarely. A sudden severe psychological stressor can precipitate this disorder. By definition, it is of short duration and it is unknown if a familial pattern is present.

A possible nonpsychotic disorder that may exist in the differential diagnosis of psychotic symptoms is paranoid personality disorder. Paranoid personality disorder is a lifelong condition characterized by distrust and suspiciousness of others. This distrust can border on the definition of a paranoid delusion but does not meet the bizarre quality or fixed nature of a delusion. The prevalence of paranoid personality disorder is greater than any of the individual psychotic disorders and tends to run in families. Schizoid and schizotypal personality disorders can also mimic psychotic disorders, particularly resembling disorganized schizophrenia.

MANAGING PSYCHOTIC DISORDERS

The management of psychotic disorders requires accurate diagnosis and participation in a multidisciplinary treatment team. The primary care physician may be involved in treating co-occuring medical conditions and managing psychotropic drug treatment. For unstable patients, a psychiatrist may be necessary to assist in hospitalizations and psychopharmacologic consultation. For many stable patients, medication management may involve minimal change over time.

Management Issues

Primary care physicians will experience unique issues while managing patients with acute and chronic psychotic symptoms.

Patient-physician relationship issues. It may be difficult to develop a positive, sustainable patient-physician relationship with patients with psychotic symptoms. Psychosis often impairs the development of trust in interpersonal relationships, and this barrier holds true for relationships with physicians. Physicians must avoid any words or behaviors that could be interpreted as threatening or demeaning to the psychotic patient. It is best to avoid any types of confrontation (eg, of delusions) if at all possible. Because psychotic patients may be uncomfortable in closed or small examining rooms, physicians should consider evaluating these patients in the largest room possible, which provides patients with the feeling they may leave if they become too uncomfortable.

Use of family and social support resources. Psychosis can prevent patients from seeking proper care for both medical and psychiatric problems. Family members and friends can be a valuable resource for primary care physicians in the day-to-day care for patients with psychotic disorders. A family member or friend may be able to encourage the patient with psychosis to seek out professional help. Additionally, a family member can assist psychotic patients in monitoring symptoms and complying with medication management.

Psychiatric assessment and collaboration. Psychiatric consultation can provide primary care physicians with assistance in the management of psychotic symptoms. At the onset of psychosis, psychiatric hospitalization can be a significant aid in the assessment and treatment planning. This is particularly true if the potential for harm to self and others exists. Because psychosis can cause behavior to be unpredictable, hospitalization may be necessary even without a specific threat to self or others. Some primary care physicians may elect to manage chronic psychotic symptoms and prefer to collaborate with a psychiatrist.

Involuntary commitment. Psychosis can present as a medical emergency that requires attention to the safety of the patient and those around the patient. Patients with psychosis often lack insight into their psychotic symptoms and are blind to the need for treatment. During the mental status evaluation, the potential for harm to self or to others must be evaluated. If there is a significant potential for harm and the patient is unwilling to enter a psychiatric hospital, legal commitment for psychiatric treatment should be considered. Note that legal statutes for involuntary commitment for mental health treatment vary from state to state. Primary care physicians may consider psychiatric consultation for processing an involuntary commitment. If a psychiatrist is not available, the local state's attorney, county sheriff, or county clerk's office can provide assistance.

Medication Management

Psychopharmacologic management of psychosis can be divided into the acute phase and the maintenance phase of treatment. Because of the psychiatric severity of psychotic symptoms, many patients with new-onset psychotic disorders are admitted to an inpatient psychiatric treatment facility for initial evaluation and treatment. If new-onset psychosis presents as an emergency, the patient will need to be treated by the primary care physician for a brief period of time until psychiatric hospitalization can be arranged. Primary care physicians may be involved in monitoring patients on long-term antipsychotic medication, especially in rural areas where access to a psychiatrist may be limited. Table 9-4 summarizes information about some of the most common antipsychotic medications.

TABLE 9-4 Antipsychotics Commonly Used in the United States

Drug (Trade name)	Dose Equivalent*	Usual Daily Dose (mg/day)† Acute	Maintenance
Chlorpromazine (Thorazine)	100	200–1000	50–400
Thioridazine (Mellaril)	100	200–800	40–400
Perphenazine (Trilafon)	10	12–64	8–24
Trifluoperazine hydrochloride (Stelazine)	5	10–60	4–30
Fluphenazine (Prolixin)	2	5–60	1–15
Thiothixene (Navane)	5	10–120	6–30
Haloperidol (Haldol)	2	5–50	1–15
Loxapine succinate (Loxitane)	10	20–160	10–60
Molindone hydrochloride (Moban)	10	40–225	15–100
Clozapine (Clozaril)	50	300–900	200–400
Risperidone (Risperdal)	1	4–8	2–6
Quetiapine (Seroquel)			
Olanzapine (Zyprexa)	2	10–20	10–20
Ziprasidone (Geodon)	20	40–200	40–160
Aripiprazole (Abilify)	2	10–30	10–30
Long-acting Injectables			
Fluphenazine decanoate			6–100‡
Haloperidol decanoate			50–200§

* Doses may vary with individualized responses. In general, lower doses are used in the elderly, when there is hepatic impairment, or when the patient has central nervous system disease.

† Approximate values. Relative potency may differ in higher dose ranges.

‡ May be given at 3- to 4-week intervals. Dosage requirements may vary widely.

§ May be given at 4-week intervals. Dosage requirements may vary widely.

Source: Modified from Gabbard GO, ed. *Treatment of Psychiatric Disorders*. Washington, DC: American Psychiatric Press; 1995.

Management of acute psychosis. Patients requiring rapid antipsychotic treatment are best treated with intramuscular drugs, which have a more rapid onset of action than oral drugs. Oral antipsychotic elixirs have an intermediate onset of action compared to that of intramuscular agents and oral tablets. Intravenous haloperidol has been used in the general hospital setting, but this route is not approved by the US Food and Drug Administration (FDA), and cardiac complications, although rare, have been reported.

Antipsychotic drugs can be broken into two classes: low-potency and high-potency drugs. Chlorpromazine (Thorazine) is the prototypical low-potency antipsychotic and haloperidol (Haldol) is the prototypical high-potency antipsychotic. Both agents are available in generic formulation. As a general rule, low-potency antipsychotics are more sedating and high-potency antipsychotics have more extrapyramidal effects. Except for clozapine, antipsychotic medications have similar efficacies.

Haloperidol is superior to chlorpromazine for intramuscular injection because of the high rate of orthostatic hypotension associated with intramuscular chlorpromazine. Intramuscular injections of haloperidol usually take effect within 30 minutes, and repetitive dosing can be used until the psychotic patient is calmed and any behavioral emergencies have been resolved. Intramuscular antipsychotics tend to have bioavailability rates two to four times higher than those of oral antipsychotics. Some psychopharmacologists recommend augmentation of the antipsychotic agent with a benzodiazepine for the acutely agitated patient. Lorazepam, which has the advantage of a relatively short half-life, may be used at 1 to 2 mg PO or IV. Combined use of these drugs may reduce the dosage of the antipsychotic needed to control the patient and reduce the risk of acute dystonic reactions.

Some newer atypical antipsychotic options exist or are in the FDA-approval process for acute treatment of psychosis. Olanzapine is available in an orally dissolvable preparation, which may have a more rapid onset of action than the tablet formulation. An injectable formulation of olanzapine is also being developed. An injectable formulation of ziprasidone hydrochloride, approved in 2002, is another alternative for rapid management of psychotic symptoms.

Management of chronic psychotic disorders. Maintenance antipsychotic treatment provides the foundation for successful ambulatory management of patients with chronic psychotic disorders. Many psychotic disorders, including schizophrenia, are conditions with periodic episodes of remission and relapse. Recurrence rates in schizophrenia approach 50% within 6 months of discontinuing antipsychotic agents, compared to a relapse rate of 15% if the medication is continued. Not only are psychotic relapses dangerous, they are also detrimental to the patient's long-term recovery and rehabilitation.

Once psychotic symptoms have been satisfactorily controlled, maintenance treatment for a period of 1 to 2 years is recommended. For patients with multiple psychotic episodes, at least 5 years of maintenance treatment are indicated. Any tapering trial of an antipsychotic drug should be done with caution. A specific reason for a trial of discontinuation should be identified, ie, the presence of significant side effects or concern about risk of tardive dyskinesia (TD). It often takes up to 3 months for recurrence of symptoms after a dosage is reduced. Because of this, it is best to reduce dosages only approximately every 3 months when attempting a discontinuation trial. For example, for a patient taking haloperidol 10 mg per day, a reduction to 8 mg per day and close observation for 3 months is a reasonable strategy for a discontinuation trial. If psychotic symptoms recur, the patient should return to the previous dose that had successfully controlled the symptoms.

Depot antipsychotic treatment provides a significant advantage in compliance with antipsychotic regimens. Depot injections of haloperidol (Haldol) or fluphenazine decanoate (Prolixin) can be administered every 2 to 4 weeks. Dosage adjustments can be made when the clinical conditions warrant a change.

Clozapine (Clozaril), risperidone (Risperdal), quetiapine fumarate (Seroquel), olanzapine (Zyprexa), ziprasidone hydrochloride (Geodon), and aripiprazole (Abilify) are six newer antipsychotic agents. These and other antipsychotic agents have been developed in an attempt to increase efficacy and reduce the adverse effects associated with earlier antipsychotic agents. Clozapine's primary disadvantage has been a low but significant risk of drug-induced agranulocytosis. Unlike other antipsychotics, the risk of TD with clozapine is extremely low. Clozapine has demonstrated a clear superiority over chlorpromazine for treatment-resistant schizophrenia. However, because agranulocytosis can be fatal, clozapine should be reserved for patients who are unresponsive to or intolerant of other antipsychotics. Olanzapine is very similar to clozapine but is thought not to have the hematologic problem. Experience with this agent is still relatively limited.

Risperidone (Risperdal) is an antipsychotic with potency similar to haloperidol but with fewer reported extrapyramidal side effects. Most studies have used a dose of 6 to 10 mg per day of risperidone; higher doses produce significant extrapyramidal effects. It is unclear whether the reduced extrapyramidal side effects of risperidone are due to the drug itself or to the lower doses used in recent trials. There is some optimism that risperidone may be associated with a lower risk of TD. Further experience with this drug is needed to confirm this.

Quetiapine (Seroquel) is a newer antipsychotic agent with potency similar to that of chlorpromazine (Thorazine). Typical doses of 300 to 600 mg per day are used for psychotic disorders. Like other newer agents, there is less risk of extrapyramidal symptoms with quetiapine.

Olanzapine (Zyprexa) has an intermediate potency profile. Typical doses of 10 to 20 mg are used. This agent shares some structural similarities with clozapine but without the risk of agranulocytosis.

Ziprasidone (Geodon) also had an intermediate potency profile. Typical doses of 40 to 160 mg per day are therapeutic. It is recommended that Ziprasidone be taken on a twice-daily basis.

Aripiprazole (Abilify) has an intermediate potency profile. Typical doses of 10 to 15 mg per day are therapeutic. Aripiprizole can be taken in a single daily dose.

Recent evidence suggests atypical antipsychotic treatment may result in significant weight gain and a possible increased risk for diabetes mellitus. Patients receiving chronic antipsychotic treatment should be monitored for evidence of weight gain. Nutritional counseling and an exercise prescription may reduce the risk for psychotropic-associated weight gain.

Management of Adverse Neurologic Antipsychotic Effects

There are five adverse neurologic conditions that may arise from use of antipsychotic medication. Their effects and management are summarized in Table 9-5.

TABLE 9-5 Adverse Neurologic Effects of Antipsychotic Medications

Adverse Effect	Key Features	Onset*	Key Treatments†
Acute dystonia	Acute, often painful dystonic reaction (torticollis, oculogyric crisis, etc)	Hours to days	• Diphenhydramine, 25–50 mg IM/IV; benztropine, 1–2 mg IM/IV • Continue PO anticholinergic for 7 days
Akathisia	Restlessness, difficulty sitting still	Usually within first 2 weeks	• Reduce antipsychotic dose • Benztropine, 1–2 mg bid; propranolol hydrochloride, 20–40 mg bid-qid; lorazepam, 0.5–1.0 mg bid-qid
Pseudoparkinsonism	Cogwheel rigidity, tremor, bradykinesia, akinesia	Usually within first 2 weeks	• Reduce antipsychotic dose • Benztropine, 1–2 mg bid; amantadine, 100 mg bid-tid
Tardive dyskinesia	Oral, lingual, buccal dyskinetic movements; may involve trunk or limbs	After several or more years	• Reduce or stop antipsychotic ‡ • Consider use of clozapine, olanzapine
Neuroleptic malignant syndrome	Hyperthermia, lead-pipe rigidity, autonomic instability, delirium	Days to weeks, may occur at any time	• Stop antipsychotic • Hospitalize, monitor closely, cardiopulmonary support

*Time after initiating antipsychotic treatment.
† Use lower doses in the elderly and those with central nervous system disease.
‡ May initially see transient worsening of symptoms with dose reduction or cessation.

Acute dystonia. Dystonia can present as a psychiatric or medical emergency. Common dystonic reactions seen with antipsychotics include acute torticollis, oculogyric crises (dystonia of the muscles of the eye), contractions of specific muscles or muscle groups in the shoulder or back, and contractions of the tongue. More rare but potentially life threatening are laryngeal or diaphragmatic dystonic reactions that impair respiration.

Patients often describe dystonic reactions as painful and frightening. Physicians must act quickly to reduce the physical and emotional distress produced by the reaction. Risk factors for dystonic reactions are young age, male gender, and use of high doses of high-potency antipsychotics. Dystonic reaction risk can be reduced by prophylactic treatment with anticholinergic drugs in high-risk individuals. For patients with acute dystonia, diphenhydramine hydrochloride (Benadryl) 50 mg IV or IM or, alternatively, benztropine mesylate (Cogentin) 2 mg IV or IM will reverse the syndrome within minutes. Rarely is a second dose of anticholinergic required. For severe dystonia, the IV route is preferred because it produces relief in 2 or 3 minutes. Once a dystonic reaction occurs, patients remain at risk for a recurrent episode for an additional 5 to 7 days. This risk of recurrence drops when prophylactic anticholinergic treatment is prescribed, ie, benztropine 2 mg bid to tid during the week following a dystonic reaction.

Akathisia. Akathisia, which means to "not sit," describes an antipsychotic side effect that can be quite distressful. Akathisia includes a psychological and physical component and will develop in up to 40% of psychotic patients in the first 2 weeks of initiating antipsychotic treatment in usual doses. For some patients akathisia may be relatively mild; for others it may be quite severe. Patients suffering from drug-induced akathisia feel restless and have a hard time remaining still. Along with these subjective complaints, they may display an actual inability to sit still or to remain calm or comfortable in any position. Akathisia appears to be more prevalent in patients with pseudoparkinsonian symptoms such as tremor and rigidity. Rapid increases in antipsychotic dose and higher absolute antipsychotic dose levels predict a greater risk for akathisia.

Because akathisia is related to the antipsychotic dose, clinicians can consider if a reduced dose of antipsychotic is possible. Alternately, substitution of a lower-potency antipsychotic can be considered. Anticholinergic agent therapy may reduce akathisia, especially in patients with concurrent pseudoparkinsonism. Other agents that support efficacy in reducing akathisia include amantadine hydrochloride beta-blockers and benzodiazepines, particularly clonazepam.

Pseudoparkinsonism. Patients with pseudoparkinsonism show motor signs and symptoms identical to Parkinson disease. These adverse effects include tremor, cogwheel rigidity (particularly of the upper extremities), akinesia, or bradykinesia. Parkinsonian symptoms may be missed or mistakenly assumed to be part of the negative symptoms of schizophrenia. Pseudoparkinsonian symptoms occur in 15% to 20% of drug-naïve patients with schizophrenia when antipsychotic medications are initiated. Treatment for pseudoparkinsonism is the same as that for akathisia, although anticholinergic medications are usually more efficacious in pseudoparkinsonism. Clozapine and risperidone are alternate agents when pseudoparkinsonism is severe and patients do not respond or are intolerant of pharmacologic treatment of the extrapyramidal symptoms.

Tardive dyskinesia. One of the most persistent of the extrapyramidal effects is tardive dyskinesia (TD) because it may be permanent and may not reverse with discontinuation of antipsychotic treatment. In contrast to acute dystonia, akathisia, and pseudoparkinsonism, TD risk is cumulative and increases with the number of years of treatment with antipsychotics. At any time, the prevalence of TD in patients receiving long-term antipsychotics is 20% to 30%. Roughly 4% to 5% of patients receiving chronic antipsychotic treatment will develop TD each year. Although TD does sometimes resolve, more serious cases can persist even after discontinuing antipsychotic treatment. It is not possible to distinguish reversible TD from irreversible TD while the patient remains on antipsychotics.

Treatment for TD is often minimally successful. If possible, antipsychotic doses should be reduced or discontinued. TD often worsens initially with drug discontinuation. Adjunctive drugs can be considered to reduce or replace the use of antipsychotics. Drugs in this category include lithium and benzodiazepines. Clinicians may consider substituting clozapine for the antipsychotic drug being used at the time TD develops. Some success for treatment of TD with benzodiazepines, vitamin E, adrenergic antagonists, and dopamine agonists has been documented. Referral to an expert or center specializing in movement disorders or TD should be considered for serious and impairing cases.

Neuroleptic malignant syndrome. Neuroleptic malignant syndrome (NMS) is the most acutely serious adverse event associated with antipsychotics and should be regarded as a medical emergency. NMS is characterized by hyperthermia, severe ("lead-pipe") muscular rigidity, autonomic nervous system instability, and cognitive impairment. Incidence estimates for NMS are approximately 0.2% to 0.5% of patients exposed to these drugs. The syndrome typically occurs within 2 weeks of initiating antipsychotics or increasing the dose of an antipsychotic. In 80% of cases, the onset is fulminant, peaking in severity in 48 to 72 hours. Mortality rates range from 4% to 20%. Major medical complications include rhabdomyolysis, neuropsychological impairment, myocardial infarction, sudden cardiac or respiratory arrest, intravascular coagulation, pulmonary embolus, and severe infection.

Treatment of NMS usually begins with hospitalization, often in an intensive care unit. Supportive care should include intravenous fluid support and efforts to maximize cardiopulmonary function. Antipsychotic drugs should be discontinued. There is no generally agreed-on approach to the pharmacologic treatment of NMS. Anticholinergic agents, amantadine, dantrolene sodium, and bromocriptine mesylate may be helpful for some individuals. If available, medical intensivists or psychiatrists knowledgeable about NMS should be involved in patient care. After recovery, another antipsychotic may need to be used. This decision should be made carefully in consultation with the patient, the family, and a psychiatrist.

Psychosocial Treatments

Chronic psychotic disorders necessitate activation of all available professional, family, and community resources. Individual long-term supportive psychotherapy forms the base for a comprehensive treatment plan. This psychotherapy focuses on practical management of daily problems and supports compliance with medical treatment and may include or be complemented by social skills and/or assertiveness training.

For the patient who lives at home or has frequent family contact, family education becomes an important treatment component. The risk for relapse in schizophrenic patients increases in families with high levels of "expressed emotion" (frequent criticism of the patient) and interpersonal discord. Family therapy should be implemented in these distressed families. Family members can benefit by joining national organizations that educate, support, and advocate for the severely mentally ill. In the United States, the National Alliance for the Mentally Ill (NAMI) has many local chapters.

Community case management approaches provide additional assistance in managing schizophrenia and other chronic psychotic disorders. Case management involves identifying a primary caregiver, such as a nurse or social worker, who coordinates a comprehensive treatment plan. Patients with high levels of social isolation may require assertive community outreach programs, in which the caregiver goes to the patient rather than the patient visiting an office or clinic. Vocational rehabilitation is often an important component of comprehensive treatment plans. Unfortunately, case management programs are not available in many areas of the United States.

SUMMARY

Psychotic signs and symptoms frequently indicate a serious psychiatric syndrome that can interfere with the management of concurrent medical disorders. The differential diagnosis of psychotic symptoms includes disorders of cognitive impairment, substance intoxication or withdrawal, and mood disorders as well as those in the psychotic disorders categories. Antipsychotic medication can be helpful in the acute and chronic management of psychotic symptoms and psychotic disorders. However, these drugs can have serious side effects and require close monitoring. Psychosocial interventions can also reduce the morbidity associated with psychotic disorders.

ADDITIONAL READINGS

American Psychiatric Association. *Diagnostic and Statistical Manual of Mental Disorders*. 4th ed. Text Revision. Washington, DC: American Psychiatric Press; 2000.

American Psychiatric Association. *Practice Guidelines for the Treatment of Psychiatric Disorders*. Compendium: 2002. Washington, DC: American Psychiatric Press; 2002.

American Psychiatric Association. *Diagnostic and Statistical Manual of Mental Disorders*. 4th ed. Primary Care Version. Washington, DC: American Psychiatric Press; 1995.

Cummings JL, Frank JC, Cherry D, et al. Guidelines for managing Alzheimer's disease: part II. Treatment. *Am Fam Physician*. 2002;65:2525-2534.

Glick ID, Suppes T, Debattista C, Hu RJ, Marder S. Psychopharmacologic treatment strategies for depression, bipolar disorder, and schizophrenia. *Ann Intern Med*. 2001;134:47-60.

Glick ID, Murray SR, Vasudeyan P, Marder SR, Hu RJ. Treatment with atypical antipsychotics: new indications and new populations. *J Psychiatr Res*. 2001;35(3):187-191.

Goldman LS. Medical illness in patients with schizophrenia. *J Clin Psychiatry*. 1999;50(suppl 21):20-15.

Kindermann SS, Dolder CR, Bailey A, Katz IR, Jeste DV. Pharmacological treatment of psychosis and agitation in elderly patients with dementia: four decades of experience. *Drugs Aging*. 2002;19:257-276.

Muench J, Carey M. Diabetes mellitus associated with atypical antipsychotic medications: new case report and review of the literature. *J Am Board Fam Pract*. 2001;14:278-282.

Perry PJ, Alexander B, Liskow BI. *Psychotropic Drug Handbook*. 7th ed. Washington, DC: American Psychiatric Press; 1997.

Sachdev P, Kruk J. Clinical characteristics and predisposing factors in acute drug-induced akathisia. *Arch Gen Psychiatry*. 1994;51:963-974.

Webster R, Holroyd S. Prevalence of psychotic symptoms in delirium. *Psychosomatics*. 2000;41:519-522.

Chapter **10**

Cognitive Disorders: Delirium, Mild Cognitive Impairment, and Dementia

Hochang Benjamin Lee, MD
Michael Ankrom, MD
Constantine G. Lyketsos, MD, MHS

Delirium, mild cognitive impairment (MCI), and dementia involve impairment in cognition and are commonly encountered in a primary care setting. Cognitive complaints, especially involving memory, are common among the elderly, and cognitive assessment is an important aspect of primary care for our rapidly aging population.

Cognitive disorders have many presentations as well as causes. Delirium is an acute impairment in level of consciousness that affects cognitive capacity. Mild cognitive impairment and dementia are more insidious in their inception and do not involve impairment in attention. Depression can closely mimic mild delirium and MCI and should be considered in the differential diagnosis of all cognitive evaluations. Table 10-1 compares the features of delirium, dementia, and depression.

TABLE 10-1 Comparative Features of Delirium, Dementia, and Depression			
	Delirium	**Dementia**	**Depression**
Definition	Impaired sensorium (reduced level of consciousness)	Global decline in cognitive capacity in clear consciousness	Disturbance in mood, with associated low vital sense and low self-attitude
Core symptoms	Inattention, distractibility, drowsiness, befuddlement	Amnesia, aphasia, agnosia, apraxia, disturbed executive function	Sadness, anhedonia, crying
Common associated symptoms	Cognitive impairment, hallucinations, mood lability	Depression, delusions, hallucinations, irritability	Fatigue, insomnia, anorexia, guilt, self-blame, hopelessness, helplessness
Temporal features	Acute or subacute onset	Chronic onset, usually gradual	Episodic, subacute onset
Diurnal features	Usually worse in the evening and night	No clear pattern	Usually worse in the morning

Assessment and treatment of cognitive disorders is complex and involves the patient, family, care providers, and health professionals. This chapter provides a synopsis on assessing and treating each cognitive disorder in a primary care setting.

DELIRIUM

Definition and Epidemiology

Delirium is a disorder of sensorium or level of consciousness. (Consciousness can be defined as a function of the nervous system that is concerned with the perceptual experience of information from the environment and from our own body.) The American Psychiatric Association's *Diagnostic and Statistical Manual of Mental Disorders*, fourth edition (DSM-IV), defines delirium as a syndrome of disturbed consciousness that results in a change in cognition (memory, disorientation, or language disturbance) or in perception from baseline and is not due to dementia. The disturbance typically develops over a short period of time (hours to days) and tends to fluctuate during the course of the day. Usually, delirium is directly caused by a general medical condition. Dementia, as discussed later, does not involve change in level of consciousness. In addition to dementia, fluent aphasia and some psychiatric conditions may be mistaken for delirium. Delirious patients can present with multiple symptoms as a result of impaired level of consciousness. Symptoms can involve alteration in cognitive abilities, mood, and behavior (Table 10-2). Although delirium is a result of attentional impairment, attentional impairment can impair other psychiatric and cognitive domains, producing symptoms associated with the affected domain. It is important to note that occasionally a patient with delirium will not meet DSM-IV diagnostic criteria and may require longer periods of observation to make a definitive diagnosis. This is especially true in patients with prolonged delirium as a result of traumatic brain injury or prolonged drug withdrawal. The Confusion Assessment Method (CAM) also provides a diagnostic algorithm using standardized (CAM) questions that can assist in the detection of delirium (Table 10-3).

Risk factors for delirium include advanced age, cognitive impairment (eg, Folstein Mini-Mental State Exam [MMSE] of ≤24), vision impairment (visual acuity of <20/70), dehydration (blood urea nitrogen [BUN]/creatinine ratio ≥18), and severe illness. Delirium occurs in 10% to 40% of hospitalized elderly over age 65, and 25% to 65% of elderly patients develop delirium during their hospital stay. The consequences of delirium

---

TABLE 10-2 Symptoms of Delirium

Cognitive
  Poor memory

  Disorientation

  Aphasia, most often word finding

Affective
  Sadness/apathy

  Anxiety/lability

Psychotic
  Fearfulness

  Hallucination

  Delusions

Behavioral
  Aggression

  Pacing

  Calling out

  Sleep impairment

  Anorexia

  Hypersexuality

TABLE 10-3 The Confusion Assessment Method (CAM) Diagnostic Algorithm

Feature 1. Acute onset and fluctuating course

This feature is usually obtained from a family member or nurse and is shown by positive responses to the following questions: Is there evidence of an acute change in mental status from the patient's baseline? Does the (abnormal) behavior fluctuate during the day, ie, tend to come and go or increase and decrease in severity?

Feature 2. Inattention

This feature is shown by a positive response to the following question: Does the patient have difficulty focusing attention, eg, being easily distractible or having difficulty keeping track of what is being said?

Feature 3. Disorganized thinking

This feature is shown by a positive response to the following question: Is the patient's thinking disorganized or incoherent, such as rambling or irrelevant conversation, unclear or illogical flow of ideas, or unpredictable switching from subject to subject?

Feature 4. Altered level of consciousness

This feature is shown by any answer other than "alert" to the following question: Overall, how would you rate this patient's level of consciousness? (alert [normal], vigilant [hyperalert], lethargic [drowsy, easily aroused], stupor [difficult to arouse], or coma [unarousable]).

Note: The diagnosis of delirium by CAM requires the presence of features 1 and 2 and either 3 or 4.

Adapted with permission from Inouye SK, van Dyck CH, Alessi CA, et al. Clarifying confusion: The Confusion Assessment Method (a new method for detection of delirium). *Ann Intern Med.* 1990;113:941-948.

include longer hospital stays and a mortality of 10% to 65%, 2 to 20 times the mortality of control patients with acute myocardial infarction or sepsis. The risk of delirium increases with the intensity of surgical intervention, occurring in 1% to 3% of cataract surgeries, 10% to 15% of general surgeries, and 28% to 61% of orthopedic surgeries.

Assessment

The diagnosis of delirium is difficult because the condition fluctuates, at times requiring multiple evaluations. Delirium can be quite obvious when a cognitively intact person becomes clearly confused and is either agitated or lethargic. The first step in evaluating a delirious patient is to assess and document the impairment in level of consciousness. A quick cognitive evaluation should assess the patient's orientation to person, place, time, and circumstance. Short cognitive screening tests such as the MMSE or attentional measures such as the digit span can be used to assess the initial state and the course of delirium. Delirium can wax and wane, resulting in different levels of orientation at different times. Language is usually preserved except in the most severe cases of delirium. Once a diagnosis of delirium is made, an investigation for precipitating underlying medical condition should be performed. Documented precipitating factors for delirium in the hospital setting include physical restraint use, malnutrition, adding three or more new medications, and bladder catheter use. Because almost any medical, physical, or chemical insult can cause delirium, the mnemonic D-E-L-I-R-I-U-M is often used to allow a standardized assessment of the confused patient (Figure 10-1). Medications are implicated in

FIGURE 10-1 Causes of Delirium

D   Dementia*

E   Electrolytes

L   Lung, liver, heart, kidney, brain†

I   Infection

RX   Drugs‡

I   Injury, pain, stress

U   Unfamiliar environment contributing

M   Metabolic§

---

* Although dementia is a predisposing factor for delirium, only subtypes like Lewy body dementia are commonly seen with delirium.

† Lung—pulmonary embolism, hypoxia, hypercarbia
Liver—hepatic failure
Heart—acute myocardial infarction, CHF
Kidney—renal insufficiency or failure
Brain—CVA especially posterior circulation strokes, acute right parietal lesions, and frontal lobe lesions, seizure, encephalopathy, subdural hematoma, hypotension, meningitis

‡ Medications, herbal supplements, and drugs of abuse including intoxication and withdrawal states

§ Hypoglycemia, hypercalcemia

between 20% and 40% of cases of delirium; especially among the elderly, opiate medications are occasional culprits. It is important to remember that the cause of delirium is often multifactorial in etiology, with studies finding that between two and six factors may contribute to a single case of delirium.

Standardized assessment tools have been created for evaluating delirium, including the CAM, Memorial Delirium Assessment Scale, Delirium Symptom Inventory, and Delirium Rating Scale-Revised (DRS-R). Standardized cognitive measurement tools like the MMSE (described in Chapter 3) can be used to document changes in cognition but can miss subtle delirium in some patients. The electroencephalogram (EEG) can demonstrate diffuse background slowing (background rhythm less than 6 Hz) consistent with metabolic encephalopathy, but this does not help in diagnosing the cause of delirium. Nor does EEG have known sensitivity or specificity to detect delirium due to normative age-related changes on EEG and changes due to underlying dementia. The EEG can also detect delirium by relative slowing (reduction of background rhythm by 3–4 Hz), but this requires a baseline EEG. It is also important to know that as many as 20% of patients with delirium have normal EEGs and that patients with dementia may have slowed EEGs in the absence of delirium. The EEG can differentiate between delirium and seizure activity and delirium and drug withdrawal states in which the EEG may be abnormally fast. Also, EEG can help follow the course of delirium. A normal EEG would argue against diagnosis of delirium although it wouldn't completely rule out mild delirium.

Delirium can present with a multitude of symptoms (Table 10-2). Classic delirium involves a patient with increased alertness and confusion; this overactive patient may be talkative, humorous, angry, or belligerent. As common, but more easily overlooked, is the hypoactive patient with delirium, whose condition may not be diagnosed until the patient is very lethargic or comatose. Both ends of this clinical spectrum may result in patients being dangerous to themselves and others. In addition to disturbances in orientation and level of consciousness, disturbances in attention, memory, planning, organization, sleep-wake cycle, thought processes, affect, perception, and activity levels have been reported.

Case Vignette

Ms Arlen, a 60-year-old schoolteacher, has moderate chronic obstructive pulmonary disease. She is admitted to the hospital with a community-acquired pneumonia complicated by an empyema. Her fever and white count begin to decrease after 2 days of treatment. However, the nurses report that she is uncooperative with self-care, refusing to ambulate, even to use the toilet; she has urinated in her bed on several occasions and seems unconcerned about doing so. She has been speaking little and demonstrates little emotional responsiveness when she does talk. Her primary care physician suspects depression, but before starting an antidepressant, the doctor conducts a more thorough mental status examination of Ms Arlen. The patient denies feeling any sadness or hopelessness about her situation, but she acknowledges that she is puzzled by all of the strangers who have been "touching me" while she has been "at the mall here this past week." Her short-term memory is significantly impaired, and she writes an illegible, unintelligible sentence when asked to do so. Hypoactive delirium is diagnosed. A subsequent investigation reveals newly developed hyponatremia and hypercapnia as likely etiologic factors.

Management

The first step in managing delirium involves rapid recognition and a search for and treatment of the precipitating medical condition. Efforts should be made to correct multiple medical abnormalities because most patients with delirium have multiple treatable causes (Figure 10-1). During the course of delirium, other important management strategies include nonpharmacologic interventions such as reassurance, communication, and supervision. Reassurance of the confused patient includes attempts to increase orientation and adjust sensory inputs by either decreasing sensory overload or decreasing sensory deprivation as appropriate. Communication with a confused patient includes maximizing the sensory modalities of hearing, vision, and touch to increase appropriate awareness of the patient's surroundings. The last intervention includes appropriate supervision to provide for the safety of the confused patient. In many cases nonpharmacologic interventions may allow time to correct the cause of the delirium. However, some delirious patients are a significant safety risk to themselves or to others and may require either medication intervention or physical restraint. Clearly, physical restraints can result in injury to the confused patient and are short-term interventions applied in the least restrictive form to maintain safety. As a result, there exist strict hospital and skilled nursing facility guidelines on the proper use and assessment of the least restrictive device for each confused patient.

Pharmacologic management of delirium has traditionally included neuroleptic antipsychotic medications or sedative/hypnotic medications of the benzodiazepine class. The indiscriminate use of psychotropic medications can complicate the assessment of mental status and impair the patient's ability to cooperate and understand treatment. An increased risk of falls is another complication. Although affective symptoms are common in delirium, psychotropic medications with anticholinergic properties may exacerbate delirium. Neuroleptic medications include haloperidol, fluphenazine, and droperidol as well as newer atypical neuroleptics such as risperidone, olanzapine, and quetiapine fumarate. These medications immediately relieve anxiety and provide sedation, with the antipsychotic effect occurring 3 to 6 days later. Risperidone and quetiapine are only available as oral agents. Olanzapine is available in intramuscular injectable form as well.

High-potency typical neuroleptic medications such as haloperidol and fluphenazine are generally preferred for pharmacologic management of delirium because of their low anticholinergic activity. The usual starting dosage for haloperidol and fluphenazine is about 2 to 5 mg every 8 to 12 hours, as needed. The elderly and those with known central nervous system dysfunction (eg, dementia, stroke) require doses as low as 0.5 mg two to three times per day. Caution should be used because these medications can cause significant acute hypotension as well as the extrapyramidal syndrome, akathisia, and neuroleptic malignant syndrome. Intravenous administration of haloperidol is generally considered safe, but infrequent, yet life-threatening cases of torsade de pointes have been reported with high doses. The efficacy of newer, atypical neuroleptic medications in managing delirium is less known, but olanzapine 5 to 10 mg and risperidone 0.5 to 1 mg every 8 to 12 hours as needed have been reported to be effective. Additionally, risperidone and olanzapine are less likely to cause extrapyramidal syndrome and neuroleptic malignant syndrome. Very little is known about the efficacy of other atypical antipsychotic medications such as quetiapine and ziprasidone hydrochloride in treating delirium.

Most randomized controlled trials that compared the efficacy of neuroleptic medications to that of benzodiazepines for treating delirium show more favorable results for neuroleptic medications. Thus, benzodiazepines are second-line agents that should be used only after neuroleptic medication has proved to be unsuccessful or unsafe. Lorazepam 1 to 2 mg or diazepam 2 to 5 mg every 8 to 12 hours as needed is the typical dosage for treating delirium. Respiratory depression is an important adverse effect of benzodiazepine. Furthermore, benzodiazepines can cause increased cognitive impairment and, in some patients, significant disinhibition or paradoxical agitation.

Some patients are unable to tolerate the effects of antipsychotic medication or find them to be ineffective. Case reports on the use of ondansetron, a 5-HT3 receptor antagonist; trazodone hydrochloride, an atypical antidepressant; donepezil hydrochloride, an acetylcholinesterase inhibitor; and valproic acid, an anticonvulsant, have been reported to be effective in specific circumstances. For patients with possible acute anticholinergic delirium, administration of intravenous physostigmine should be considered.

Patients with delirium require close follow-up for response to medical and symptomatic interventions. Patients can be followed clinically or with general cognitive measures such as the MMSE, with delirium-specific measures such as the Delirium Rating Scale (DRS), or with EEG. Not only is it important to document the resolution of delirium, one must attempt to withdraw symptomatic interventions once they are no longer necessary. Patients who develop delirium may also have an underlying dementia or psychiatric disorder and should be appropriately evaluated once the delirium has resolved.

MILD COGNITIVE SYNDROME

Definition and Epidemiology

Cognitive impairment is now known to occur in the absence of dementia in as many as 20% of people over age 65. Here the term *mild cognitive syndrome (MCS)* is used broadly to refer to cognitive impairment that is neither global nor of sufficient severity to meet criteria for dementia. MCS might be purely amnestic, or it might also involve cognitive impairment in other spheres, such as language or executive dysfunction. Other terms used for MCS include mild cognitive impairment (MCI), cognitive impairment no dementia (CIND), or age-associated memory impairment.

The clinical entity of MCS lies on the boundary of normal aging and early dementia. It refers generally to complaints of memory or other cognitive dysfunction in elderly people, which may have a high probability of evolving toward dementia. The cognitive deficits in an MCS patient are detectable; yet unlike those in a patient with dementia, the deficits are not severe enough to impair daily activities or are not global in their scope, affecting only a few cognitive functions, typically memory. The best characterized subset of MCS is MCI. There are several multicenter treatment trials for MCI, and criteria for diagnosis are listed in Table 10-4. Based on these criteria, an MCI patient has full ability to carry out daily activities, scores within the normal range in the MMST, and does not have global cognitive impairment. At the same time, MCI differs from normal senescence because an MCI patient has complaints of worsening memory (preferably corroborated by family members), as well as objective memory impairment at a level that is at least 1.5 standard deviations below average for age and education on neuropsychological tests of new learning and memory. However, various studies have noted that patients with MCI, although having primarily memory complaints, commonly showed deficits on tasks in language, orientation, and praxis. In fact, patients with purely amnestic MCI likely represent only a small proportion of elderly people with cognitive deficits.

Due to recent characterization of MCS, its incidence and prevalence are not well known but have varied according to the definition of MCS used. In the Canadian Study of Health and Aging, the classification of CIND had a prevalence rate of 17%; however, this definition of MCS is likely to be broader than that generally accepted in the United States. MCI appears to be prodromal to Alzheimer dementia (AD) as has been well documented in several studies. Compared to healthy control subjects who convert to AD at a rate of less than 1% per year, studies have shown that MCI patients progress to AD at a

---

TABLE 10-4 Criteria for Amnestic Mild Cognitive Impairment

- Memory complaint, preferably corroborated by an informant
- Impaired memory function for age and education
- Preserved general cognitive function
- Intact activities of daily living
- Absence of dementia

Source: Petersen RC, Doody R, Kurz A, Mohs RC, et al. Current concepts in mild cognitive impairment. *Arch Neurol.* 2001;58(12):1985-1992.

rate of 10% to 15% per year. It is unclear whether individuals with other forms of MCS, using broader definitions, also are at higher risk of progression to AD.

Differential Diagnoses of "Memory Problems"

Geriatric depression often presents with a chief complaint of "memory problems" in a primary care setting. Once adequately treated with psychotherapy and/or pharmacotherapy, a substantial portion of elderly depressed patients do recover cognitively. This cognitive phenomenon of geriatric depression once led to coining of the term *pseudodementia*. However, the relationship between depression and cognitive impairment in the elderly is quite complex. A depressed elderly patient has a higher risk of developing dementia, and depressive symptoms might represent a prodrome of dementia. Also, depression is common among patients with dementia, and depression could be superimposed on dementia. In any case, geriatric depression should be treated vigorously, and the clinician should closely follow the associated cognitive deficits.

Numerous reversible medical conditions cause subtle cognitive impairment. Table 10-5 lists medical conditions that could cause deficits in memory. In particular, any injuries to diencephalic and medial temporal structures may cause amnestic symptoms. The most common etiology of such injury is thiamin deficiency due to alcohol dependence. Identification and treatment of the underlying medical condition may reverse the cognitive deficits. If a toxic substance is the cause, stopping or tapering use may reverse

TABLE 10-5 Medical Causes of Deficits in Memory

Thiamin deficiency (Korsakoff syndrome)

Hypoglycemia

Hypoxia

Injury to brain (ie, thalamic and temporal lobe)

    Seizures

    Head trauma

    Cerebral tumors

    Cerebrovascular diseases

    Surgical procedures on the brain

    Viral encephalitis (ie, herpes simplex virus)

    Multiple sclerosis

Alcohol

Neurotoxins

Benzodiazepines

Sedative hypnotics

Opiate medications

Many over-the-counter medications (eg, anticholinergic medications)

the condition. For those who have permanent brain injury, supportive measures should be employed.

Even after medical causes of cognitive impairment and depression are ruled out, it may be difficult to definitively diagnose MCI in a primary care setting. Neuropsychological testing can be very useful in identifying and quantifying subtle deficits. When interpreting results from neuropsychological testing, clinical judgment always takes precedence because education, age, cultural background, and illnesses may influence test performance and different subtypes of MCI have substantial overlap between them.

Management

Because the diagnosis of MCS may forewarn the onset of senile dementia, earlier detection may mean earlier intervention for dementia. Several clinical trials have been initiated to test the use of cholinesterase inhibitors, antioxidants, and anti-inflammatory drugs in patients with MCS, typically using the MCI definition. Cholinesterase inhibitors have symptomatic effects that can relieve hypothetical depletion of acetylcholine neurotransmission, which may occur in MCI. Previous epidemiological studies had suggested that hormones, particularly estrogens, were associated with delayed onset of the appearance of AD. More recent evidence, based on the Women's Health Initiative Memory Study, however, has cast strong doubts on the benefits of hormone replacement therapy on cognition. Thus, estrogens should probably be avoided as treatments of cognitive symptoms. Clinical trials on the effect of cyclooxygenase-2 (COX-2) inhibitors in MCI patients with the rationale that reducing inflammation in the brain could delay the onset of AD are ongoing. Antioxidants such as vitamin E and ginko biloba are also in clinical trials.

The decision to treat MCS or MCI with cholinesterase inhibitors involves weighing potential benefits against the potential financial cost for a patient who will likely remain on medication for several years. Because patients with MCI are likely to convert to dementia of AD at some point, early use of cholinesterase inhibitors in MCI may mean longer symptomatic relief of cognitive deficits due to AD. If judiciously prescribed, side effects from cholinesterase inhibitors can be minimized. Thus, cholinesterase inhibitors should be considered unless side effects or financial cost is an impediment for the patient.

Several studies have suggested that antioxidants such as vitamins C and E may be helpful in delaying either the onset or the progression of AD. Given that both vitamin E and vitamin C have very few side effects, they should be considered for MCS and especially MCI patients who may already be on other nutritional supplements. Use of COX-2 inhibitors and hormone replacement therapy to delay the onset of dementia in MCS patients awaits results from the clinical trials.

DEMENTIA

Definition and Epidemiology

Dementia is defined as a global decline of cognitive capacity in clear consciousness. There are three elements to the definition of dementia. First, *global* means that multiple areas of cognition are impaired. Unlike aphasia or amnestic syndrome, dementia means that more than one area of cognition is impaired. In addition to impairment in memory, other cognitive domains such as language, abstraction, calculation, perception, and judgment are impaired. Second, *decline* means deterioration from a previous level of cognitive capacity. This element distinguishes dementias from other cognitive disorders, such as mental retardation and learning disorders, that are present from birth. Also, the level of decline should be severe enough to impair one's daily activities. This level of decline distinguishes dementia from MCS. Finally, *in clear consciousness* means that level of consciousness is not impaired. This element distinguishes dementia from delirium.

Dementia syndromes can be largely divided into two types based on the pattern of impairment in cognitive domains: cortical type and subcortical type. In cortical dementia, cognitive functions that are located in the cortex, such as memory, language, gnosis, and praxis, are impaired. Thus, cortical dementias such as AD are characterized by amnesia, aphasia, apraxia, and agnosia (the four As). In subcortical dementia, primary cognitive deficits are localized to deeper brain structures. Patients with subcortical dementia such as Huntington disease (HD) typically have difficulty coordinating cognition. As a result, they have difficulties with memory, slowed thinking, impaired decision making, and reduced complexity of thought (dysmnesia, delay, dysexecutive, and depletion—four Ds). Table 10-6 summarizes the distinction between cortical and subcortical dementia.

Dementias are frequently accompanied by various behavioral and psychiatric disturbances such as delusion, hallucination, depression, anxiety, and agitation. These disturbances are generally irreversible because of underlying progressive degenerative diseases. A sizable number of patients (5% to 10%) do have causes for which restorative treatment is available (see Table 10-7). However, the actual reversal of decline in cognitive function depends on the extent of damage to the brain because neurons rarely regenerate. Nevertheless, even when the disease process is determined to be irreversible, cognitive and associated psychiatric symptoms can be managed effectively with proper evaluation and treatment. Also, with evolving knowledge from basic research and with development of new intervention strategies, more effective treatments are likely to be available over the next several years.

TABLE 10-6 Cortical vs Subcortical Dementia

	Cortical	Subcortical
Key feature	Loss of core ability (capacity) to "do" cognition	Loss of ability to coordinate cognition
Mnemonic features	The four As: Amnesia Apraxia Agnosia Aphasia	The four Ds: Dysmnesia Dysexecutive Delay Depletion
Typical symptoms	Can't recall or recognize Repeats questions Can't do things Doesn't "know" things Trouble with language	Needs cues to remember Slowed thinking/movement Can't plan and execute Less flexible Less initiative
Examples	Alzheimer disease Lewy body disease Frontotemporal degeneration	Parkinson disease Huntington disease Normopressure hydrocephalus

TABLE 10-7 Causes of Dementia

Degenerative Brain Diseases	Traumatic Brain Injuries
Alzheimer disease	Closed head injury
Parkinson disease	Open head injury
Pick disease	Subdural hematoma
Frontotemporal degeneration	**Vitamin Deficiencies**
Huntington disease	Vitamin B_{12} deficiency (subacute combined sclerosis, pernicious anemia)
Progressive supranuclear palsy	
Spinocerebellar degeneration	Vitamin B_6 deficiency (pellagra)
Multiple sclerosis	Vitamin B_1 (thiamin) deficiency
Multiple Infarct Disease	**Endocrine Diseases**
Binswanger disease	Hyperthyroidism
Subcortical leukoareosis	Hypothyroidism
Thalamic infarct	Growth hormone deficiency
Cerebral Vasculitides	Hyperparathyroidism
Lupus erythematous	Cushing disease (hyperadrenalism)
Giant cell arteritis	Addison syndrome (hypoadrenalism)
Infectious Diseases	**Cerebral Tumors**
Syphilis (general paresis of the insane)	Intrinsic brain tumor
Tuberculosis	Metastatic cancer
HIV disease (AIDS dementia complex)	**Toxin Exposure**
Prion disease (Creutzfeldt-Jakob disease [CJD])	Alcohol
	Heavy metals (lead, arsenic, mercury)
Fungal encephalitides	Volatile hydrocarbons
Viral encephalitides	Medications
Psychiatric Disorders	**Others**
Major depressive disorder	Normopressure (communicating) hydrocephalus
Schizophrenia	

Although dementia can afflict the young, it is primarily a syndrome of the elderly. Before age 65, the prevalence of dementia is low (0.5% to 1%). However, over age 65, the prevalence increases dramatically—5% to 8% of people suffer from dementia. For those 75 years and older, 18% to 20% suffer dementia. For individuals over age 85, more than one third may suffer from dementia.

Assessment

Assessment for dementia is composed of two steps. The first step is to determine presence or absence of dementia. To assess for decline in cognitive capacity, a baseline cognitive level must be established.

A standard recommendation is that all patients older than age 65 have one and possibly an annual standardized cognitive assessment done during the routine medical checkup. The MMSE is a basic, yet extremely useful tool for primary care physicians, given its short length and reliability (see Table 3-9 in Chapter 3). Although a score of 24 is often used as a cutoff for diagnosis of dementia in some epidemiologic studies, a decline of more than 3 points from a stable baseline is a clinically significant change that warrants a dementia evaluation. Also, a collateral source, such as a family member, is critical for filling in the gaps in evaluation of a patient with cognitive difficulty.

Once the presence of dementia is determined through history and clinical exam, laboratory investigations may elucidate its underlying cause. Table 10-8 lists common laboratory and imaging studies used to evaluate dementia. Atypical course and symptoms may require laboratory investigations that are less frequently used but that may point to specific, yet unusual etiology of dementia (Table 10-9).

Additionally, the patient's family and personal environment should be assessed. The following questions should be asked: How are the patient's needs and wants provided for and by whom? To what extent do family and/or care providers have insight into the patient's condition? Which care providers require help in caring for the patient? What resources are available to them to do this? How are family members and other care providers coping? What financial and human resources are available to the patient?

TABLE 10-8 Common Laboratory Investigations for the Evaluation of Dementia Syndromes

Urinalysis and microscopy

Blood tests

    Complete blood count

    Serum electrolytes, including magnesium calcium

    Serum chemistries, including liver function tests

    Thyroid function testing

    Serum B_{12}, RBC folate assays

    Erythrocyte sedimentation rate

    Serologic tests for syphilis

*Chest x-rays

*Electrocardiogram

*Toxicology screens

    Urine toxicology

    Serum toxicology (alcohol, salicylates, other)

*Computed tomography or magnetic resonance imaging of brain

---

*To be considered; not universally needed.

TABLE 10-9 Less Common Laboratory Investigations When Specific Etiology Is Suspected for Atypical Course and Symptoms

Test	Indication
EEG	Possible seizures: CJD
Lumbar puncture	Onset of dementia <6 months, rapidly progressive dementia
Heavy metal screen	History of potential exposure
HIV test	History of potential exposure
Lyme disease titer	History of potential exposure or compatible clinical picture
Ceruloplasmin, arylsulfatase, electrophoresis	Wilson disease, metachromatic leukodystrophy, or multiple myeloma
Slit lamp exam	History and exam suggest Wilson disease
Apolipoprotein E testing	Need to increase likelihood that AD diagnosis is correct
Genetic testing for Alzheimer genes or other dementia genes	Family history is strong and confirmation clinically necessary
PET	Need to increase likelihood that AD diagnosis is correct

Referral to geriatric psychiatrists or behavioral neurologists should be considered when the diagnosis is uncertain, the case is atypical, there are associated complex behavioral or psychiatric symptoms, or the initial management of symptoms has failed.

Cortical Dementia

Alzheimer disease. AD is marked by insidious onset of symptoms and slowly progressive decline in cognitive capacity. A definite diagnosis of AD requires demonstration of neuritic plaques and neurofibrillary tangles in the brain, primarily in the temporal and parietal lobes, through autopsy. However, the clinical diagnosis of probable AD (see Table 10-10) by an experienced clinician is more than 90% accurate. The dementia of AD is a classic cortical dementia with impairments in memory (amnesia), coordination dexterity (apraxia), language (aphasia), and perception (agnosia). The diagnosis is most often made by the primary care physician, but the presence of atypical features such as neurologic signs or evidence of psychiatric disease should suggest the need for specialty consultation.

In the United States, 3% to 5% of persons 65 years or older suffer from AD. For persons 85 years of age or older, the prevalence of Alzheimer disease increases to 20% to 25%. The incidence of AD at age 65 is around 0.25% per year. However, it doubles every 5 years so that the incidence is 1% per year at age 75 and approaches 4% per year at age 85.

In the early stages of AD, widespread loss of neurons occurs most prominently in the entorhinal and hippocampal areas of the temporal lobe. This loss spreads throughout the

TABLE 10-10 Criteria for Probable Alzheimer Disease

A. Dementia

   1. Decline on examination and objective testing

   2. Deficits in two or more areas of cognition

B. Gradual progression

C. Level of consciousness intact

D. Onset after age 40

E. No other cause after workup

Source: McKhann G, Drachman D, Fostein MF, Katzman R, Price D, Stadlan E. Clinical diagnosis of Alzheimer's disease: report of the National Institute Neurologic and Communicative Disorders and Stroke/Alzheimer's Disease Related Disorders Association workgroup under the auspices of DHHS task force on Alzheimer's disease. *Neurol.* 1984;34:939-944.

temporal region and into the parietal and frontal regions of the brain. These changes lead to the shrinkage of the brain, which occurs at a faster rate than age-associated atrophy. The two pathologic elements prominent in AD are the extracellular accumulation of neuritic or senile plaques consisting of beta-amyloid deposition and the intracellular deposition of neurofibrillary tangles, made up of hyperphosphorylated tau protein. These pathologic elements are found in some individuals at autopsy without the individual having manifested any symptoms of dementia or memory loss.

It is still unclear whether neuritic plaques and neurofibrillary tangles cause neuronal deaths or if the opposite is true. Nevertheless, widespread neuronal death and the associated loss of acetylcholine are thought to be the cause of memory loss and other cognitive symptoms. In addition to acetylcholine, depletion of other neurotransmitters, including serotonergic, dopaminergic, glutaminergic, and gabanergic neurotransmitters, may underlie depression, psychosis, agitation, and other behavioral symptoms in AD.

Twin studies, with demonstrated high rates of concordance, reveal that heredity plays an important role in the causation of the disease. Relatives of people with AD are more likely than the general population to develop the disease. Autosomal dominant genes for transmission of AD have been recently discovered. Genes on chromosome 21 (the APP gene), 1 (the presenilin-2 gene), and 14 (the presenilin-1 gene) have been implicated in causation of familial AD. Other genes on chromosome 19 (the apolipoprotein E gene) and chromosome 12 (the alpha-2M gene) are associated with increased risk and possible acceleration of the age of onset of AD.

The onset of cognitive symptoms is usually insidious for patients in their 70s and 80s and is slowly progressive. A crude rule of thumb is that a patient with Alzheimer dementia loses 3 to 4 points a year on the MMSE. Progression of the disease lasts 8 to 10 years on average but can be as brief as 2 years or as long as 22 years, depending on the individual. The course of a patient's condition is the best predictor of his or her future decline.

In the early stage, memory impairment predominates and personality changes may occur in some patients. At this early stage, which lasts approximately 3 to 4 years, activities of daily living (ADL) are not usually impaired, but instrumental activities of daily living (IADL) such as shopping, keeping up with bills, cooking, and driving may be impaired. In later stages, patients develop deficits in language (aphasia) and in recognizing people, places, and situations (agnosia) and deteriorate in their ability to do everyday activities. Eventually, the impairment in memory, language, perception, and coordination worsens to the point that the patient becomes fully dependent on others for basic ADL such as bathing, dressing, eating, and mobility.

More than 90% of Alzheimer patients develop noncognitive psychiatric symptoms, including depression, delusions, hallucinations, sleep disturbance, aggression, and agitation, all of which are common and often require either pharmacologic or behavioral intervention or both.

Noncognitive neurologic symptoms also develop in the later stages of AD, including hyperreflexia, apraxic gait, and frontal release signs (grasp and snout reflexes). Some patients may develop parkinsonian symptoms. As motor symptoms worsen in the very late stages, patients may become immobile and incontinent. They also may become unable to chew or swallow.

Dementia with Lewy bodies. The clinical triad of fluctuating cognitive impairment, persistent hallucinosis, and parkinsonism characterizes dementia with Lewy bodies (DLB). Table 10-11 lists the DLB criteria used by the Newcastle-Upon-Tyne group in England.

The population prevalence of DLB has been controversial because different groups have estimated that 5% to 25% of all dementia is due to this entity. Between 5% and 18% of all elderly patients coming to autopsy suffer from Lewy body disease. The mean age at onset is 75 years, with a slight male excess. There is wide variety in the duration of illness, with a mean of 3.5 years.

The Lewy body, an intracellular inclusion body, is the hallmark of DLB. Unlike Parkinson disease (PD), the Lewy bodies in DLB are present outside the substantia nigra as well. Dense presence of Lewy bodies in the brain stem, in the entorhinal cortex, and in other areas of the temporal lobes has been demonstrated. This presence parallels neuronal loss in these areas. Autopsy studies have shown that in a substantial proportion of DLB cases, neuritic plaques and neurofibrillary tangles of AD are present as well. The overlap

---

TABLE 10-11 Criteria for Dementia of Lewy Body Disease

A. Fluctuating cognitive impairment

   1. Memory and one other area affected

   2. Episodic confusion followed by lucid intervals

B. One of the following

   1. Visual or auditory hallucinations, paranoid delusions

   2. Mild extrapyramidal symptoms, neuroleptic sensitivity, unexplained falls, transient clouding, or loss of consciousness

C. A and B sustained over a period of months

D. No other cause after workup

E. No evidence of vascular dementia

Source: McKeith IG, Perry RH, Fairbairn AF, Perry EK. Operational criteria for SDLT. *Psychol Med.* 1992;22:911-922.

between AD and DLB appears to be substantial, and the nosological relationship between them remains to be elucidated.

Shifting levels of attention and alertness that occur in 50% to 75% of the patients make characterization of cognitive deficits in DLB difficult. Attentional deficits and visuospatial dysfunction are generally prominent. Rarely, nonepileptic "unresponsive spells" may occur and complicate the clinical picture. Cognitive impairment may occur as a progressive deterioration or as an episodic confusional state resembling intermittent delirium. In general, DLB patients perform better than those with AD on tests of verbal recall but do worse on tests of copying and drawing.

The most prominent noncognitive psychiatric symptom is visual hallucinations, present in up to 80% of patients. This typically coexists with perceptual difficulties and misidentification. Other psychotic symptoms such as auditory hallucinations and paranoid delusions are also often seen. Up to 40% of patients with DLB suffer from depression. Parkinsonian symptoms are present in up to 80% of DLB patients. Typical symptoms are bradykinesia and rigidity. Tremor is uncommon. Frequent falls are generally due to orthostatic change.

Managing psychosis and behavioral disturbances is complicated by sensitivity to neuroleptic medication among DLB patients. Use of neuroleptic medications could result in prolonged delirium and even death. Yet low doses of quetiapine and clozapine have been effective anecdotally in managing psychosis and agitation in DLB patients. Reduction of cholinergic activity has been also associated with poor performance in cognitive testing and hallucination. Thus, cholinergic enhancers such as cholinesterase inhibitors might be useful in improving both cognitive and noncognitive functions.

Frontotemporal dementia. Frontotemporal dementia (FTD) refers to a group of dementias that predominantly affect the frontal and temporal lobes. Table 10-12 lists

---

TABLE 10-12 Criteria for Frontotemporal Dementia

A. Progressive personality change and breakdown in social conduct

    1. Restless, distractible, disinhibited, or pathetic, slowed, amotivated

    2. Hypochondriasis with bizarre complaints

    3. Stereotyped behavior

    4. Echolalia and perseveration

    5. Variable memory disturbance

B. Normal neurologic examination

    1. May have frontal release signs

C. Supportive features

    1. Family history of dementia

    2. Reduced frontal lobe blood on functional imaging

    3. Normal EEG

Source: Hooten RM, Lyketsos CG. Fronto-temporal dementia: a clinicopathological review of four post-mortem studies. *J Neuropsychiatry Clin Neurosci*. 1996;8:10-19.

diagnostic criteria for FTD. Many different names that have been associated with this entity, including Pick disease, lobar atrophy, frontal lobe dementia, and frontal lobe degeneration.

It is unclear what the population prevalence is for FTD, but autopsy studies report that 3% of all patients with dementia and 10% of patients with dementia who die before age 70 have findings consistent with FTD. Substantial familial aggregation of FTD in different parts of the world have been reported, particularly linked to chromosome 17. The average age of onset is 54 and average duration of disease is 7 years; onset occurs earlier and the progression is faster than in AD.

Various subtypes exist, but in general neuronal loss, astrocytosis, and vacuolization of the superficial layers of the frontal and temporal cortices are seen. In some cases, pathological findings of intranuclear inclusion called Pick bodies are present in the dying neurons and diagnosis of Pick disease would be more specific than FTD. The etiology of Pick bodies is unknown.

Changes in personality, executive functions, and behavior are the earliest symptoms. Apathy, disinhibition, intrusiveness, explosiveness, irritability, and aggression are also commonly seen. Dysphasia occurs early because the temporal lobe is affected. Depression, delusions, and hallucinations can be seen but are less frequent than in other comparable dementias. Motor functions such as gait disorders, rigidity, and bradykinesia develop later in the illness.

Case Vignette

Mr Bruce, a 56-year-old college professor with well-controlled high blood pressure, comes to see his primary care physician, Dr Nelson, at the urging of his wife "because he has turned into a lump around the house, I think he is depressed." Mr Bruce has been eating and sleeping more than usual during the previous 3 months, and although his energy level is adequate, he reports having little motivation to prepare for class, hold office hours, talk to colleagues, or go out socially. He denies difficulty concentrating, and his MMSE score is 29/30. Chemistry screening panel, complete blood count, and a thyroid-stimulating hormone are all normal. A selective serotonin uptake inhibitor (SSRI) is prescribed, but when Mr Bruce returns a month later, there has been no change despite his taking the antidepressant. Dr Nelson prescribes a different SSRI for a month. This too fails to affect his depressive symptoms, and his wife notes that he has begun to sing childhood songs to himself in public and make sexually suggestive comments to her friends, both highly atypical behaviors for this normally straitlaced man; he has no other symptoms suggestive of mania. A general neurologic examination is normal, and his MMSE remains 29/30. A computerized tomography (CT) scan of his head reveals minimal atrophy, most prominently in the frontal lobes. Neuropsychological assessment reveals slightly diminished performance on memory tasks but prominent deficits on tests of executive (frontal lobe) functioning. Frontotemporal dementia is suspected, and he is referred to a neuropsychiatrist for a consultation, who concurs with the diagnosis. Over the next 6 months Mr Bruce begins to demonstrate further disinhibited behavior along with clear-cut memory problems and his self-care begins to decline.

Prion dementias. Two forms of the prion dementia are known. Creutzfeldt-Jakob disease (CJD) (rapidly progressive type) is a sporadic, nonfamilial form of dementia that has received much attention lately due to recent publicity related to mad cow disease. CJD could be due either to spontaneous mutation of the prion protein or to infection with mutated prion protein. There are also familial forms of CJD. A rare form of prion dementia is the Gerstmann-Straussler-Scheinker (GSS) syndrome (slowly progressive type), which follows an autosomal dominant pattern of transmission. Both forms of dementia are extremely rare. CJD affects approximately one person per million. GSS syndrome is even rarer, and the population prevalence is unknown.

Prion proteins are normal brain proteins that are encoded by a gene on chromosome 20. Spontaneous alteration of the normal form of the prion protein leads to conformational changes where alpha helix (soluble) protein formation is converted to beta sheets (insoluble). Deposits of the beta sheet form of the prion protein lead to plaque formation. Subsequently, neuronal injury and death with formation of characteristic spongiform patterns occur in CJD. Specific mutations in the human prion protein, which makes the protein more vulnerable to spontaneous formation of beta sheets, has been implicated in GSS syndrome.

CJD generally has a rapid onset and course, leading to death within 1 to 2 years. Early symptoms include executive dysfunction, aphasia, amnesia, and apraxia. Motor symptoms such as myoclonus, spasticity, and ataxia tend to occur concurrently. The GSS syndrome runs a slower course, at times over many years, but symptoms are identical. Noncognitive psychiatric disorders such as depression, mania, delusions, and hallucinations are often associated with both forms, but their prevalence is not known.

Subcortical or Mixed-Pattern Dementia

Dementia due to Parkinson disease. Parkinson disease (PD) is a degenerative neurologic illness characterized by bradykinesia, resting tremor, pill-rolling tremor, masklike faces, cogwheel rigidity, and shuffling gait. More than one third of patients with PD become demented and an additional 50% may have mild cognitive impairment.

PD affects about 1 per 1000 in the population. This prevalence is age dependent, rising from approximately 0.5 per 1000 at age 60 to approximately 1.3 per 1000 at age 75. Onset of PD after age 60 is more likely to lead to dementia. Treatment-resistant PD is also a risk factor for developing dementia.

The etiology of PD is unknown in most cases. A small percentage of cases are familial. Loss of dopamine-producing cells in the substantia nigra is the basic pathological change in PD. The degree of dopamine loss correlates with the degree of the motor symptoms. In dementia of PD, pathological findings of AD and PD are seen, but the exact relationship between them is not known. Also, Lewy bodies are found in nucleus basalis, locus coeruleus, the raphe nuclei, and the cortex and contribute to the development of dementia.

The cognitive symptoms due to dementia of PD follow a subcortical pattern. Patients have difficulty spontaneously recalling information but can pick the correct response when given a right and wrong choice. Executive function, attention, and speed of thought process are impaired as patients lose the ability to coordinate thoughts.

As many as 60% of patients with PD develop depression. Also, up to 30% of PD patients experience visual hallucinations. Paranoid or persecutory delusions are also frequent, and most are complications of pharmacotherapy for PD with dopaminergic agents such as bromocriptine mesylate, amantidine hydrochloride, or levodopa.

Dementia due to Huntington disease. Huntington disease (HD) is an autosomal dominant familial disease with complete penetrance, characterized by choreiform motor disorder, mood disorder, and dementia. An offspring of a parent with HD has a 50% chance of inheriting the condition.

The population prevalence is 1 per 10,000 live births. The average onset of the clinical symptoms is the late 30s to early 40s. The average patient lives approximately 10 years after onset of symptoms.

Specific mutation (expansion of CAG triplet repeat) in a gene located on the short arm of chromosome 4 causes HD. Even in preclinical patients who carry the mutant gene, progressive shrinkage of the caudate nucleus is seen bilaterally.

The defining symptoms of HD are its motor symptoms: impairment of voluntary movement leading to poor coordination of fine motor skills and dyskinesia in the form of choreic, brief, dancelike, nonrepetitive, involuntary, and athetoid movements of the face, limbs, and trunk. The dementia due to HD is initially characterized by a subcortical pattern: apathy, slow speed of thought-processing, executive function impairment, and attention deficits. Then, more global impairments such as amnesia, aphasia, agnosia, and apraxia are seen.

Depression is common in up to one third of HD patients and occasionally presents as the initial symptom. Relatively high rates of mania, up to 10%, are seen. Other noncognitive symptoms such as irritability, explosiveness, and agitation are common. Delusions, hallucinations, and personality disturbance occur in up to 10% of HD patients. These noncognitive symptoms tend to worsen with progression of the disease.

Vascular dementia. Vascular dementia is caused by either vascular insufficiency to deep brain areas leading to degeneration of subcortical white matter or small- and/or large-vessel thromboembolic events in the brain. The diagnostic criteria of the National Institute for Neurologic Disorders and Stroke–Association International pour la recherdie et l'Enseignmenment en Neurosciences (NINDS-AIREN) for vascular dementia are listed in Table 10-13.

Vascular dementia accounts for 15% to 30% of all dementias. As many as 10% of new stroke patients suffer from dementia in 6 months, and one third of patients develop dementia in 4 years. The same risk factors for stroke, such as hypertension, hypercholesterolemia, and diabetes, increase likelihood of developing dementia after stroke.

Vascular dementia is a distinct form of dementia, although some have questioned whether it is an entity at all because of its heterogeneity. There is a large overlap between vascular dementia and AD. In fact, pathological diagnosis usually fails to confirm the clinical diagnosis: Dementia that is clinically diagnosed as vascular dementia is often diagnosed at autopsy as AD or mixed AD and vascular dementia. Nevertheless, in the purer form of vascular dementia cognitive impairment is presumed to be caused by tissue injury from ischemia with diverse pathologic patterns ranging from complete cortical death to mild subcortical hypoperfusion. In general, the more brain tissue affected, the greater the likelihood and severity of vascular dementia. There are two subtypes of vascular dementia. The first is primarily due to long-standing vascular insufficiency in deep brain areas leading to degeneration of the subcortical white matter. Binswanger disease is the classic example of this subtype, and brain imaging demonstrates extensive white matter change. Memory disturbance, executive dysfunction, apathy, and amotivation are prominent symptoms. The other subtype is related to stroke. Thrombotic or embolic strokes that cause perfusion defect in large or small cerebral blood vessels cause neuronal death and associated symptoms. The pattern of symptoms depends on the location of

TABLE 10-13 Criteria for Vascular Disease Causing Dementia

A. Dementia

   1. Decline by examination and objective testing

   2. Deficits in memory plus two other areas of cognition

   3. Functional impairment

B. Cerebrovascular disease by history, examination, or imaging

C. A relationship between A and B

   1. Dementia onset within 3 months of cerebrovascular accident

   2. Cognitive change is stepwise, abrupt, or fluctuating

   3. Strokes that affect critical areas

D. Supportive features

   1. Early presence of gait disturbance

   2. Early presence of urinary frequency or incontinence

   3. Typical neurologic examination findings

   4. Consciousness intact

Source: Romain GC, Tatemichi TK, Erkinjuntti T, et al. Vascular dementia: diagnostic criteria for research studies, report of the NINDS-AIREN international workshop. *Neurol.* 1993;43:250-259.

injury. Common symptoms include amnesia, receptive or expressive aphasia, constructional or other types of apraxia, and dysfunctions associated with injury of the frontal lobes, including executive disturbance.

Vascular dementia progresses classically in a step-wise pattern, but a slow, progressive course as in AD is not uncommon. The likelihood of vascular dementia increases with advanced age, which also increases the likelihood that pathological findings of both vascular disease and AD would be found at autopsy. In fact, vascular dementia frequently resembles AD in its clinical course and pathological findings. There is no clinical gold standard for the clinical distinction between AD and vascular dementia. Strong association between vascular risk factors and AD suggests a potential causal relationship between them, but the true direction of causality has not been determined.

Several noncognitive psychiatric symptoms are associated with vascular dementia. The most prominent is depression in 50% to 60% of patients, which has been shown to increase morbidity and mortality among poststroke patients. Delusions and hallucinations are often seen in patients with vascular dementia, particularly those with strokes of the nondominant hemisphere. Apathy, psychomotor retardation, and disinterest have been associated with vascular dementia. Personality change is also common.

Controlling the risk factors for cerebrovascular disease reduces the incidence and progression of vascular dementia. Underlying illness such as diabetes, hypertension, and hypercholesteremia should be treated. Antihypertensives, statins, and anticoagulation medications are beneficial if indicated. For significant carotid artery stenosis, carotid enarterectomy should be considered to both prevent future strokes and prevent the chronic cerebral ischemia that lead to vascular dementia. Given the general resemblance of course and comorbidity with AD, anticholinesterase treatment should be also considered.

Other dementias. Table 10-7 lists other rare forms of dementia such as normopressure hydrocephalus (with triad of symptoms: gait apraxia, subcortical dementia, and incontinence), supranuclear palsy, Wilson disease, and HIV dementia.

MANAGEMENT OF DEMENTIAS

Dementias are chronic diseases with protracted courses, substantial morbidity, complicated presentations, and serious effects on families and caregivers. Once dementia is diagnosed and the etiology determined with reasonable certainty, a comprehensive treatment plan should be developed.

Ideally, a multidisciplinary team that includes the patient's primary care physician, a specialist (geriatrician, psychiatrist, or neurologist) if needed, as well as a social worker, occupational therapist, and nurse should develop a consensual, comprehensive treatment plan that can be followed and adapted over the years of treatment. The diagnosis, prognosis, and treatment plan must be communicated to the family in a clear, concise manner, preferably at a family conference. Written family guidelines and effective information pamphlets are helpful and widely available through the local Alzheimer's Association.

The patient should be involved in the treatment plan at the early stage of dementia because this may be neither practical nor possible in the later stage. Lack of awareness of cognitive deficits is a common symptom of dementia, and dementia patients without insight into their illness may resist necessary treatment. Also, cognitive impairment interferes with higher processing, such as judgment. There is no evidence that confrontation with patients who lack insight about their condition is useful. Instead, gentle persuasion with help from a trusted caregiver such as a spouse or child is preferred in implementing a treatment plan.

The goals of the treatment plan are listed in Table 10-14. To accomplish these goals, consider the four pillars of dementia care (Table 10-15), which serve as the foundation of treatment planning for all dementia patients.

TABLE 10-14 Goals of Treatment for Dementia Patients
1. Disease treatment (stabilization)
2. Resolution (or improvement) of cognitive symptomatology
3. Resolution of noncognitive symptomatology (depression, psychosis, agitation, etc)
4. Adequate provision for patient's needs and wants
5. A future with dignity and respect
6. Effective adaptation to stressors and other environmental changes
7. Good general health and physical well-being
8. Effective coping and adaptation amongst family members and other caregivers

TABLE 10-15 The Four Pillars of Complete Dementia Care
A. Supportive care for the patient
B. Supportive care for the family/caregiver
C. Disease treatment
D. Symptom treatment
1. Cognitive symptoms
2. Mental and behavioral symptoms

Supportive Care for the Patient

There is no cure in the treatment of dementia. More often than not, nonpharmacologic interventions are more important than pharmacologic interventions.

Safety and level of care evaluations. The risks of living at home increase for the AD patient as the dementia progresses. Common risks are medication misuse, wandering, falls, and accidents. An occupational therapist should assess the level of care necessary to ensure independent living and safety. The evaluating physician should make recommendations for supervision, companion, daycare, or placement in an assisted living facility to ensure the patient's safety in conjunction with the occupational therapy evaluation.

Driving is a major concern in patients with dementia. One third of all seniors who die during motor vehicle accidents have AD, and drivers with cognitive impairment present public risks to all. Eventually, all patients with progressive dementia must stop driving. Local departments of motor vehicles offer driving evaluations for safety. Also, some local hospitals offer driving evaluations, which may be less threatening to dementia patients.

Decision-making capacity. Because all dementia patients lose certain aspects of capacity, they should be evaluated for their decision-making ability. Designation of decision-making agents is important to ensure that financial and medical decisions are made according to the patient's wishes. By working closely with the patient's family and counseling them, the primary care physician can ensure the smooth transfer of decision-making responsibility from the patient to a surrogate.

Wills, medical and financial powers of attorney, and advance directives must be addressed during the early stage of dementia to ensure that the patient's wishes are respected. In rarer cases, guardianship may be necessary.

Other essential aspects of supportive care. Insight into their impairment is intact among one third of AD patients. The need to discuss their diagnosis and counsel them in a compassionate manner cannot be overemphasized. Their input along with that of their family should be incorporated in the treatment plan.

Local senior centers and adult daycare programs offer structure to daily life and provide respite for the care provider. Also, some studies have shown that cognitively stimulating activities and regular physical exercise are beneficial in delaying the onset or progression of AD. Often, local senior and adult daycare centers offer such programs.

Medical comorbidity is a serious problem for patients with dementia and is a major cause of morbidity and death. Small metabolic perturbation or even minor surgery can lead to functional decline or behavioral exacerbation. On the average, AD outpatients take four other medications for comorbid medical conditions. Because patients with dementia are less likely to articulate their somatic symptoms, meticulous medical care and close communication with the caregiver are important.

Supportive Care for the Caregiver

AD creates unique problems for the patient's family, especially for the primary caregiver. Coping with the patient's ongoing need for care is made more difficult by the progressive deterioration caused by the disease. Caregivers often feel alone and lost because their lifestyle and social relationships have been affected. Referring caregivers to local support or advocacy groups such as the Alzheimer's Association can be very reassuring. Sometimes the caregiver may suffer from a psychiatric disorder and need evaluation and treatment. Referral should be made when appropriate.

All caregivers should be educated about the diagnosis and symptoms of dementia and dementia care and its benefits through interaction with the clinician and a support group such as those run by the local Alzheimer's Association. Reading materials such as the *36 Hour Day* (Mace and Rabins, 1999) and brochures are a good source of education and support for families stricken by the diagnosis of dementia. A recent study showed an 18-month delay in institutionalization when caregivers received adequate counseling, education, and support. (See Chapter 18 for additional information on providing caregivers with strategies for managing the behavioral and psychological symptoms of dementia.)

Regardless of the strength in relationships, no caregiver can provide 24-hour supervision, 7 days a week to a patient with dementia. Caregivers need respite, a critical factor in preventing institutionalization. As the disease progresses, senior centers, adult daycare programs, and hired aides provide caregivers with the necessary respite.

Disease Treatment

Disease treatment is targeted at the very etiology or process of progression in dementia. There is no known cure for dementia, but several epidemiological studies have suggested that pharmacologic agents may delay either onset or progression of AD.

Management of the vascular process is important in managing the progress of the disease. Treatment of hypertension, hypercholesterolemia, and diabetes may delay cognitive decline, based on population studies. Treatment of hypertension has been associated with a 32% to 41% decline in two population studies. Also, a total serum cholesterol level below 200 has been associated with slower cognitive decline in AD in observational studies. Active pharmacologic intervention for vascular disease risk factor is highly recommended.

Vitamin E, an antioxidant, may delay cognitive decline; one randomized trial showed an approximately 6-month delay to the next level of care. Previous epidemiological studies have suggested that nonsteroidal anti-inflammatory drugs, antihyperlipidemic agents (ie, HMG-CoA reductase inhibitors), or hormone replacement might have a role in delaying the onset of cognitive decline among the elderly. Indeed, there are several ongoing double-blind placebo trials for these agents. However, due to concerns about risk and uncertainty about dosing, they are not currently recommended for treating AD.

Symptom Treatment

Symptom treatment is targeted at the associated symptoms of dementia such as cognitive decline, depression, psychosis, agitation, and other psychiatric symptoms. The goal of symptom treatment is not to stop the disease process but to relieve the associated symptoms in order to comfort both the patient and the care provider and to improve their life quality.

Cognitive enhancers. The most widely used strategy in managing cognitive symptoms in AD is cholinesterase inhibition. Its efficacy in other forms of dementia such as dementia of Lewy body disease, mixed Alzheimer dementia with the vascular component, and vascular dementia is probable. However, the role of cholinesterase inhibitor (CI) in either stabilizing or delaying the progression of dementia is very controversial. Few studies are available for other forms of dementia.

- Cholinesterase inhibition: Currently, the four CIs approved for use in the United States are tacrine hydrochloride, donepezil hydrochloride, rivastigmine tartrate, and galantamine hydrobromide. All inhibit acetylcholinesterase and leave more acetylcholine in the synaptic cleft, which increases activity in remaining neurons. They do not inhibit cell loss, but modest improvements in cognitive performance in one third of patients have been demonstrated. Also, they may improve functional ADLs and delay placement in the nursing home.
- Tacrine hydrochloride (Cognex): Tacrine hydrochloride was the first CI approved for indication of AD in the United States. Its nonselective binding of both peripheral and central cholinesterase causes frequent side effects such as gastrointestinal (GI) upset, exacerbation of chronic obstructive pulmonary disease, bradycardia, and liver enzyme elevation. Tacrine hydrochloride has a short half-life of 4 to 6 hours, which requires frequent dosing. This drug is rarely used.
- Donepezil hydrochloride (Aricept): Donepezil hydrochloride is a reversible, noncompetitive CI that binds selectively to block acetylcholinesterase and may cause fewer peripheral side effects. A long half-life of 70 hours allows daily dosing. Double-blind placebo trials have shown modest clinical benefits in cognition and possible delay in loss of ADLs and placement in a nursing home. The starting dose is 5 mg; an increase to 10 mg after 6 to 8 weeks is recommended if there is no response. Mild GI side effects are noted. The trial should be at least 3 months, at which point the clinician and family should decide if benefits outweigh costs.
- Rivastigmine tartrate (Exelon): Rivastigmine tartrate is also a reversible, noncompetitive CI that has similar efficacy in treating cognitive symptoms. Its shorter half-life means twice-a-day dosing. More frequent GI side effects on therapeutic dosing of 6 to 12 mg a day has been noted. However, its binding on butyl cholinesterase may be beneficial in delaying the progression of AD.
- Galantamine hydrobromide (Reminyl): Galantamine hydrobromide is another noncompetitive CI that has similar efficacy in treating cognitive symptoms compared to other CIs. It does have additional effects in modulating nicotinic receptors, which may affect progression of AD. The starting dose, 4 mg twice a day, is titrated up to 8 to 12 mg twice a day, depending on efficacy and tolerability. Mild GI side effects are comparable to those with donepezil hydrochloride.

Precursor loading. Loading patients with choline and lecithin has not been shown to be effective.

Selective postsynaptic cholinergic agonist. Oral xanomeline has improved cognition and reduced behavioral abnormalities in patients with mild to moderate AD. However, excess peripheral side effects (cardiovascular and GI symptoms) led to discontinuation of its development. Whether the potentially better tolerated transdermal form of xanomeline will offer any significant advantages over conventional therapy (eg, acetylcholinesterase inhibitors) remains to be determined.

Pharmacologic treatment for noncognitive psychiatric symptoms. Some of the more common noncognitive psychiatric symptoms can be treated as follows:

- *Depression:* Depressive symptomatology is relatively common in dementia, affecting as many as 25% to 30% of patients. It may also lead to earlier institutionalization and death, aside from mental suffering. The SSRIs are thought to be the first line followed by a trial of agents with dual effects on the serotonin and norepinephrine transporters such as venlafaxine hydrochloride or nefazodone hydrochloride.
- *Delusions and hallucinations:* Few randomized controlled trial studies are available, but people with these conditions have benefited from low-dose neuroleptic medication. The newer, atypical neuroleptic agents such as risperidone and olanzapine have less side-effect potential and are the first line before trial of other agents.
- *Problem behaviors such as agitation and aggression:* The most common etiologies for such behaviors include medical illnesses (eg, urinary tract infection, pneumonia), delirium, environmental stressors, psychiatric disorders, and the underlying dementia. If no underlying etiology beside dementia is apparent, a trial of low-dose risperidone (0.25 to 1 mg) or olanzapine (2.5 to 5 mg) could help. Other agents such as mood stabilizers (eg, divalproex sodium [Depakote] and carbamazepine [Tegretol]) have been helpful. The role of cholinesterase inhibitors in problem behavior is unclear but may also be considered.

SUMMARY

Delirium, minimal cognitive impairment, and dementia are cognitive disorders that are frequently encountered in a primary care setting. Delirium is a serious illness that afflicts those who are elderly, suffer from brain disease, or are taking multiple medications. Early diagnosis and identification of all contributing causes of delirium will avoid potentially fatal outcome for the patient. Mild cognitive impairment and dementia put a tremendous burden on the patient, family, health system, and society. The total costs of care for dementia patients in the United States were calculated to be $76 billion annually in the late 1990s. Although effective prevention strategy and cure for dementia are not available, a comprehensive care plan that involves both the patient and the family improves the quality of life for patients and their families.

ADDITIONAL READINGS

American Psychiatric Association. Practice guideline for the treatment of patients with Alzheimer disease and other dementias of later life. *Am J Psychiatry.* 1997;154:5, Suppl:1-39.

American Psychiatric Association. *Practice Guidelines for the Treatment of Patients with Delirium.* Washington, DC: American Psychiatric Association; 1999.

Burns A, Levy R. *Dementia*. London, England: Chapman and Hall Medical; 1994.

Folstein MF, Folstein SE, McHugh PR. "Mini-mental state." A practical method for grading the cognitive state of patients for the clinician. *J Psychiatr Res*. 1975;12:189-198.

Hooten RM, Lyketsos CG. Fronto-temporal dementia: a clinicopathological review of four post-mortem studies. *J Neuropsychiatry Clin Neurosci*. 1996;8:10-19.

Inouye SK, van Dyck CH, Alessi CA, et al. Clarifying confusion: The Confusion Assessment Method (a new method for detection of delirium). *Ann Intern Med*. 1990;113:941-948.

Inouye SK. Prevention of delirium in hospitalised older patients: risk factors and targeted intervention strategies. *Ann Med*. 2000;32:257-263.

Lishman WA. *Organic Psychiatry*. Oxford, England: Blackwell Scientific; 1996.

Mace N, Rabins P. *The 36-Hour Day*. 3rd ed. Baltimore, Md: The Johns Hopkins University Press; 1999.

McKeith IG, Perry RH, Fairbairn AF, Perry EK. Operational criteria for SDLT. *Psychol Med*. 1992;22:911-922.

McKhann G, Drachman D, Fostein MF, Katzman R, Price D, Stadlan E. Clinical diagnosis of Alzheimer's disease: report of the National Institute Neurologic and Communicative Disorders and Stroke/Alzheimer's Disease Related Disorders Association workgroup under the auspices of DHHS task force on Alzheimer's disease. *Neurol*. 1984;34:939-944.

Mittelman MS, Epstein C, Pierzchala A. *Counseling the Alzheimer's Caregiver*. Chicago, Ill: AMA Press; 2003.

Petersen RC, Doody R, Kurz A, Mohs RC, et al. Current concepts in mild cognitive impairment. *Arch Neurol*. 2001;58(12):1985-1992.

Rabins P, Lyketsos CG, Steele CD. *Practical Dementia Care*. New York, NY: Oxford University Press; 1999.

Romain GC, Tatemichi TK, Erkinjuntti T, et al. Vascular dementia: diagnostic criteria for research studies, report of the NINDS-AIREN international workshop. *Neurol*. 1993;43:250-259.

Chapter **11**

Sleep Disorders

Ravi T. Chandran, MD
Bharat Jain, MD

In the past decade, disorders of sleep and wakefulness have become increasingly recognized as pervasive throughout society. The National Commission on Sleep Disorders (1992) reported that more than 40 million Americans suffer from sleep-wake disorders. Approximately 37% of working adults complain of excessive daytime somnolence (EDS) that disrupts their daytime functioning. Sleep disturbances have a close association with mental illness: 40% of patients with insomnia and 45% of patients with hypersomnia have an underlying psychiatric disorder.

Despite a high prevalence of sleep disorders with associated morbidity, there is limited awareness among health care providers and the public of these disorders. Nearly two thirds of patients have not been asked by their physician if they have sleep problems. It was unknown until recently that specific causes and treatments for sleep complaints were present and that only 33% to 50% of the diagnosed patients were treated. In addition, only one in five individuals reports a sleep problem to his or her physician. Primary care physicians must play an active role in recognizing, treating, and educating patients with sleep disorders. Table 11-1 lists some of the abbreviations related to sleep disorders that are used in this chapter.

TABLE 11-1 Abbreviations Commonly Used in This Chapter

AASM	American Association of Sleep Medicine
CPAP	Continuous positive airway pressure
DIMS	Disorders of initiating and maintaining sleep
EDS	Excess daytime somnolence
MSLT	Multiple sleep latency test
OSAS	Obstructive sleep apnea syndrome
PLMS	Periodic leg movements of sleep
PSG	Polysomnogram
REM	Rapid eye movement
REMSBD	Rapid eye movement sleep behavior disorder
RLS	Restless legs syndrome
SDC	Sleep disorders center

SLEEP PHYSIOLOGY AND COMMON SLEEP PROBLEMS

Awareness about the importance of sleep and its effect on the human organism is growing. Adult humans spend approximately one third of their lives sleeping, yet we do not have a clear understanding of the functions of sleep. We do, however, know that almost every system in the body undergoes changes during sleep. It is important to be aware of the various stages of sleep and the changes that occur during sleep to understand how they may affect the various sleep disorders.

Basic Sleep Physiology

In healthy adults sleep and wakefulness normally alternate in two major periods, with a range of 4 to 12 hours of nocturnal sleep. There are significant differences in how much sleep is required for a person to feel alert and refreshed throughout the day. Sleep itself is organized in a regular pattern of brain activation with rapid eye movement (REM) sleep and relative quiescence (nonrapid eye movement, NREM) sleep. NREM sleep is divided into four stages. As sleep progresses from "lighter" stage 1 through "deeper" stage 4, the electroencephalogram (EEG) becomes more synchronized (ie, lower frequency, higher amplitude) and the arousal threshold increases.

The organization of sleep throughout the night is referred to as the *sleep architecture.* Sleep architecture of an adult is characterized by short sleep latency and high sleep efficiency (the ratio of total sleep time to total time in bed). NREM and REM sleep alternate in cycles of about 90 to 100 minutes. The bulk of the slow-wave sleep (stages 3 and 4) occurs in the first few hours of the night. REM sleep cycles every 90 to 100 minutes, with the REM periods becoming progressively longer as the night progresses.

Age is a powerful determinant of a person's sleep physiology. Total sleep time drops from a high of 17 to 18 hours in a neonate to about 6.5 hours in old age. Sleep state also changes dramatically with increasing age. A newborn spends about 50% of total sleep time in the REM state; this decreases and stabilizes at about 20% after puberty and throughout adulthood. Slow-wave sleep, which is associated with growth hormone secretion, decreases steadily from childhood to old age. Finally, the transition from wake to sleep (stage 1 sleep) increases in the elderly and sleep efficiency declines. Thus, even in a healthy elderly person, sleep is lighter and less robust.

Common Sleep Problems

The primary care physician's sleep evaluation should include the following information:

- *Current sleep-wake schedule*: Patients should be asked about the occurrence of physical or emotional events during sleep, particulars of the physical environment for sleep, and daytime sequelae of sleep loss or disturbance.
- *Psychiatric history*: Because many sleep disorders have a psychiatric component, a thorough psychiatric history should always be taken before initiating treatment. The major psychiatric conditions associated with disturbances in sleep or wakefulness must be carefully diagnosed. These include depression, dysthymia, mania, dementia, schizophrenia, anxiety disorders, and alcoholism and drug abuse. Standardized measures of mood and psychological functioning can be used to examine the sleep disorder patient. These include the Minnesota Multiphasic Personality Inventory and the Beck Depression Inventory.
- *Comprehensive medical history*: Because sleep disorders may be a sign of disease in the liver, heart, brain, kidney, or endocrine systems, attention should be directed to any signs of major systemic illness. Furthermore, sleep may exacerbate preexisting medical conditions such as seizure disorders, heart and lung disorders, and migraine headaches.

Sleep disorders medicine has not reached the point where a diagnosis is based on the pathophysiological mechanisms. Symptoms still form the basis of diagnostic nomenclature. Typically, the complaints will fall into three broad areas:

- *Insomnia:* "Doctor, I cannot sleep."
- *Hypersomnia:* "Doctor, I sleep too much."
- *Parasomnia:* "Doctor, strange things happen to me at night."

Because patients rarely present with sleep complaints, an exploration of sleep-wake patterns is an important component of any general review of systems. A discussion with the bed partner can help identify primary snoring, sleep apnea, periodic leg movements of sleep (PLMS), and any abnormal behavior during sleep. The following four questions will help screen for sleep disorders:

- *Disorder of initiating and maintenance of sleep*: Do you have trouble sleeping, either falling/staying asleep or getting enough sleep?
- *Disorder of EDS*: Do you feel excessively sleepy when engaged in usual daytime activities or when trying not to fall asleep?
- *Sleep-associated breathing disorder*: Do you snore or note any abnormalities in breathing during sleep?
- *Periodic leg movements of sleep or parasomnia*: Does your bed partner notice any unusual movements during sleep?

This symptom-based approach does not separate true disorders of sleep from other medical conditions that affect sleep, resulting in disorders with similar symptoms. For example, obstructive sleep apnea syndrome (OSAS) is not a true sleep disorder but a disorder of respiratory-related physiology that causes EDS. For diagnostic coding purposes, one would use the classification by the American Association of Sleep Medicine (AASM), which has been incorporated into the *Diagnostic and Statistical Manual of Mental Disorders*, fourth edition (DSM-IV), and the International Classification of Diseases (ICD-9-CM). In 1990, the widely used International Classification of Sleep Disorders (ICSD) was produced by the AASM. The ICSD consists of four major categories: the *dyssomnias*, which include DIMS, disorders of EDS, and the circadian rhythm sleep disorders, which are also discussed in this chapter; the *parasomnias*, which are disorders that do not primarily cause a complaint of insomnia or EDS; *disorders associated with medical or psychiatric disorders*; and the *proposed sleep disorders*, which are disorders for which there is insufficient information to confirm as a sleep disorder. This chapter summarizes the clinical descriptions of dyssomnias, parasomnias, and disorders. For each disorder, issues pertinent to differential diagnosis, management in the primary care setting, and indications for referral to a sleep disorders center are discussed.

Evaluation at a Sleep Disorders Center

Referral for expert evaluation and management is recommended for many of the problems discussed in this chapter. Referral is made to physicians who are expert in managing sleep disorders or to a sleep disorder center (SDC) accredited by AASM.

When a patient is evaluated at an SDC, the sleep problem is carefully reviewed and, if indicated, a polysomnogram (PSG) followed by a multiple sleep latency test (MSLT) is performed. The all-night PSG involves noninvasive simultaneous measurement of brain activity, eye movements, submental and anterior tibialis muscle activity, respiratory airflow and effort, cardiac rhythm, and blood oxygen saturation. Esophageal pressure and pH monitoring and penile tumescence (see Chapter 12) may be performed. An MSLT involves taking four to five 20-minute naps in the daytime to objectively assess EDS. The MSLT is usually scheduled for the day after the overnight PSG. The usual schedule for the patient in the sleep lab would be 8:30 PM to 7:00 AM for the PSG and 8:00 AM to 4:30 PM for the MSLT. A PSG along with an MSLT is considered for any patient with EDS and no underlying cause or when the history suggests sleep apnea, PLMS, or narcolepsy.

The maintenance of wakefulness test (MWT) was developed to clinically assess a patient's ability to maintain wakefulness under soporific conditions. Results from an MWT can be used to determine if the patient's ability to maintain wakefulness falls outside of the normal range. This is of particular value for determining efficacy of treatment. An MWT is often performed for medico-legal reasons related to licensure issues for public transportation equipment operators such as pilots and truck drivers.

Patients with parasomnia often require a PSG to determine the sleep stage in which an abnormal movement or behavior occurs and to exclude seizure disorder. In insomniac patients, an SDC referral is considered when attempts at improving sleep hygiene do not help. A PSG is performed when insomnia is refractory to psychiatric/behavioral treatments or when PLMS or sleep apnea is suspected. A PSG adds, refutes, or fails to support the clinical impression in 49% of patients with chronic insomnia.

DISORDERS OF INITIATING AND MAINTAINING SLEEP

Insomnia is the single most common sleep problem. A Gallup Poll survey carried out by the National Sleep Foundation in 2002 found that 58% of adults in the United States reported having insomnia. The prevalence increases with age and is more common in women and those with chronic illnesses. Nonetheless, only 5% of the insomniacs specifically visited their physician to discuss the sleep problem; 26% mentioned their sleep problem when visiting for a different reason.

An insomnia complaint to primary care physicians, who provide 65% of all office-based treatment of insomnia, should indicate a possible underlying illness. However, insomnia has typically been managed inappropriately. Some physicians think of insomnia as a neurotic complaint with little validity, and only 53% of insomniacs are treated. Others are pessimistic about the success of treatment. However, an adequate understanding of insomnia can prevent overlooking treatable disorders and inappropriate use of hypnotic drugs.

Differential Diagnosis

Insomnia is a *symptom* and not a disease; therefore, a detailed sleep history is the first step in evaluating this symptom. The history includes the type of insomnia problem (sleep onset, sleep maintenance, early awakening), when it began (childhood, recently, at time of major life stress), when it occurs (every night, weeknights only, at times of stress), what has been done when and by whom, and previous response to treatment. A sleep diary kept for 1 to 2 weeks helps establish the type, perceived severity, and periodicity of insomnia. Keep in mind that adults vary greatly in the amount of sleep they need each day in order to feel rested.

There are transient and chronic forms of insomnia. Transient insomnia characteristically has an identifiable stressor and lasts less than 3 weeks. It is the most common sleep disorder, with the affected individuals rarely seeking medical help. These patients exhibit nocturnal arousals or early-morning awakenings, with daytime consequences of fatigue and drowsiness.

Chronic insomnia lasts several months or longer and has many etiologies. Patients are likely to report memory problems, difficulty concentrating, impaired social relationships, and fatigue-related automobile or on-the-job errors and accidents. Patients with untreated insomnia that persists for more than 1 year are 40 times more likely to develop major depression. The first task in confronting this symptom is to search for the following possible etiologies:

- *Psychiatric-psychological problems.* More than 40% of all insomnias fall into this category. Screening questions for depression, anxiety, adjustment problems, and job/marital stress should be asked.
- *Medical issues.* Such discomforts as pain, dyspnea, and nocturia can cause insomnia. Medical disorders accounting for insomnia increase with age.
- *Drugs and alcohol.* Several medications can cause insomnia (see Table 11-2). Alcohol consumption allows one to fall asleep easily but causes a fragmented sleep after it is metabolized. Poor sleep can also occur when tranquilizers, sedating antidepressants, alcohol, opiates, marijuana, or cocaine are discontinued after regular use.
- *Poor sleep hygiene.* Such habits as excessive coffee, alcohol, or tobacco use; lack of exercise; consumption of heavy meals or exercise before bedtime; irregular sleep-wake habits; and focusing on the bedroom clock can result in insomnia.
- *Circadian factors.* A shift in sleep-wake schedule causes an inability to fall asleep until early morning hours, but sleep is sound thereafter. Alternatively, the patient falls asleep in the early evening hours and wakes up early.
- *Periodic leg movements of sleep.* Sleep disruption can occur from restless leg movements, or PLMS. A PSG will confirm these disorders.
- *Central sleep apnea.* This infrequent cause of chronic insomnia is characterized by an absence of respiratory effort and airflow during sleep and frequently becomes apparent on the PSG.

TABLE 11-2 Drugs That May Cause Insomnia

Nonprescription

• Decongestants	• Alcohol
• Caffeine, theobromine	• Cocaine
• Nicotine	• Methamphetamine

Prescription

• Oral contraceptives	• Antimetabolites
• Aminophyllines	• Beta-blockers
• Calcium channel blockers	• Diuretics
• Corticosteroids	• Thyroid hormones

- CNS stimulants (methylphenidate, pemoline, dextroamphetamine, etc)
- Stimulating antidepressants (fluoxetine hydrochloride, venlafaxine hydrochloride, etc)
- Beta-agonists (sympathomimetics)

- *Psychophysiological insomnia.* Patients with this type of insomnia are conditioned to being awakened rather than relaxed by the bedroom environment. Patients report better sleep when not in their own bed (eg, while on vacation) or when they are not trying to sleep (eg, while watching TV, reading, or driving). Although this is a diagnosis of exclusion, the symptoms characteristically begin during a time of stress and are aggravated by a fear of inability to sleep even after the resolution of stress. These patients develop conditioned anxiety about falling asleep or about the consequences of sleep loss. The anticipatory anxiety perpetuates the insomnia.

Management

Transient insomnia. Patients with transient insomnia recover either when the stressor subsides or by adapting to the stressor. Short-term use of a hypnotic medication such as short-acting benzodiazepines (eg, triazolam), zolpidem tartrate (Ambien), or zaleplon (Sonata) is often helpful. These hypnotic agents should be taken 10 to 60 minutes before bedtime, following the guidelines suggested in Table 11-3. These drugs, however, result in only a 10- to 30-minute average reduction in sleep onset and a 20- to 40-minute increase in total sleep time. Unlike the benzodiazepines, zolpidem tartrate and zaleplon have no muscle-relaxant or anticonvulsant properties and are thought to be less likely to induce tolerance and rebound insomnia.

There is usually no reason to prescribe barbiturates or other hypnotics (eg, glutethimide, meprobamate) to treat insomnia because they have a far higher toxic-to-therapeutic dose ratio. Over-the-counter sleeping pills, which include antihistamines as the most common ingredient, have few beneficial effects and possess undesirable anticholinergic and EDS effects.

Chronic insomnia. Managing chronic insomnia is more difficult than treating transient insomnia and usually requires referral to an SDC. Treatment is directed toward the underlying cause(s) and aims to improve sleep hygiene (Table 11-4). For the insomniac with no clear-cut etiology, behavioral therapies such as stress management and stimulus control to minimize the conditioned frustration, anxiety, and hyperarousal associated

---

TABLE 11-3 Guidelines for Use of Hypnotics Treating Insomnia

- Avoid using hypnotics in patients suspected of having pulmonary conditions, CNS disease, or sleep apnea.

- Watch for interaction with alcohol and drugs (eg, H_2 blockers, anticonvulsants).

- Use the lowest effective dose. In patients over age 65, use half the young adult dose.

- Warn patients about:

    Risk of dependence/withdrawal effects

    Hangover effects with long-acting hypnotics

    Rebound insomnia after stopping shorter-acting hypnotics.

- Dispense no more than 20 tablets at a time and monitor side effects.

- When a hypnotic is indicated for longer than 2 weeks, limit use to three times per week to prevent tolerance.

TABLE 11-4 Sleep Hygiene Measures

- Maintain a regular sleep-wake schedule and avoid routine daytime naps.
- Exercise regularly but not before bedtime.
- Avoid taking heavy meals before bedtime.
- Do not use alcohol and sleep medications.
- Avoid caffeinated beverages and smoking, especially later in the day.
- Make the bedroom conducive to sleep (avoid noise and light/temperature extremes).
- Eliminate stimulating activities in the bedroom (watching TV, reading, phone calls).
- Schedule time to wind down and relax before bedtime.
- Go to bed when sleepy and leave the bedroom if unable to sleep within 30 minutes.
- Write down troubling recurring thoughts affecting sleep with a plan of action.

with sleeping should be considered. Stimulus control therapy may be especially useful for psychophysiological insomnia. The goals of stimulus control are to improve the patient's sleep-wake rhythm, strengthen the image of the bed as a cue for sleep, and weaken the image of the bed as a cue for other activities that may interfere with sleep (eg, eating, reading, watching TV). The following is an outline of stimulus control instructions:

1. Lie down intending to go to sleep only when you are sleepy.
2. Do not read, watch TV, eat, or worry in bed. Sexual activity is the only exception.
3. If you find yourself unable to fall asleep after 10 minutes, get up immediately and go do something else. Return to bed when sleepy.
4. If you still can't fall asleep, repeat step 3. Do this as often as necessary throughout the night.
5. Set your alarm and get up at the same time every morning irrespective of how much sleep you got through the night.
6. Do not nap through the day.

Another behavioral approach attempts to consolidate sleep by restricting the amount of time an individual is permitted to be in bed. Sleep-restriction therapy is considered for those who report sleeping fewer than their usual number of hours at night. The patient is instructed to limit the time in bed to the time actually spent sleeping. A sleep diary helps to determine the patient's sleep-wake schedule. However, the physician should be aware that sleep restriction may make the patient sufficiently sleepy to risk injury, although the risk is short term and self-limited. The sleep restriction should therefore be started on a weekend to prevent sleepiness-related accidents. The time in bed is increased in 30-minute increments to maintain a sleep efficiency (time asleep:time in bed) of at least 85%. Clinically, sleep restriction is often easier to apply and more effective for a broader range of patients than stimulus control.

Other behavioral therapies such as progressive muscle relaxation, biofeedback techniques, autogenic training, hypnosis, guided imagery, and meditation are sometimes effective, although there is not enough data to offer clear guidelines for their use.

These treatments can be provided through sleep disorders programs or by behavioral therapists.

Pharmacotherapy is used only as an adjunct to the measures listed. Long-term use is contraindicated because tolerance tends to develop. In addition, the long-term benefits and risks in patients who are elderly, frail, or have psychiatric or substance abuse disorders have not been carefully evaluated. Some patients may benefit from long-term hypnotic use; ongoing surveillance is advised for these patients. The patient must be warned about temporary worsening of the sleep disorder when the hypnotic is withdrawn.

Patients with insomnia frequently take melatonin, a pineal hormone that is a marker in the process of resetting the human 24-hour circadian clock. The popular press has reported many outlandish claims about melatonin as a treatment for insomnia or aging. Statistics show that consumers were so convinced by this information that 20 million of them bought this supplement in 1995. Also of concern is the fact that such nutritional supplements are not evaluated by the US Food and Drug Administration in terms of their safety or supposed benefits. Consequently, there is limited information regarding their safety, side effects, drug interactions, and long-term effects, as well as concerns that they may cause coronary vasospasm and affect the gonadal hormones. Caution is necessary with using melatonin until further information is available.

DISORDERS OF EXCESSIVE DAYTIME SOMNOLENCE

EDS is found in 1% of general hospital inpatients and more than 4% of industrial workers. In the 2002 sleep poll mentioned earlier, 37% of respondents reported sleepiness to the extent that it interfered with their daytime function and 53% reported sleepiness while driving in the past year. Although insomnia is more common, EDS can greatly affect a patient's lifestyle and overall health. EDS symptoms may represent a potentially serious medical disorder. It can be incapacitating and may result in job loss, injury, marital and family problems, and poor school performance. If EDS poses a major risk for operating a motor vehicle and the patient is noncompliant, the physician should consider reporting the patient's condition.

EDS has a wide spectrum of presentation, ranging from mild sleepiness with minor decrements in daytime functioning to industrial or motor vehicular injuries due to uncontrollable sleep attacks. One should differentiate true EDS symptoms from such common symptoms as fatigue and lack of motivation. To clarify the diagnosis, the focus is placed on situations where sleepiness occurs (eg, reading, driving, watching television) and where inappropriate sleep occurs (eg, while driving short distances, in conversation). Corroboration from a spouse, roommate, coworker, or close friend is useful because patients often underestimate the severity of their symptoms. The Epworth Sleepiness Scale (ESS) and the MSLT can be used to quantify the subjective and objective degrees of EDS, respectively. In the ESS, the patient is asked to rate the likelihood of falling asleep in the following eight situations on a scale of 1 to 3:

- Sitting and reading
- Watching TV
- Sitting, inactive in a public space
- As a passenger in a car for an hour without a break
- Lying down to rest in the afternoon when circumstances permit

- Sitting and talking to someone
- Sitting quietly after lunch without alcohol
- In a car, while stopped for a few minutes in traffic

A patient is considered sleepy if he or she scores more than 10 on this scale. EDS is evaluated by asking the screening questions in Table 11-5. Because more than one cause for EDS may be operative, eg, a patient with obstructive sleep apnea who is taking medications with a sedative effect (Table 11-6), *all* potential etiologies are evaluated. If a patient is diagnosed with EDS, a SDC referral should be considered because these patients often require diagnostic testing such as PSG and MSLT.

TABLE 11-5 Taking a History With a Complaint of Hypersomnolence

- *Insufficient sleep:* Do you sleep much longer on weekends?

- *Medical conditions:* Do you have hypothyroidism, kidney/liver failure, etc?

- *Medication-related:* What medications have you used chronically in the past few months?

- *Sleep apnea:* Have you been told that you stop breathing or that you snore while asleep?

- *Narcolepsy:* Have you ever fallen or lost control of your muscles when very excited?

- *Periodic leg movements of sleep:* Do your legs feel restless when you relax or do you kick during sleep?

- *Sleep-wake cycle disorder:* Does your sleep occur at inappropriate times?

TABLE 11-6 Drugs That Can Cause Hypersomnia

Nonprescription
- Histamine$_1$ antagonists

- Sleeping remedies

Prescription
- Sedative-hypnotics

- Sedating tricyclic antidepressants

- Trazodone hydrochloride, nefazodone hydrochloride, mirtazapine

- Anticonvulsants

- Centrally acting alpha adrenergic antagonists

- Some SSRI antidepressants

- Antipsychotics (especially low-potency ones)

Obstructive Sleep Apnea Syndrome

Obstructive sleep apnea syndrome (OSAS) is the most serious disorder associated with EDS and is seen in 2% of women and 4% of men. Repeated episodes of upper airway obstruction and oxygen desaturation during sleep characterize OSAS. Although OSAS can

TABLE 11-7 Risk Factors Associated With Obstructive Sleep Apnea Syndrome

- Obesity (BMI >28 kg/m^2)
- Male gender
- Positive family history
- Race (African American, Hispanic, and Pacific Islander)
- Parkinson disease
- Hypothyroidism
- Acromegaly
- Marfan syndrome
- Down syndrome

occur at any age, most patients present between the ages of 40 and 60 years. The risk in females increases with obesity and postmenopausal status. Although obesity is often associated with OSAS, about 15% to 20% patients are not overweight. Risk factors are shown in Table 11-7. OSAS is significantly underreported by the medical community. A 1991 survey of patient charts from 10 internal medicine and family practice clinics in northern California found no mention of sleep apnea.

Case Vignette

Mr Otto, a 45-year-old, severely obese (313 lb) male, presents with a primary complaint of EDS. His problem started when he was in his early 30s. He had lost many jobs for "laziness" (falling asleep 5 to 10 times every day). His personal life was in ruins: two of his previous wives left him, preferring divorce to living with a sleepy, obese, heavy snorer. During the PSG, Mr Otto fell asleep soon after the lights were turned off. He quit breathing soon thereafter and awakened 35 seconds later gasping for air. This cycle repeated itself for the next 10 hours of sleep. Throughout the night he did not sleep for more than 3 minutes at a time. His oxygen saturation, which was 92% while awake, repeatedly fell below 50%. During the second PSG the following night, his respiratory disturbances were eliminated with the use of continuous positive airway pressure (CPAP) at 13 cm H_2O. In the morning, the patient answered a questionnaire and reported that he felt well rested. Mr Otto was instructed to use the CPAP machine every night and warned that the symptoms would recur if he stopped using it. In addition, he was advised to attain ideal body weight and abstain from using alcohol or any other sedatives. He was also cautioned against driving or using any heavy machinery. At a follow-up visit 1 year later, Mr Otto felt the best that he had in years, having lost more than 50 lb and doing well at work.

Most patients with OSAS are unaware of their loud snoring and breathing difficulty during sleep. A typical snoring pattern involves loud snores or brief gasps alternating with episodes of silence that last 20 to 30 seconds. The apneic event is often associated with loud snores and vocalizations that consist of gasps, moans, or mumblings. These patients typically feel unrefreshed and experience grogginess, morning headaches, and dryness of the mouth. Memory lapses, depression, impaired concentration, irritability, and anxiety are commonly associated with OSAS. Patients may experience loss of libido and erectile ability. Although patients are often unaware of their breathing problem and frequently overlook their symptoms, the bed partner may notice apneic episodes and loud snoring, which often results in the patient's presentation.

OSAS may be an independent risk factor for hypertension. There is a dose-response relation between severity of OSAS and blood pressure and this is independent of known confounding factors. Treatment of OSAS often results in reduction of daytime systemic blood pressure. OSAS is also associated with arrhythmias, ischemic heart disease, pulmonary hypertension, and cerebrovascular disease. The presence of OSAS is associated with a clear but moderately increased prevalence of stroke; the odds ratio for the severest OSAS is 1.58 times that of the mildest OSAS. Among patients who suffer a stroke, OSAS is extremely common and reported to occur in 43% to 91% of patients. The presence of OSAS is also associated with a 2.38 relative odds for congestive heart failure independent of other known risk factors. A small study has reported that treatment of OSAS resulted in dramatic improvements of left ventricular function (37% to 49%). A larger randomized trial will be required to confirm this finding. The diagnosis of OSAS requires a PSG because the predictive value of clinical findings is low.

OSAS is treated by correcting such associated medical conditions as obesity and hypothyroidism. Drugs likely to worsen OSAS (Table 11-8) should be avoided. CPAP is the mainstay of therapy for moderate to severe OSAS. Although very effective, CPAP may be difficult for some patients to use. Oral and dental appliances, which offer better compliance, are an option for patients with mild to moderate OSAS. However, a PSG should be obtained to evaluate its effectiveness. Surgical measures are considered when clear anatomic problems of the upper airway (severe nasal obstruction, tonsillar hypertrophy, redundant pharyngeal tissue, retrognathia) can be remedied. Permanent tracheostomy is the treatment of last resort.

Narcolepsy

An infrequent though important cause of EDS is narcolepsy, a disorder that characteristically presents with cataplexy (sudden weakness of the weight-bearing muscles in association with laughter or anger), sleep paralysis, and hypnogogic hallucinations. Narcolepsy occurs in 0.03% to 0.06% of the population; there is no sexual preponderance and peak onset is around 14 years of age. A statistically significant association between narcolepsy and certain subtypes of the human leukocyte antigens, HLA, DR2, and DQ1, was

TABLE 11-8 Drugs Affecting Obstructive Sleep Apnea Syndrome

Favorable Effects	Unfavorable Effects
Thyroid hormones	Alcohol
Tricyclic antidepressants	Sedative-hypnotics
Fluoxetine hydrochloride	Anesthetic agents
Buspirone hydrochloride	Narcotics
Progestational agents	

reported in the 1980s. The association between narcolepsy and certain HLA haplotypes has generated speculation that narcolepsy may be an autoimmune disorder. For example, HLA-DR2 is associated with autoimmnue diseases that affect the central nervous system, including multiple sclerosis and opyic neuritis. Narcoleptics with cataplexy frequently (>85%) have HLA DQB1*0602, a subtype of DQ1, irrespective of the ethnic group, although this allele is also present in 12% to 38% of the general population. In 1999, the genetic defect was localized to the hypocretin (or orexin) receptor gene. Decreased levels of hypocretin were found in the cerebrospinal fluid and brain tissue of narcoleptics. This discovery will change the approach to managing EDS.

Case Vignette

Mr Fox, a 35-year-old driver, was referred to an SDC for evaluation of EDS. His symptoms started when he was 20 years old. Inappropriate sleep occurred while driving, eating, or in conversation. Because a short nap offered considerable relief, Mr Fox took a few naps per day despite adequate sleep at night. A few years later he noticed that he would collapse and fall during periods of laughter or excitement. Such cataplectic attacks became increasingly bothersome. Three or four times a week he felt suddenly unable to move while falling asleep (sleep paralysis) or vividly sensed the presence of other persons in the room when he knew he was alone (hypnogogic hallucinations). Mr Fox's physical and neurological examinations were unremarkable. Sleep in the laboratory was poor and fragmented with many awakenings. The MSLT revealed a mean sleep onset latency of approximately 2 minutes (normal, 10 to 15) with a sleep onset REM period occurring with three of the five naps (REM latency is normally 75 to 90 minutes). After the evaluation, Mr Fox experienced considerable relief from using modafinil 200 mg twice a day for his daytime somnolence and protriptyline hydrochloride 5 mg twice a day for cataplexy. He was excused from hazardous duties and allowed two 20-minute naps per day at work.

EDS is usually the first symptom of narcolepsy. Cataplexy may appear either simultaneously with EDS or following a delay of as many as 30 years. Psychosocial dysfunction is considerable, leading to poor school and job performance. The rates of depression and automobile injuries are also higher than normal in these patients. Diagnosis is based on the clinical features, findings on the MSLT, and after excluding other causes of EDS on the PSG. First-degree relatives of a narcoleptic are at 20 to 40 times greater risk of having narcolepsy. HLA typing for DQB1*0602 allele helps in detecting those at a higher risk.

Treatment involves avoiding sleep deprivation by following proper sleep hygiene and taking strategically timed naps. Modafinil, a nonamphetamine approved in 1999, is the current drug of choice for EDS. It is a better-tolerated drug with fewer side effects than other central nervous system (CNS) stimulants such as pemoline, methylphenidate, or dextroamphetamine sulfate. It can, however, decrease the efficacy of oral contraceptives and should be used with caution by women taking these pills. Tolerance is a major problem for all stimulants, and patients are advised to take weekend drug "holidays." Tricyclic antidepressants such as protriptyline hydrochloride have been used for cataplexy. Gamma hydroxybutyrate, a naturally occurring metabolite of the human nervous system, has recently been approved for treatment of cataplexy.

OTHER SLEEP DISORDERS

These disorders are not as common as those associated with insomnia and EDS. However, many medical and psychiatric disorders are associated with disturbances of sleep and wakefulness, and addressing these symptoms can frequently help in hastening recovery from the underlying disorder. The primary care physician therefore needs to be aware of these disorders to help in the proper management and referral to the sleep disorders center.

Disorders of the Circadian Rhythm

Disorders of the circadian rhythm include transmeridian jet travel, shift work, and advanced/delayed sleep phase syndrome. Approximately 24% of the US adult population performs shift work, with 2% to 5% of these workers experiencing insomnia and/or EDS.

A sleep-wake cycle is governed by circadian rhythms. The suprachiasmatic nucleus, the body's circadian pacemaker, is stimulated by light and synchronizes sleep-wake cycle with the environment. The sleep-wake cycle is also influenced by environmental time cues called *zeitgebers* ("time-givers"). For example, jet lag syndrome occurs when movement to the new destination is so fast that the internal body time of the traveler is no longer synchronized with the external time. Realignment of the cycle to the *zeitgebers* may be slow and generally takes a day to readjust for each time zone crossed. Jet lag is associated with varying degrees of difficulty with sleep, excessive sleepiness, decrements in subjective daytime alertness, and performance and somatic symptoms (largely related to gastrointestinal function). The risk factors for jet lag are listed in Table 11-9. Following a schedule of the destination time zone and using short-acting sedative hypnotics to consolidate sleep lessen jet lag. Hypnotics help by preventing any further increase in sleep debt, not by resetting the clock in our brains. Recent studies now validate that melatonin could reduce jet lag by setting the clock.

Delayed sleep-phase syndrome results in a sleep cycle shift that causes sleep-onset insomnia and difficulty with rising early enough in the morning (eg, sleeping from 3:00 AM to noon). It may interfere with work attendance. In contrast, early sleep onset with early morning awakening is associated with advanced sleep-phase syndrome (eg, sleeping from 7:00 PM to 3:00 AM). Unlike with other sleep disorders, these patients report good-quality sleep once they fall asleep. Exposure to bright light may also benefit patients with delayed and advanced sleep-phase syndrome. Light therapy in the early morning shifts the sleep

---

TABLE 11-9 Predisposing Factors for Jet Lag

- Eastward travel
- Increased number of time zones crossed
- Sleep loss before and during travel
- Minimal environmental stimulation
- Caffeine or alcohol consumption
- Older age

phase backward in patients with a delayed sleep-phase syndrome; when administered in the early evening period, light shifts the sleep phase forward in patients with advanced sleep-phase syndrome.

Shift work may also disrupt sleep and results in impaired performance, somatic distress, and accidents. The incidence of physical illness (particularly stress-related illness such as ulcers) as well as psychiatric illness may be increased in shift workers. Shift workers frequently suffer from chronic sleep deprivation, sleeping 1 to 2 hours less than normal each day. Sleep difficulty in shift workers can be reduced by maintaining a forward rotating schedule, staying on a particular shift for at least 2 weeks, following adequate sleep hygiene, and avoiding concurrent use of caffeine, nicotine, alcohol, or sedatives. In addition, domestic and social factors that protect the shift worker from interruptions of daytime sleep patterns and social isolation may be helpful. Application of light (more than 2500 lux) at appropriate times can reset the circadian clock. Light input from the retina to the suprachiasmatic nucleus causes an alerting response that drives sleep away. Increasing the light levels under which shift workers work and darkening the places where they sleep can improve the quality of sleep. Until industries adopt the above physiological principles in scheduling workers, those who cannot adapt to shift work must change jobs to find relief.

Abnormal Behaviors Associated With Sleep (Parasomnias)

Parasomnias (events around sleep) are a group of sleep disturbances that range from being common to very rare. Non-REM sleep-associated disorders such as sleepwalking or sleep terrors occur in the first third of the sleep period and are associated with amnesia on awakening. They are more frequent in children and are generally benign in nature. In children, treatment frequently involves reassurance and measures to decrease the risk of accidents. If the problem is disrupting, a low-dose anxiolytic agent such as triazolam may be used at bedtime. In contrast, these behaviors in adults necessitate evaluation for a possible serious underlying problem.

In REM sleep behavior disorder (REMSBD) there is intermittent loss of normal REM sleep muscle atonia and the appearance of aggressive or emotional behavior (eg, hitting, diving off the bed in fright) associated with dream mentation that can be recalled by the patient when he or she is awakened. REMSBD, which is apparently rare, almost exclusively occurs in adults and should be differentiated from seizure activity. Approximately 60% of cases are idiopathic; advanced age is an apparent predisposing factor. Injury to oneself or one's bed partner (lacerations, ecchymosis, fractures) and damage to surroundings is the major complication. Social consequences that involve the relationship with the bed partner may be significant.

If REMSBD is suspected, referral to an SDC for diagnosis with a PSG and planning treatment are required. A systematic evaluation includes (*a*) review of sleep-wake complaints from the patient and the bed partner; (*b*) neurological and psychiatric examination; and (*c*) a PSG that includes videotaping of behavior. If structural neurological disease is suspected, brain-stem auditory-evoked potentials, EEG, and brain imaging should be considered. Diagnostic criteria for REMSBD include lack of evidence for seizure activity and increased muscle activity during REM. REMSBD is treated using short-acting benzodiazepines.

Restless Legs Syndrome and Periodic Leg Movements of Sleep

Restless legs syndrome (RLS) is characterized by an uncomfortable sensation in the legs that is described as pins and needles, creeping or crawling sensation, or internal itch and typically occurs with rest and disrupts sleep. Although 16% of respondents in the 2002 sleep poll experienced RLS, less than 4% were diagnosed and only 1% were treated. Periodic leg movements of sleep (PLMS) are stereotyped movements of the legs that are seen in 23% to 30% of elderly patients with sleep difficulties. Patients with PLMS are frequently unaware of their leg movements; information regarding PLMS is usually obtained from the patient's bed partner. PLMS may cause arousals, fragmented and nonrestorative sleep, insomnia, and hypersomnolence. In patients with RLS, daytime neurological and electromyographic examination is frequently normal and myoclonic movements may be seen prior to the onset of sleep and during sleep on the PSG.

Tricyclic antidepressants, monoamine oxidase inhibitors, and antipsychotics can induce or aggravate RLS, as does withdrawal from such drugs as anticonvulsants, benzodiazepines, barbiturates, and other hypnotic agents. Anemia, uremia, and COPD have been associated with RLS. Although RLS may last throughout a patient's life, it is usually a benign condition that neither reflects deterioration of an underlying illness nor preempts the appearance of a more sinister pathology. PLMS can accompany narcolepsy and OSAS.

Case Vignette

Mrs Rohm, a 68-year-old woman who has been otherwise healthy and active, presents with complaints of restless legs. She can never sit down and relax—the restlessness in her legs seems to take over. During the night hours, she cannot lie still in bed and spends her evenings walking the floors. Lately, this does not seem to help. For many years Mrs Rohm thought her problem was unique to her. She has seen many different physicians, but nothing seems to have helped. Her physical exam, including the neurological exam, is within normal limits. She undergoes a PSG, which demonstrates periodic leg movements while she is awake and sleeping. Her primary care physician prescribes pergolide mesylate 0.15 mg at bedtime, with resolution of her symptoms.

The goal in managing these types of cases is to avoid anything that overly stimulates the nervous system, including caffeine, chocolate, and smoking, and to limit the use of centrally active stimulants, such as decongestants, antihistamines, and appetite suppressants. Selective serotonin reuptake inhibitors (SSRIs) should be avoided unless they are the only effective treatment (bupropion hydrochloride and nefazodone hydrochloride may be better tolerated). Application of counterstimuli such as socks, stretching, hot baths or showers, and ice packs also relieves the discomfort. The treatment of choice for RLS is a dopaminergic agent such as pergolide mesylate and levodopa/carbidopa (Sinemet). Clonazepam may be used in patients with PLMS after coexisting sleep-disordered breathing and narcolepsy have been excluded.

Psychiatric Illness and Sleep Disorders

Most psychiatric disorders are associated with sleep disturbances. Insomnia may be one of the earliest symptoms of acute psychosis and often persists for long periods. Poor sleep is observed in 90% of patients with affective disorders. Major depression usually produces initial and maintenance insomnia, including early morning awakening. EDS is observed in approximately 15% to 20% of patients with atypical depression and seasonal affective disorder. In a large epidemiological study, 14% of patients with insomnia and 9.9% of patients with hypersomnia met all criteria for major depression. A sleep study of patients presenting with sleep disorders may document specific abnormalities associated with depression. These include early onset of REM sleep, increased number of eye movements, reduction in slow-wave sleep, and poor sleep continuity.

Treatment of a mood disorder frequently results in resolution of the sleep complaint. When pharmacological treatment is anticipated, sedating antidepressants such as nefazodone hydrochloride, mirtazapine, or doxepin hydrochloride may be preferred if insomnia is present. Patients should be screened for RLS because these medications can worsen this syndrome by further disrupting the patient's sleep. If the patient has hypersomnia, stimulating antidepressants (eg, fluoxetine hydrochloride, venlafaxine hydrochloride) may be started.

Anxiety disorders are found in 25% of subjects complaining of insomnia and hypersomnia. It is important to differentiate these disorders from sleep terrors for successful treatment. Benzodiazepines may be considered in treating anxiety disorders. In patients with panic disorder, sleep is remarkably normal except during panic attacks. Although these patients may have trouble sleeping following these episodes, they report only vague dread or fear.

Patients with a history of alcohol abuse frequently report a fragmented, short, and shallow sleep. Although alcohol promotes sleep, disrupted and fragmented sleep can occur later in the night from withdrawal. Alcohol may exacerbate sleep-related breathing disorders in some patients. Recovering alcoholics may experience insomnia and objective sleep disturbances for a year or longer. These disturbances often predispose a patient to renewed drinking. It is unwise to treat abstinent alcoholics with benzodiazepines because they are cross-tolerant with alcohol. Management involves following general sleep hygiene principles and treatment of underlying psychiatric syndromes.

Medical Disorders Affecting Sleep

Several medical conditions are associated with disrupted sleep. Patients with COPD experience difficulty initiating sleep, frequent awakenings, dyspnea, nocturnal cough, morning headaches, and unrefreshing sleep. In cardiac patients, dyspnea and chest pain can disrupt sleep. The pain or discomfort of sleep-related gastroesophageal reflux disease may cause sleep fragmentation, and sleep disturbances among uremic patients is reported to be high. Disturbed sleep and EDS are the most common complaints, followed by symptoms consistent with RLS and OSAS.

Patients with dementia frequently experience sleep disturbances that range from increased awakenings and nocturnal wanderings to agitation and confusion. Their circadian sleep-wake cycle flattens. Management involves treating underlying metabolic, neurologic processes and recognizing the sensitivity of delirious patients to medication side effects. Behavioral management includes maintaining proper sleep hygiene, strengthening the circadian rhythm, and avoiding the "sundowning" syndrome by keeping the patient awake during the day using bright light exposure and providing more environmental cues in the evening. Safety precautions should be maintained at night for agitated patients.

Between 60% and 90% of patients with Parkinson disease have sleep complaints such as insomnia, EDS, and RLS. These sleep disturbances are related to bradykinesia, rigidity, tremor, leg cramps, and nocturia. Depression, dementia, REMSBD, circadian rhythm disturbances, and sleep apnea may be seen in some patients with Parkinson disease. L-Dopa and anticholinergic agents can mitigate sleep problems in these patients.

Seizures occur during sleep or following an arousal in nearly 80% of cases. Sleep-related seizures can masquerade as enuresis, sleep terrors, or somnambulism, although the waking EEG may be normal. If a sleep-related seizure is suspected, an experienced EEG technician should run a full EEG with a split-screen video recording for the entire night.

Chronic and acute pain is incompatible with good sleep. Chronic pain syndromes are often associated with depression; consequently, these patients may benefit from antidepressant medication such as amitryptyline hydrochloride at bedtime. Patients with fibromyalgia often feel unrestored even after an adequate sleep and complain of morning stiffness, aches, and increased sensitivity to pain. On the PSG there may be evidence of intrusion of alpha waves into the sleep patterns, PLMS, or sleep apnea. Psychotropic medications have been variably successful.

Sleep Deprivation

Sleep deprivation is a common yet unrecognized modern epidemic. According to the 2002 sleep poll, people are sleeping only 6.9 and 7.5 hours during weekdays and weekends, respectively. In current society sleep is treated as a waste of time. Over the past 25 years, people have added 1 month to their average annual work/commute time by reducing sleep. Insufficient sleep results in decreased productivity and accidents secondary to daytime sleepiness, irritability, concentration and attention deficits, fatigue, and reduced vigilance and motivation. Quality of life also suffers; people cut back on activities they enjoy, claiming they just do not have the energy. Sleep deprivation can adversely affect immune function and contributes to intensive care unit psychosis. Management consists of educating the patient about sleep hygiene and maintaining adequate sleep.

SUMMARY

Sleep complaints and disorders are commonly encountered in primary care settings, and patients look to their physicians for advice about improving sleep. Physicians must be familiar with the clinical picture of common sleep disorders and aware of when evaluation at a sleep disorders center is warranted. The primary care physician can manage many sleep disorders once a definitive diagnosis is made. A summary of initial management and typical treatments is shown in Table 11-10.

TABLE 11-10 Summary of Sleep Disorder Management

Suspected Disorder	Initial Management Step	Treatment
DIMS		
Transient insomnia	Care by primary care physician	Short-term hypnotics, sleep hygiene, emotional support
Chronic insomnia	SDC referral if sleep hygiene fails	Behavioral therapy or treatment of underlying psychiatric condition
EDS		
OSAS	SDC evaluation	CPAP, surgery, etc
Narcolepsy	SDC evaluation	Stimulants ± tricyclics
Disorders of sleep-wake cycle	PCP care	Environmental manipulations, light therapy
Parasomnias	SDC evaluation	Benzodiazepines
Restless legs syndrome	PCP care	Dopaminergic agent
Periodic leg movements of sleep	PCP care	Clonazepam

DIMS = disorders of initiating and maintaining sleep

EDS = excess daytime somnolence

OSAS = obstructive sleep apnea syndrome

SDC = sleep disorders center

CPAP = continuous positive airway pressure

ADDITIONAL READINGS

Chokroverty S, ed. *Sleep Disorders Medicine: Basic Science, Technical Considerations and Clinical Aspects.* Boston, Mass: Butterworth-Heinemann; 1999.

Kryger M, Roth T, Dement WC, eds. *Principles and Practice of Sleep Medicine.* 3rd ed. Philadelphia, Pa: WB Saunders Co; 2000.

Malone S, Liu PP, Holloway R, Rutherford R, Xie A, Bradley TD. Obstructive sleep apnea in patients with dilated cardiomyopathy: effects of continuous positive airway pressure. *Lancet.* 1991;338:1480-1484.

Mendelson WB, ed. *Human Sleep: Research and Clinical Care.* New York, NY: Plenum Press; 1987.

Thorpy MJ. *The International Classification of Sleep Disorders: Diagnostic and Coding Manual.* Rochester, Minn: American Sleep Disorders Association; 1997.

Chapter **12**

Sexual Disorders

R. Taylor Segraves, MD, PhD

Diagnosing and effectively treating sexual disorders can be a very rewarding aspect of clinical practice. For many individuals, their sense of masculinity or femininity, self-esteem, and sense of personal adequacy are integrally related to their sexual function. Similarly, sexual behavior is generally essential for maintaining intimacy and stability in long-term relationships. Thus, when a patient has a sexual disorder, effective intervention into that patient's sexual life can have multiple beneficial effects.

Effective intervention is based on a thorough differential diagnosis. In many cases the diagnosis can be made confidently, based on a careful history of the complaint by the primary care physician, without the need for specialty referral. A thoughtful sexual history, combined with a proper physical examination and some basic laboratory investigations, is often enough for the clinician to determine if the problem has primarily a psychogenic or a biogenic etiology. This workup also helps determine whether the problem requires a referral or can be effectively treated by the primary care physician.

Although sexual dysfunction occurs in about 10% of family practice patients, it often remains undetected and, as a result, goes untreated. This is primarily due to the physician's failure to elicit the sexual history and failure to perform a genital examination. Many primary care physicians have received additional training to treat patients with sexual dysfunction; however, for most physicians this is not necessary because numerous specialists are readily available. Every primary care physician, however, should discuss sexual issues with patients in order to provide them with adequate care.

This chapter describes the appropriate workup for a patient with a sexual dysfunction. Each of the various diagnoses delineated by the *Diagnostic and Statistical Manual of Mental Disorders*, fourth edition (DSM-IV), for sexual dysfunction is discussed. This is followed by a brief survey of the paraphilias. The degree of coverage of each topic reflects two factors—the frequency with which these problems are seen by the primary care physician and the actual empirical knowledge base. In particular, sexual disorders in women have been less well studied than those in men; consequently, we can say far less about these conditions with scientific certainty.

CONSULTATIONS AND REFERRALS

Because not all mental health professionals are experienced in treating sexual disorders, it is critical to choose the correct psychiatric or mental health specialist for cases of sexual dysfunction. Previous studies indicate that most patients do not comply with a recommended referral to mental health specialists. For example, if a urologist introduces the psychiatrist to a patient in the urology clinic, compliance with psychiatric treatment recommendations appears to be greatly improved.

The primary care physician must realize that the results of psychiatric treatment are as variable as the etiologies. Disorders that are related to deficiencies in experience and/or the consequence of anticipation anxieties can be expected to have better prognoses than disorders that are the result of anxieties over gender identity. If a patient is using a sexual symptom to punish a partner or to manage ambivalence concerning intimacy, the results of therapy will be much more difficult to predict. In these cases, the prognosis may relate to factors that are difficult to precisely define, such as the couple's motivation and readiness to change, the therapist's artistry as much as the therapist's professional knowledge and qualifications, and the match between the therapist's personality and the patient's personality.

Ultimately, the primary care physician must establish a relationship with one or two experienced mental health professionals to whom he or she can refer patients.

EVALUATION

Sexual History

A sexual history should be taken routinely when performing a comprehensive evaluation. There are at least two reasons for this. First, the history can act as a screening test to determine if the patient has a sexual dysfunction. Second, it gives the patient permission to discuss any fears about sexual problems he or she could develop in the future. If the patient has a complaint related to sexual function, the focused sexual history is similar to the history one would obtain for any other complaint.

The physician must determine the specific nature of the chief complaint, its development over time, and the situations in which the problem occurs. Determining whether the problem is primarily one of impaired sexual desire, arousal, or orgasm can assist in the differential diagnosis, even though many sexual problems involve more than one phase of the sexual response cycle. The physician should also briefly inquire how frequently the patient is sexually active, the nature of the relationship with the usual sexual partner, and a brief description of a typical sexual encounter. If the patient has difficulty describing a typical encounter, the patient could describe his or her last sexual encounter. With minor modifications, this basic format can be adapted to fit a variety of clinical presentations. The key elements of the sexual history are shown in Table 12-1.

Because a sexual history is used to gather basic information concerning the chief complaint, the interview should not be overly structured, so as to establish a dialogue with the patient and not inhibit the spontaneous flow of information. An attempt to economize on time by using numerous detailed questions can often result in an incomplete history and consequently be an inefficient use of time. Sexual history questionnaires can be given to patients to help specify the problem, but ultimately, critical information is obtained by face-to-face interview. Unfortunately, many individuals are reluctant to divulge their difficulties or to be specific regarding their sexual practices due to the symbolic meaning of sexual behavior.

Sexual behavior can be influenced by a variety of biological, psychological, interpersonal, cultural, and social variables, making it difficult to determine the specific

TABLE 12-1 Elements of the Sexual Disorder History

- Nature of complaint
- Course of complaint over time
- Situations in which problem occurs
- Frequency of sexual activity
- Nature of relationship with sexual partner(s)
- Description of a typical sexual encounter

etiology of a sexual problem. It is vitally important to ask about the use of prescribed medication, over-the-counter and illicit drugs, and alcohol because these are common causes of sexual dysfunction. As a general rule, sexual problems that are situation-specific, meaning restricted to one partner or situation, are psychogenic. Complaints that occur in all situations are more likely to be biogenic in etiology. The latter usually require more sophisticated diagnostic evaluation and consultation. As in all of clinical medicine, there are exceptions to this general rule.

Physical Examination

Evaluation of a patient with a sexual dysfunction should include a complete general physical and mental status examination. This serves to confirm or rule out diagnoses suspected during the history. Although various physical problems can cause sexual dysfunction, it is somewhat unusual for a sexual complaint to be the first or only symptom of a previously undiagnosed disease. In most cases the disease process will be manifest in symptoms other than a sexual dysfunction and be picked up earlier. The mental status exam helps to rule out depression, mania, or other psychiatric diagnoses that could impact a patient's sexual function.

The physician should examine the patient for evidence of chronic or debilitating disease, especially endocrinopathies, which could interfere with libido. Additionally, a search for surgical scars, indicating a procedure that may have interrupted the nerve supply to the genitals, should be conducted. A lower body neurological exam should also be performed to rule out spinal cord pathology or evidence of a peripheral neuropathy. This exam includes checking anal sphincter tone, the bulbocavernosus reflex, and saddle sensation.

The focused genital examination in men and women should include checking the femoral pulses, checking for hernias, evaluating the secondary sexual characteristics for appropriate sexual development, and looking for obvious excoriations, which could suggest the presence of a venereal disease.

In men, the genital examination begins with the foreskin of the penis to check for phimosis or paraphimosis. Then check the glans for signs of ulcers, scars, nodules, inflammation, or discharge. The scrotum is then checked for the presence of a varicocele or hernia. Finally, the testes are checked for size and consistency and for the presence of any nodules.

In women, the genital exam begins with a visual inspection of the external genitalia to observe for lesions of the vulva; an enlarged clitoris, which could suggest masculinizing conditions; or swelling in the vulva or the vagina, which could suggest a chronic infection of the Bartholin's gland, cystocele, or rectocele. The internal examination with a speculum allows for observation of cervical abnormalities or the presence of purulent cervical discharges. A bimanual examination can detect possible tumors or adnexal masses. In postmenopausal women, especially those who are not on estrogen replacement therapy, the vaginal mucosa will commonly be thin and dry.

Laboratory Investigations

After completing the sexual history and the physical exam, general laboratory investigations should be performed to help arrive at the correct diagnosis. These include a complete blood count, multipanel chemical tests, and venereal disease reaction level (VDRL) tests. Additional tests such as cervical cytology, thyroid function tests, HIV, urine toxicology, and specific endocrinological tests such as luteinizing hormone (LH), follicle-stimulating hormone (FSH), prolactin, or testosterone should be performed as necessary based on the history and physical examination. Further investigation with tests such as nocturnal penile tumescence and bilateral internal iliac angiography should only be performed following consultation with a specialist.

SPECIFIC SEXUAL DISORDERS
Hypoactive Sexual Desire

Case Vignette

Mrs Carl, a 33-year-old married woman in good health, comes to see her primary care physician, Dr Lyle, because of a markedly decreased interest in sexual activity over the past 12 months. Mrs Carl and her husband used to have intercourse three to four times per week, about half the time at her initiation, and she would masturbate at the same frequency when he was traveling on business. One year ago she discovered that he was having an extramarital affair, which he ended after she confronted him. They have had a tense relationship since that time, and they currently have sex one to two times per week, always at his initiation; she no longer masturbates, saying, "I just don't think about sex anymore—ever." When her husband initiates sexual activity, she becomes aroused and reaches orgasm as readily as she had before. She presented to her doctor 9 months ago because of depression over the affair, and citalopram hydrobromide was prescribed with good therapeutic response. Mrs Carl's menstrual periods remain regular. Physical examination is normal, with no evidence of pelvic abnormalities or symptoms suggestive of an endocrinopathy. TSH, LH, and prolactin levels are all normal. Dr Lyle tells Mrs Carl to discontinue her citalopram hydrobromide and refers her and her husband for couple's therapy. Three months later she returns, reporting a level of sexual interest almost that of a year previously.

Patient complaints of low libido are among the most frequent sexual complaints that primary care physicians hear. In one multicenter study involving 906 patients presenting for treatment of sexual problems, 65% were diagnosed as having a primary diagnosis of hypoactive sexual desire disorder, with the problem being far more common in female patients. Unfortunately, these are some of the most complex and perplexing complaints to diagnose. The etiology can vary from interpersonal discord to major endocrinopathies. Psychogenic desire problems are commonly agreed to be the most difficult sexual problems to treat and also the ones with the poorest prognosis. However, once identified, the primary care physician can readily manage many treatable etiologies. Other problems may require consultation with an endocrinologist or psychiatrist.

The first thing the physician needs to clarify is whether the problem is situation-specific or generalized. This question is based on the assumption that most biogenic etiologies for decreased sexual desire are present in all situations. If a patient complains of decreased sexual desire for the spouse but normal sexual desire for a neighbor, this is unlikely to be an organic problem. Similarly, if the patient reports a sustained sexual fantasy life and frequent masturbatory activity, it is highly likely that the problem is related to interpersonal difficulties with the present partner or other psychological factors, because the biologic urge for sexual activity is intact. These patients often benefit from a referral to a mental health specialist.

Situational low sexual desire. Chronic interpersonal discord and marital separation are common precipitants for situational low sexual desire, as well as for periods of high utilization of nonpsychiatric medical services for psychiatric illness. These situations generally benefit from brief targeted couples therapy. Other, less common causes of acquired libido problems include a history of childhood sexual abuse or an atypical sexual arousal pattern. Although these individuals usually have a lifelong history of decreased libido, they often present with a complaint of a period of normal sexual function followed by a period of decreased libido. It is unclear why a problem related to a remote event or a chronic situation would have a sporadic presentation. However, some patients with a history of sexual abuse present with intermittent libido problems, perhaps related to fluctuations in levels of experienced intimacy and safety. These individuals are likely to require extremely high levels of interpersonal intimacy in order to experience sexual desire and are likely to benefit from referral to a mental health specialist. Occasionally, individuals will experience atypical arousal patterns that are only manifest during periods of high stress.

Generalized low sexual desire. Situations in which the loss of libido is generalized are the result of a variety of factors. Depression should be ruled out, because it is treatable and should not require referral to a specialist. Another treatable problem not requiring referral is drug-induced libido reduction. In these cases, a careful history will establish that the problem began after drug initiation or dose increase. Drugs commonly associated with decreased libido include psychiatric and antihypertensive drugs. Among psychiatric drugs, the selective serotonin reuptake inhibitors (SSRIs) (eg, fluoxetine hydrochloride, sertraline hydrochloride, paroxetine hydrochloride) are commonly associated with decreased libido. Lowering the dose, decreasing frequency of dosing, or substituting with an antidepressant with a lower likelihood of sexual side effects (eg, bupropion or nefazodone) are likely to resolve the problem. Among antihypertensive agents, angiotensin-converting enzyme inhibitors such as captopril, enalapril maleate, and lisinopril appear to have a very low incidence of sexual side effects. A list of drugs associated with decreased libido is found in Table 12-2.

Hypogonadism and hyperprolactinemia, treatable causes of low libido in males, can be diagnosed and treated by the primary care physician. In one clinical series, a primary complaint of low libido in males was associated with hypogonadism approximately 15% of the time. There is now unequivocal evidence that androgens are necessary for maintaining sexual interest. Hypogonadal men occasionally develop erectile problems secondary to decreased libido, but androgens per se are not needed for normal erectile function. If low serum bioavailable testosterone is present, LH levels should be assessed. Low to normal LH levels are suggestive of pituitary or hypothalamic defects, whereas high LH levels indicate testicular failure.

In postmenopausal females, especially postoophorectomy, decreased libido is often related to decreased androgen production and may be responsive to androgen-estrogen replacement. Transient stress can be associated with low libido. In these cases, watchful waiting is the preferred course prior to referral to a mental health specialist. Of course, any general medical problem associated with fatigue or chronic pain may in turn be associated with decreased sexual desire. Aging is associated with decreased sexual desire

TABLE 12-2 Drugs Associated With Decreased Libido

acetazolamide	diazepam	methazolamide
alprazolam	dichlorphenamide	methyldopa
amitriptyline hydrochloride	digoxin	paroxetine hydrochloride
amoxapine	ethoxzolamide	phenelzine
chlorpromazine	fenfluramine hydrochloride	primidone
chlorthalidone	fluoxetine hydrochloride	protriptyline hydrochloride
cimetidine	fluphenazine	reserpine
clofibrate	haloperidol	sertraline hydrochloride
clomipramine hydrochloride	hydrochlorothiazide	spironolactone
clonidine hydrochloride	imipramine hydrochloride	thioridazine
clorazepate dipotassium	lithium	thiothixene

and activity in men. This reduction does not appear to be solely the result of decreased gonadal function or changes in bioavailable testosterone levels. In females aging is also associated with a decline in libido and sexual interest, although there appear to be minimal differences between pre- and postmenopausal women in sexual responsiveness.

Some clinicians advocate the use of androgens to treat low libido in premenopausal women. Considerable evidence indicates that supraphysiological levels of exogenous androgens increase libido in women. However, the indications, dosages, duration, and risks of such treatment remain unclear. For these reasons, androgen therapy in premenopausal women with low libido should be regarded as experimental.

Lifelong low sexual desire. This condition is usually difficult to diagnose and treat. One exception is the patient with minimal sexual experience and excessive guilt concerning the experience of sexual pleasure. A respectful discussion of the problem with the patient often helps the patient to feel less guilty about experiencing sexual pleasure. Highly religious individuals should be referred to an understanding pastoral counselor. If a mental health referral is made, anticipate a good prognosis with brief psychotherapy.

An issue to confront early in the evaluation is whether the patient genuinely wants his or her sexual circumstances to be different. If the partner prompts the request for treatment, the patient is not likely to change. Many patients who are ambivalent about change do not make an initial appointment with a therapist. Even if the primary care physician makes the appointment for the patient, it is unlikely that the patient will show up for the appointment or follow through with psychotherapy.

An unusual arousal pattern such as fetishism, arousal requiring a specific nonanimate object, or arousal predominantly to someone of a different sex or age from the regular partner are unsuspected causes of decreased libido. In these situations, the patient's masturbatory fantasies will give clues to etiology. These situations are often difficult to diagnose because the patient is embarrassed to reveal the specifics of the situation. It is important to remember that fetishism is not always a fixed problem. Patients who report adequate sexual function in stable relationships will report the interruption of this pattern, by fetishism, only during periods of high external stress.

Female patients with a history of sexual abuse are likely to experience decreased libido characterized by extreme ambivalence toward any male activity that could be interpreted as aggressive. Lifelong patterns of low libido in both sexes are often psychogenic and often require referral to a mental health specialist. Unfortunately, the prognosis in these cases is often poor, and there is minimal controlled evidence documenting the efficacy of such therapy. Most clinicians who specialize in treating sexual problems have encountered at least a few individuals with markedly low libido in which an etiology cannot be established and an unknown organic etiology is suspected. There is evidence to suggest that a minority of women with lifelong low libido have abnormalities in androgen metabolism. The suggested approach to differential diagnosis is outlined in Table 12-3.

Sexual aversion disorder. Sexual aversion disorder differs from hypoactive sexual desire disorder in that the patient has an extreme aversion to and avoidance of almost all genital contact with a sexual partner. Some individuals experience panic attacks when confronted with a sexual situation. Unfortunately, there is a paucity of controlled inquiry concerning this disorder. Some clinical reports suggest that individuals with this disorder respond to behavior therapy in combination with pharmacotherapy to control panic attacks. Typically, such cases should be referred to a mental health specialist.

Male Arousal (Erectile) Disorders

The number of men who suffer from erectile problems appears to be highly correlated with increasing age. Various studies suggest that fewer than 10% of men in their 30s suffer from erectile problems. A recent epidemiological study found that 52% of men ages 40 to 70 complained of difficulty with erections. Additionally, the number of men reporting total inability to obtain erections tripled between the ages of 40 and 70.

With the development of sophisticated diagnostic procedures during the last decade, there has been a rapid advance in knowledge concerning the physiology of erection.

TABLE 12-3 Differential Diagnosis of Hypoactive Sexual Desire Disorder

| Lifelong | Acquired | |
	Situational	Generalized
Childhood sexual abuse	Relationship discord	Depression
Restrictive sexual attitude	Childhood sexual abuse	Drug-induced
Atypical arousal pattern	Atypical arousal pattern	Postoophorectomy
		Androgen deficiency
		Hyperprolactinemia
		Other debilitating condition

Various diagnostic algorithms have been proposed; however, in many patients, a careful, logical approach to the sexual history can often preclude the need for expensive procedures that can cause patient discomfort and morbidity. A simplified decision tree for the differential diagnosis of erectile dysfunction is shown in Figure 12-1.

As with most sexual disorders, the time course of the symptom should be identified. A major decision point for erectile disorders is whether the problem is lifelong or acquired. Most lifelong erectile problems are assumed to be psychogenic in etiology and to have a poorer prognosis than acquired erectile problems. In general, such patients are able to masturbate but unable to obtain and maintain erections in partner-related activity. Organogenic lifelong erectile problems are felt to be infrequent, although accurate epidemiological data are lacking. In these cases, a history of difficulty with erections both during masturbation and in partner-related activity is to be expected.

Lifelong problems. Patients who experience a lifelong history of erectile problems often have congenital vascular problems. Focal cavernosal arterial blockade secondary to trauma and occurring at a prepubescent age is another possible cause of lifelong erectile problems. Injection of vasoactive substances into the corpora cavernosum has been suggested as a diagnostic procedure in these cases, although evidence concerning this is controversial. Theoretically, patients with arterial blockade do not obtain erections with large doses of vasoactive substances, whereas patients with venous leakage problems can obtain erections of brief duration. Given the uncertainty of a diagnosis of lifelong erectile dysfunction and the radically different treatment approaches that a urologist is likely to take, as compared to a psychiatrist, to treat this problem, referral to a sexual dysfunction center where urologists and psychiatrists work as a team to make a diagnosis should be considered.

Acquired problems. Acquired erectile problems are far more common than lifelong erectile problems. When making the differential diagnosis of acquired erectile problems, the physician attempts to establish if the problem is generalized or situational, based on the assumption that adequate erectile function under any situation establishes the physiological capacity for normal sexual function. A question from the sexual history that is

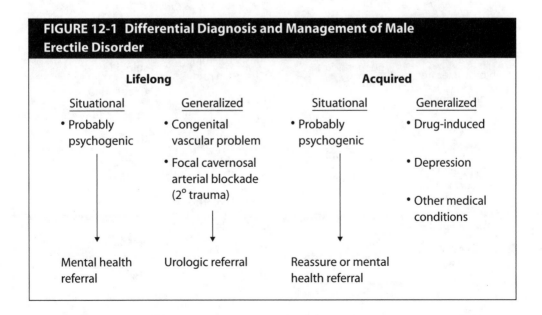

FIGURE 12-1 Differential Diagnosis and Management of Male Erectile Disorder

Lifelong		Acquired	
Situational	Generalized	Situational	Generalized
• Probably psychogenic	• Congenital vascular problem	• Probably psychogenic	• Drug-induced
	• Focal cavernosal arterial blockade (2° trauma)		• Depression
			• Other medical conditions
Mental health referral	Urologic referral	Reassure or mental health referral	

highly predictive of psychogenic erectile dysfunction is whether normal erections are present when the patient wakes up in the morning. If acquired psychogenic erectile dysfunction is the presumptive diagnosis, the chronicity of the problem needs to be established. Patients who complain of briefer duration often respond to reassurance that the problem does not appear to have a physical basis, that such problems are commonly experienced by many men, and that they are most often self-limited.

Chronic psychogenic erectile problems are much less likely to remit without extensive intervention. Patients without severe marital discord who comply with treatment recommendations can be expected to achieve about a 70% success rate with brief behavioral therapy. An alternative strategy is pharmacotherapy. Oral vasoactive drugs such as sildenafil citrate have been used to treat psychogenic erectile problems. However, the consequences and long-term efficacy of this type of intervention have not been studied extensively to date, and it is usually used only if less invasive interventions such as reassurance and counseling are unsuccessful. Assessment of the patient's relationship with his partner is recommended, because restoration of erectile function has been reported to cause marital discord in some couples.

If the problem is generalized, depression and drug use must be ruled out as treatable etiologies. Table 12-4 lists drugs frequently associated with erectile problems. Antihyper-

TABLE 12-4 Drugs Associated With Erectile Dysfunction

acetazolamide	dichlorphenamide	isocarboxazid	prazosin
amiodarone hydrochloride	digoxin	ketamine	primidone
amitriptyline	disopyramide phosphate	ketoconazole	propranolol
amoxapine	disulfiram	labetalol hydrochloride	protriptyline
atenolol	doxepin hydrochloride	lithium	ranitidine hydrochloride
baclofen	ethoxyzolamide	maprotiline hydrochloride	reserpine
bendrofluazide	fluphenazine	methantheline bromide	sertraline hydrochloride
bethanidine sulfate	fluoxetine	methazolamide hydrochloride	spironolactone
bupropion	guanethidine sulfate	methyldopa	sulpiride
chlorpromazine	guanoclor	nifedipine	thiabendazole
chlorthalidone	guanoxan sulfate	nortriptyline hydrochloride	thioridazine
cimetidine	haloperidol	paroxetine hydrochloride	thiothixene
clofibrate	hydralazine hydrochloride	perhexiline	tranylcypromine sulfate
clomipramine hydrochloride	hydrochlorothiazide	phenelzine	trazodone hydrochloride
clonidine hydrochloride	imipramine hydrochloride	pimozide	verapamil hydrochloride
desipramine hydrochloride	indomethacin		

tensive and psychotropic agents are the most common offenders. Chronic alcohol abuse may also be associated with erectile dysfunction.

Neurological and vascular diseases also cause erectile dysfunction. Neurological conditions associated with erectile dysfunction include multiple sclerosis, diseases of the temporal lobe, diabetic neuropathy, alcoholic neuropathy, and neuropathy after cancer chemotherapy or radiation therapy. Other causes include interruption of the innervation of the penis by surgical procedures. Erectile problems may also be the result of major vascular diseases, which can be detected by palpating the femoral arteries, or the result of microvascular disease, which is difficult to detect. Table 12-5 lists organic etiologies of erectile problems. A step-wise approach to treating organogenic impotence should be taken, beginning with oral phosphodiesterase inhibitors or a vacuum erection device. If these treatments are unsuccessful or unacceptable to the patient, intraurethral or intracavernosal prostaglandin E-1 therapy should be considered. Referral for evaluation for penile prosthesis implantation is the last step in this approach.

Phosphodiesterase type-5 inhibitors (eg, sildenafil citrate) are contraindicated in patients taking nitrates. In patients with unstable angina, uncontrolled hypertension, recent myocardial infarction, or severe valvular disease, referral for specialized cardiac evaluation is recommended prior to use of sildenafil citrate. Common side effects include transient headache, flushing, dyspepsia, nasal congestion, and transient visual disturbances.

The US Food and Drug Administration (FDA) is investigating other phosphodiesterase type-5 inhibitors. Apomorphine, which works centrally by stimulating erectogenic pathways in the paraventricular nucleus of the hypothalamus, is also being investigated for the treatment of erectile dysfunction.

Assessment. Current evidence suggests that testosterone is not necessary for erectile function. However, hypogonadism is associated with decreased libido, and erectile failure could occur secondary to the decreased libido. A reliable estimate of libido is difficult to ascertain in some men. For this reason, serum androgen levels should be routinely assessed in cases of erectile failure without obvious etiology. Similarly, although hyperprolactinemia is infrequently encountered, it can give a misleading presentation, which

TABLE 12-5 Organic Etiologies of Erectile Dysfunction

aortic vascular disease	peripheral neuropathy
aorto-iliac reconstruction	proctocolectomy
arteriosclerosis	radiation therapy to pelvic floor
chronic alcoholism	radical prostatectomy
colectomy	renal failure
cystoprostectomy	retroperitoneal sympathectomy
diabetes mellitus	severe debilitation
laminectomy	spinal cord injury
lumbar sympathectomy	temporal lobe lesions
multiple sclerosis	urethral rupture
pelvic fracture	

suggests the need to determine serum prolactin as well. Despite a careful history, diagnosis will be unclear in a sizable minority of patients. In these situations, additional tests of erectile capacity and specific tests of vascular and neurologic integrity are often useful (see Table 12-6). Since the introduction of sildenafil, which has efficacy in erectile impairment from multiple etiologies, many clinicians question the need for additional procedures to establish a precise etiological diagnosis. Generalized approaches are useful when making the differential diagnosis between biogenic and psychogenic problems. The most common approach relies on the observation that most men have spontaneous erections during rapid eye movement sleep. Thus, it will be helpful to measure duration and rigidity of nocturnal erections (nocturnal tumescence testing). However, the absence of nocturnal erections does not establish an organic etiology. Diminished nocturnal erections are often a manifestation of major depressive disorder. The presence of nocturnal erections of adequate duration and turgidity essentially establishes the diagnosis of psychogenic erectile dysfunction.

Portable recording devices, which are used to measure nocturnal erections, are less expensive alternatives to sleep laboratory studies and are useful if the physician remembers that the absence of nocturnal erections may be related to poor sleep patterns. Because there are numerous ways to measure nocturnal sleep erections, methodological issues confound the interpretation of results. For example, there is no general agreement concerning the degree of turgidity and duration of nocturnal erections necessary to support normal erectile function during waking hours. Also, many men over the age of 60 who are sexually functional are likely to have diminished or absent nocturnal erections. A few specialized sexual disorders clinics use visual sexual stimulation or vibratory sexual stimulation for the differential diagnosis of erectile problems. However, these procedures have their limitations. Not all men respond to visual erotic material in a laboratory setting, and response to vibratory stimulation has received little study to date and has not been used extensively in the United States. Again, the presence of adequate erections of sufficient duration is compatible with a psychogenic diagnosis, while their absence conveys less diagnostic information.

TABLE 12-6 Testing for Erectile Dysfunction

General Screening Approaches (unclear etiology)
- Nocturnal tumescence testing
- Visual sexual stimulation
- Vibratory sexual stimulation
- Intracavernosal injection of vasoactive drugs

Specific Etiological Testing
- Penile brachial index
- Duplex ultrasound scanning
- Cavernosometry and cavernosography
- Angiography
- Intracavernous injection of vasoactive drugs
- Evoked potential studies

Some clinicians use erectile response to intracavernous injection of vasoactive agents as a diagnostic procedure, based on the assumption that a good erectile response establishes normal function. The specific doses and vasoactive agents have not been standardized. It is generally assumed that 80 mg of papaverine hydrochloride will produce a full erection within 10 to 15 minutes of injection and will last 15 to 30 minutes. To minimize the risk of priapism with this procedure, some researchers advocate smaller doses of papaverine hydrochloride combined with self-stimulation or vibration. It is assumed that the absence of a full erection 30 minutes after injection is consistent with an arterial inflow problem, which should be confirmed by selective internal pudendal arteriography. It should also be noted that an adequate response does not rule out a neurogenic etiology and that normative data are lacking to establish the parameters of a normal response.

Penile blood pressure can also be used as a general screening test. It is believed that the ratio of penile systolic blood pressure to brachial blood pressure should be 0.8 or higher in normal situations and that a value of 0.6 or lower is compatible with vasculogenic impotence. However, this test has a low specificity, and both false positives and false negatives have been reported using the penile-brachial index. Detection of the deep penile arteries with a nondirectional Doppler is difficult and often leads to false readings. Duplex sonography is more reliable, but inconsistent results are likely in the flaccid penis.

Pulsed Doppler with high-resolution ultrasonography after intracavernosal injection of vasoactive substances is the standard diagnostic tool for evaluating arterial inflow to erectile function. The measurement of peak systolic velocity is a function of time and the probe angle. A value of 25 mm/sec is considered to be the lower level of normal. One would expect to see a 60% to 70% increase in the cavernous artery. Unfortunately, convincing reference values do not exist.

Venous problems should be suspected if the patient is able to obtain full erections that are suddenly lost or if the patient responds substandardly to vasoactive intracavernosus injection. Venous competence can be evaluated using dynamic infusion cavernosometry followed by cavernosography. With dynamic cavernosometry, the rate of infusion necessary to both produce and maintain a full erection is measured. The infusion rate to produce full rigidity is approximately 180 mL/min and the rate to maintain an erection is approximately 80 mL/min. Unfortunately, this assessment has not been proved reliable. Cavernosography can be used to visualize the location of the abnormal venous drainage. However, some men with normal erectile function can appear to have abnormal drainage.

Various techniques are used to evaluate neurological function. However, none of these techniques has sufficient normative data for clear interpretation, except in extreme cases. These techniques include vibrotactile thresholds, conduction velocity in the dorsal nerve of the penis, somatosensory conduction time from the pudendal nerve to the sensory cortex, time between stimulation of the penile nerves until the bulbocavernosus muscle contracts, autonomic nerve stimulating the urethral wall and recording the time for the anal reflex to occur, and cystometrography.

Female Arousal Disorders

Female arousal problems are usually associated with diminished libido. Female difficulties with vaginal lubrication, independent of problems with libido, are uncommon in premenopausal women. In postmenopausal women, problems often involve atrophic

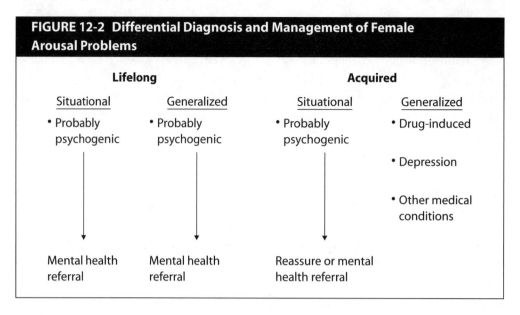

FIGURE 12-2 Differential Diagnosis and Management of Female Arousal Problems

Lifelong		Acquired	
Situational	Generalized	Situational	Generalized
• Probably psychogenic	• Probably psychogenic	• Probably psychogenic	• Drug-induced
			• Depression
			• Other medical conditions
↓	↓	↓	
Mental health referral	Mental health referral	Reassure or mental health referral	

vaginitis associated with decreased estrogen. These problems are usually alleviated by estrogen replacement. If estrogen replacement is not an option, such as in a patient with a history of breast cancer, commercially available water-based lubricants are often helpful. Normal libido and the lack of adequate lubrication in a premenopausal female should suggest problems with inadequate sexual stimulation.

Many women require relatively continuous psychological or physical stimulation to maintain arousal and vaginal lubrication. A woman who is aware of her decreased vaginal lubrication is likely to become apprehensive about what is happening and begin excessive self-observation. Shifting attention away from erotic stimuli to internal thoughts in turn interferes with lubrication. The effects of pharmacologic agents on female arousal are less well studied than the effects of such drugs on male erectile function. Presumably, the drugs that affect vasocongestion of male erectile tissue also interfere with vasocongestion of the perivaginal vasculature. Anticholinergic drugs and antihistaminic drugs have been reported as frequent offenders. The steps for making a differential diagnosis of female arousal problems and then managing these problems are shown in Figure 12-2. Studies of the efficacy of vasoactive agents (eg, sildenafil) in treating female arousal difficulties have usually been negative.

Premature Ejaculation

Case Vignette

Mr Adams, a 28-year-old married man in good health, comes to see his primary care physician, Dr Wales, at the urging of his wife, who tells him, "You come too fast, I need more time to get turned on, please get this fixed." Mr Adams reports that his first sexual encounters, which were in high school, involved fellatio and mutual masturbation, so that although he realized he ejaculated quickly, "it wasn't much of a problem at the time." Subsequently, his sexual contacts involved vaginal intercourse, and each of his girlfriends in college required manual stimulation to reach orgasm after he ejaculated within 30 to 60 seconds after penetration. This pattern continued with his last girlfriend, who is now his wife. He has tried distracting himself by thinking about nonsexual things, but this doesn't help. In college he occasionally masturbated before going on a date, but this seemed "ridiculous" to him, and it only helped delay his subsequent ejaculation a little bit. Physical examination was unremarkable.

This is one of the more common sexual complaints of younger male patients. One community survey found that 36% of self-described happily married men expressed dissatisfaction with how rapidly they ejaculated. Fortunately, this problem is readily treated by the primary care physician. Although usually assumed to be psychogenic, most cases are idiopathic. Men vary both in their propensity to rapid sexual arousal and in their ability to modulate arousal levels in sexual interactions. Clearly, an occasional episode of rapid ejaculation after an episode of abstinence or after encountering a new sexual partner is not diagnostic of a sexual disorder. The primary care physician can use two different types of treatment with these cases.

One approach is to use behavioral retraining of the ejaculatory reflex. In the most commonly used approach, the start-stop technique, the patient and his partner are told to refrain from coitus for a number of weeks. The partner is instructed to stimulate the patient either manually or orally, with the patient not attempting to avoid ejaculation but attempting to monitor his level of arousal. When the patient feels that ejaculation is imminent with further stimulation, he signals for stimulation to stop. This is repeated three times; on the fourth time, the patient is told not to signal but enjoy the experience of ejaculation. If the patient and his partner comply with these instructions, the patient will begin to experience greater latency after stimulation and prior to ejaculation with repeated trials. After the patient is able to undergo 5 to 10 minutes of manual stimulation without ejaculation, the partner is told to sit on top and insert the penis into her vagina. The same start-stop rhythm is again used to establish ejaculatory control with vaginal penetration. In cases of severe premature ejaculation, ie, ejaculation prior to penetration or immediately thereafter, this behavioral approach may not work.

An alternative approach is to achieve ejaculatory delay using pharmacologic agents. Double-blind studies have demonstrated the efficacy of using clomipramine hydrochloride, sertraline hydrochloride, fluoxetine hydrochloride, and paroxetine hydrochloride to control rapid ejaculation. These agents inhibit the reuptake of serotonin; the inhibitory effect of serotonin on ejaculation is felt to be the mechanism responsible for this effect. Of the SSRIs, clomipramine hydrochloride is the preferred agent because it can be taken on an as-needed basis.

One double-blind study demonstrated that men with severe premature ejaculation could be successfully treated with 25 to 50 mg of clomipramine hydrochloride taken approximately 6 hours prior to planned coital activities. This dose level is associated with minimal side effects. If the patient does not have an opportunity for coitus as planned, he can repeat the dose prior to the next planned event. If planning coitus in advance is difficult, clomipramine hydrochloride at doses of 25 to 50 mg can be taken on a daily basis. Current evidence suggests that premature ejaculation will return when the drug is discontinued. Alternative strategies include chronic dosing with 100 to 150 mg sertraline hydrochloride or 20 to 40 mg paroxetine hydrochloride. It appears that ejaculatory delay will occur after 3 or 4 weeks of taking the drug. If the SSRIs are ineffective, an alternative strategy (reported in a single case study) is to use 1 to 3 mg lorazepam taken 1 or 2 hours prior to coitus. None of these strategies has FDA approval.

Anorgasmia and Ejaculatory Delay

The primary care physician must establish whether anorgasmia is lifelong or acquired and, if acquired, whether it is situation specific or generalized. Lifelong anorgasmia in males is infrequently encountered in clinical practice; consequently, a large knowledge base concerning treatment of this syndrome is lacking. Masters and Johnson reported only 17 couples with retarded ejaculation out of 510 couples. Lifelong anorgasmia is usually assumed to be the result of severe psychological inhibition. Sexual desensitization therapy coupled with masturbatory training is usually used to treat anorgasmia. Table 12-7 schematically shows the differential diagnosis of anorgasmia. In general, this schematic can be used for males with delayed or absent ejaculation, as well.

Lifelong anorgasmia in females is far more common and has a much better prognosis. It appears to be related to a combination of inexperience and anxiety or guilt regarding the experience of sexual pleasure. If the female has just begun sexual activity, it is possible that the orgasmic reflex will become active with continued sexual experience in a supportive relationship. The lack of orgasm is likely to be related to the relative lack of sexual experience in both the female and her partner. The prognosis in these cases is generally favorable.

Behavioral sex therapy, which is the treatment of choice, usually involves systematic desensitization to prohibitions about the experience of sexual pleasure and instruction on how to achieve orgasm with masturbation. If the patient cooperates with treatment, failure to achieve orgasm with masturbation is infrequent. Some women who achieve orgasm with masturbation are then able to experience orgasm during coitus. Women who are unable to achieve orgasm in coitus can experience orgasm during some form of shared sexual activity with the partner. Numerous studies have addressed the frequency with which women reach orgasm during coitus as a continuum. At one extreme is the rare female who can reach orgasm through sexual fantasy alone. Approximately 20% to 30% of women experience orgasm during coitus without simultaneous manual clitoral stimulation. Many women require direct manual clitoral stimulation to reach orgasm, and approximately 5% of women report a lifetime inability to reach orgasm.

Acquired problems relating to orgasm for women are more common than lifelong problems. If the acquired problem is generalized, various possible organic etiologies including pharmacologically induced anorgasmia and ejaculatory disorder in the partner should be considered. Depressive illness often interferes with orgasmic capacity. Other common causes of acquired difficulty with orgasm involve damage to the nerves mediating orgasm. These include diseases such as diabetes mellitus and multiple

TABLE 12-7 Female Orgasm Disorder		
	Acquired	
Lifelong	**Situational**	**Generalized**
Minimal sexual exposure	Relationship discord	Depression
Restrictive sexual attitude	Poor sexual technique	Drug-induced
		Organic etiology
		Situational stress

sclerosis as well as surgical procedures such as colorectal surgery, which can damage these nerves.

Drug-induced orgasm disorders are frequently related to antihypertensive medication and psychiatric drugs such as antidepressants, antipsychotics, and minor tranquilizers. Anorgasmia and delayed ejaculation are common side effects of SSRIs. However, anti-depressant-induced anorgasmia can usually be reversed by substituting a drug with less adverse impact on sexual function, such as bupropion or nefazodone. Tables 12-8 and 12-9 list drugs and physical conditions commonly associated with orgasm and ejaculatory problems.

Person-specific acquired anorgasmia is usually related to interpersonal discord and requires referral. Anorgasmia becomes a problem because it is upsetting to the patient or the patient's partner. "Orgasmic failure only becomes a problem . . . if her partner's offended narcissism causes him to complain and he puts her under pressure, or she herself sets unrealistic orgasmic standards" (see Arentiwicz and Schmidt, p 24). Marital therapy or sex therapy with a marital focus are the preferred treatment approaches.

TABLE 12-8 Drugs Associated With Orgasm and/or Ejaculation Difficulties

alprazolam	fluvoxamine maleate	perphenazine
amitriptyline	guanethidine	phenelzine
amoxapine	haloperidol	protriptyline
bethanidine	imipramine hydrochloride	sertraline hydrochloride
chlordiazepoxide		thioridazine
chlorpromazine	isocarboxazid	thiothixene
chlorprothixene	lorazepam	tranylcypromine
clomipramine hydrochloride	maprotiline	trazodone
	mesoridazine besylate	trifluoperazine hydrochloride
desipramine	methyldopa	
doxepin	naproxen	venlafaxine hydrochloride
fluoxetine hydrochloride	nortriptyline	
fluphenazine	paroxetine hydrochloride	

TABLE 12-9 Organic Causes of Orgasm and Ejaculation Disorder

- Cerebral vascular accident
- Peripheral nerve injury
- Multiple sclerosis
- Tabes dorsalis
- Cord injury
- Sympathectomy
- Retroperitoneal lymphadenectomy
- Proctocolectomy
- Aortic-iliac surgery
- Cystectomy
- Diabetes mellitus

In men with acquired generalized ejaculatory incompetence, the possibility of organic factors should be considered. A physical exam that includes testing peripheral sensation to touch, pinprick, and vibration; testing reflex contraction of the anal sphincter with a digital insertion in the rectum; testing the bulbocavernosus reflex; and testing the cremasteric reflex should be performed. A careful history should exclude anorgasmia induced by drug and alcohol abuse. In rare cases, pituitary adenoma may be encountered. Retarded ejaculation can be distinguished from retrograde ejaculation by examining a postejaculatory urine sample. There are minimal data regarding the treatment of acquired psychogenic ejaculatory incompetence in men.

Dyspareunia

Dyspareunia, a term of ancient Greek origin, literally means difficult mating. Male dyspareunia (pain during coitus) is usually physical in etiology and is a rather uncommon complaint in primary care settings. Common causes include dermatological lesions, urethritis, phimosis, balanitis, chordee, plaques, and Peyronie disease. Sexual arousal that does not culminate in ejaculation can lead to prostatic engorgement and referred pain. Some men report postcoital pain, which appears to be related to spasms of the perineal muscles. Dyspareunia has also been reported with certain psychotropic agents such as imipramine hydrochloride and thioridazine. Urethral strictures from gonorrhea can be associated with painful orgasm in the male.

For cases of female dyspareunia, the primary care physician must first rule out insufficient lubrication secondary to inadequate sexual stimulation. Causes of dyspareunia in the female can be divided into those that affect the outer vagina and those that affect the inner vagina. Pain attributed to the outer one third of the vagina suggests an intact hymen, scarring, trauma, vaginismus, or urethritis. Pain from deep thrusting is compatible with scarring of the uterus, bladder, or adnexae; endometriosis; or ectopic pregnancy. Psychogenic dyspareunia is often a diagnosis by exclusion: It is often associated with a history of childhood sexual abuse.

Female dyspareunia, a common complaint in primary care settings, can be difficult to adequately treat. The verbal report of the pain intensity often bears little correlation with physical findings. Management is best handled by a multidisciplinary team (eg, gynecologist, psychiatrist, psychologist, pain medicine physician) if one is available. A careful history will suggest possible etiological factors. If the problem is acquired, the situation or event that preceded its onset, such as childbirth or a vaginal infection, should be determined. Other clues include accompanying symptoms such as vaginal dryness, pain, or paresthesias in the genital or pelvic area, which is often indicative of pudendal neuralgia. In cases of situational dyspareunia, precipitants in the relationship should be identified.

Vaginismus

Vaginismus, which is the spastic contraction of the outer one third of vaginal musculature when penetration is attempted, has either psychological or organic etiologies. The common factor appears to be the woman's fear that vaginal penetration will be painful. In some cases, this anxiety is based on painful past experiences with penetration. Dyspareunia often precedes development of vaginismus. Any cause of pelvic pain can be associated with vaginismus. Lifelong histories of vaginismus in sexually inexperienced women are often purely psychogenic. Such cases have a good prognosis with behavioral therapy, which usually involves the insertion of vaginal dilators of gradually increasing size over a period of weeks to months until the vaginal muscle spasm subsides completely. A sex therapist or a trained gynecologist often performs this therapy. Acquired vaginismus is infrequently encountered in most clinical practices. Note that vaginismus is an early sign of spasticity in the perineal muscles as the result of peripheral nerve or spinal cord lesions such as in multiple sclerosis.

Paraphilias

Paraphilias refers to a miscellaneous group of sexual behaviors that are either illegal or strongly socially disapproved. These behaviors are encountered somewhat infrequently in a typical primary care practice. Their infrequent appearance combined with the some-what unusual nature of the sexual arousal pattern described by these patients continues to confuse many practitioners concerning appropriate treatment. Behaviors that do not cause serious disruption to a patient's life and that do not cause harm to others, such as fetishism and transvestism, are often better left untreated, unless the atypical sexual arousal pattern is a source of considerable distress to the patient. The patient's partner is often the major force to insist on treatment. Table 12-10 lists definitions of common paraphilias. Case definitions require that the sexual arousal be intense and recurrent for at least 6 months' duration.

Other types of paraphilias such as pedophilia, exhibitionism, voyeurism, and frot-teurism, which involve others in nonconsenting behavior, are more likely to receive treatment. This treatment is frequently court ordered, and the patient is only partially compliant with treatment. Because these patients are concerned about being incarcerated, they often underreport the frequency and variety of sexual offenses committed. Treatment of these disorders usually involves a multifaceted approach. Typically, an attempt will be made to reduce the sex drive in order to control the behavior and spare future victims. In Scandinavia, this usually involves castration. In other European countries and Canada, cyproterone acetate is used to diminish libido. In America, medroxyprogesterone acetate is a widely used antiandrogen used to treat sex offenders. Recently, successful use of SSRIs to treat paraphilias has been reported.

TABLE 12-10 Definitions of Common Paraphilias

- Exhibitionism: sexual arousal to exposure of one's genitals to unsuspecting strangers

- Fetishism: intensive sexual arousal to nonliving objects (eg, female undergarments)

- Frotteurism: sexual arousal to touching or rubbing nonconsenting persons

- Pedophilia: sexual arousal to sexual activity with children

- Sexual masochism: sexual arousal to the act of being humiliated, beaten, or bound

- Sexual sadism: sexual arousal to the act of causing psychological or physical suffering to the sexual partner

- Transvestic fetishism: sexual arousal in a heterosexual male to acts involving cross-dressing

- Voyeurism: sexual arousal by observing an unsuspecting person in the nude or disrobing

The other major form of treatment involves behavior therapy. Therapy includes any or all of the following: (1) identifying behavior that precedes the unwanted behavior and teaching the patient ways to interrupt the behavioral sequence leading to unwanted sexual behavior; (2) social skills training so that the patient will be able to find less problematic forms of sexual gratification; (3) counterconditioning the sexual arousal pattern; and (4) cognitive restructuring of the person's perception of his behavior.

SUMMARY

Although patients may be reluctant to mention sexual complaints to their physicians, primary care physicians do commonly encounter these conditions. In most cases, a careful history and physical examination will clarify the diagnosis and even the specific etiology. These procedures also suggest the most appropriate type of specialty referral for additional evaluation or treatment. Primary care physicians play an important role in managing many acquired sexual disorders through patient education, pharmacologic treatment, and behavioral or other focused psychotherapies.

ADDITIONAL READINGS

Arentiwicz G, Schmidt G. *The Treatment of Sexual Disorders: Concepts and Techniques of Couple Therapy.* New York, NY: Basic Books; 1983:24.

Binik YM, Bergeron S, Khalife S. Dyspareunia. In: Leiblum SR, Rosen RC, eds. *Principles and Practice of Sex Therapy.* New York, NY: Guilford Press; 2000:154-180.

Graziottin A, Castoldi E, Montorsi F, Salonia A, Maga T. Vulvodynia: the challenge of unexplained genital pain. *J Sex Marital Ther.* 2001;27:503-512.

Leiblum SR. Sexual pain disorders. In: Gabbard GO, ed. *Treatments of Psychiatric Disorders.* 3rd ed. Washington, DC: American Psychiatric Press Inc; 2001:1935-1950.

Riley A, May K. Sexual desire disorders. In: Gabbard GO, ed. *Treatments of Psychiatric Disorders.* 3rd ed. Washington, DC: American Psychiatric Press Inc; 2001:1849-1872.

Sadovsky R, Miller T, Moskowitz M, Hackett G. Three year update of sildenafil citrate (Viagra) efficacy and safety. *Int J Clin Pract.* 2001;55:115-128.

Segraves RT, Althof S. Psychotherapy and pharmacotherapy for sexual dysfunction. In: Nathan PE, Gorman JM, eds. *A Guide to Treatment that Works.* 2nd ed. New York, NY: Oxford University Press; 2002:497-524.

Chapter **13**

Eating Disorders and Obesity

Joel Yager, MD
Brenda Erickson, MD

Anorexia nervosa and bulimia nervosa, as they are recognized today, were first described in the late 1870s and 1950s, respectively. Binge eating disorder as a discrete entity is still being delineated and refined from the larger, ill-defined group of compulsive overeating disorders. Increased awareness of these problems is largely the result of media attention to female celebrities with eating disorders. Ironically, the media's ubiquitous pressure for women to be slim has almost certainly contributed to the increasing prevalence of these disorders while highlighting their deleterious effects on physical and psychological health.

Obesity, per se, is a medical condition that is not considered to be a mental disorder; the mental health of obese patients generally parallels that of other populations. Therefore, review of obesity in this chapter is limited. However, obesity's relationship to mental disorders bears attention. Obesity is common in patients with binge eating disorder—substantial self-disparagement and psychological impairment are common in severely obese individuals, and many contemporary psychotropic medications used for psychosis and bipolar disorder result in significant weight gain.

This chapter reviews assessment, diagnosis, clinical features, etiologic theories, and treatment of anorexia nervosa, bulimia nervosa, and binge eating disorder. The chapter concludes with a discussion concerning the management of obesity.

ROLE OF THE PRIMARY CARE PHYSICIAN

Primary care physicians can play a major role in preventing, detecting, and managing patients with eating disorders. The physician should be suspicious of teenage and young adult patients who are excessively concerned about dieting and physical appearance and should educate them about good nutrition, healthy attitudes toward the body, dangers of unrealistic dieting, and eating disorders. Because these disorders are so prevalent, physicians should routinely question all young female patients about their desired weight, dieting habits, and exercise patterns. In young women in particular, depression, anxiety, perfectionism, obsessive-compulsive symptoms, and emotional lability should trigger attention to eating disorder symptoms as well as to mood disorders, substance use, and sexual issues.

After an eating disorder is detected, patients require a full physical exam and screening laboratory tests. Blood chemistry studies for all patients with eating disorders should include electrolytes, blood urea nitrogen (BUN), creatinine, thyroid-stimulating hormone (TSH), complete blood count (CBC), and urinalysis. Malnourished and severely symptomatic patients require serum calcium, phosphorus, and liver function tests, and an electrocardiogram should be performed. For patients who have been underweight longer than 6 months, dual-energy x-ray absorptiometry (DEXA), particularly of the lumbar spine and femoral neck, and estradiol levels (testosterone level in males) are advised. For specific unusual indications, nonroutine assessment may include serum amylase level in cases of persistent or recurrent vomiting, luteinizing hormone (LH) and follicle-stimulating hormone (FSH) levels for persistent amenorrhea at normal weight, and stool for phenolphthalein for patients with suspected laxative abuse. Brain magnetic resonance imaging (MRI) and computerized tomography (CT) scans are not routinely indicated.

The primary care physician should work with a registered dietitian and mental health professional, both knowledgeable about eating disorders, to ascertain whether the problem can be managed on an outpatient basis. This multidisciplinary approach can be highly successful with motivated patients. The primary care physician's role is to educate and counsel the patient and monitor the patient's weight and laboratory tests. Monitoring of patients with anorexia nervosa should include weekly or twice weekly visits to the office for stripped postvoiding weigh-ins and ongoing monitoring of any physiological abnormalities of concern. For example, marked orthostatic changes, severe bradycardia, and hypothermia are physiological indications for urgent hospitalization. Rapid weight loss in children and adolescents, even in the absence of marked physiological changes, may warrant hospitalization.

For patients with bulimia nervosa and mood or anxiety disorders associated with the eating disorder, the primary care physician should also prescribe and monitor a course of antidepressant therapy. The extent to which the primary care physician is willing and/or able to assume a more involved role with the psychological and familial issues varies with the clinician's comfort and expertise as well as the complexity of the patient and family situation.

Every patient with a serious eating disorder merits consultation with a psychiatrist knowledgeable in this area who can inform the patient, family, and referring physician about the nature, severity, prognosis, and available treatment options. The primary care physician can expect explicit guidance from the consultant for psychosocial and medical management. Specific indications for mandatory consultation include failure of the patient to respond to initial management attempts, deteriorating psychological and/or physical status, severe depression, suicidality, and/or marked family disturbances.

EPIDEMIOLOGY OF EATING DISORDERS

The prevalence of clinically significant eating disorders among adolescent and young adult women is about 4% and may be as high as 8% for more broadly defined syndromes. These disorders are much less prevalent in other populations, although rates are increasing in males, older women, and ethnic minorities. Women constitute 90% to 95% of cases of anorexia nervosa (AN) and bulimia nervosa (BN), with the age of onset typically in teenage and early adult years; BN and binge eating disorder (BED) are more common than AN. In the community at large the prevalence of BN is estimated to be 1% to 2%; BED, 2% to 5%; and AN, less than 1%. Eating disorders–associated symptoms are extremely common and include:

- body image distortion;
- extreme fear of being fat;
- the desire to reduce body fat to levels below those ordinarily considered healthy;
- restrictive and fad dieting;
- stimulant and cocaine abuse for anorectic effects;
- purging by means of vomiting, laxative abuse, diuretic abuse;
- compulsive exercise; and
- poor self-esteem.

Some of these symptoms occur subclinically in a majority of certain female subgroups, eg, college sororities, gymnastics teams, ballet groups, or cheerleading squads. Obesity, defined as being 20% above recommended weight, is very prevalent, occurring in 30% to 40% of some American subpopulations. Mild obesity accounts for about 90% of the obese, moderate obesity (weight 40% to 100% above recommended weight) accounts for approximately 9.5%, and severe or very severe, "morbid" obesity accounts for about 0.5%.

DIAGNOSING EATING DISORDERS

Case Vignette

Wendy, a 16-year-old high school sophomore, is brought to her physician's office by her parents because she has been losing weight. They report that her weight was 140 pounds (63 kg) 6 months earlier and that she began to diet, planning to lose about 5 kg over several months. She lost this amount in 3 weeks, yet continued to maintain a severely reduced intake, largely subsisting on diet soft drinks and raw vegetables, until she reached her current weight of 95 pounds (43 kg). She is 5'4" (163 cm) tall, so her BMI has gone from 24 kg/m² to 16 kg/m². Wendy readily admits that she lost this weight and seems rather proud of it, adding that she wants to lose an additional 10 to 15 pounds "because I'm still a little too fat." She says she has stopped menstruating, "but that's fine with me." She reports a good mood and "tons of energy"; she works out at least five times a week for at least an hour each time "to get rid of even more calories." She denies ever forcing herself to vomit after eating or using diuretics or laxatives. Physical examination reveals a somewhat cachectic-appearing young woman with a pulse of 60 bpm and a blood pressure of 85/63 mm Hg. She has lanugo hair and Tanner stage 5 sexual development. Anorexia nervosa is diagnosed and negotiations about a suitable treatment plan are started.

Current diagnostic criteria for AN and BN (based on *Diagnostic and Statistical Manual of Mental Disorders*, fourth edition [DSM-IV]), are shown in Tables 13-1 and 13-2. BED,

---

TABLE 13-1 Diagnostic Criteria for Anorexia Nervosa

- Refusal to maintain weight above a minimally normal weight for age and height, leading to body weight 15% below expected, or failure to gain weight as expected during growth, leading to body weight 15% below expected.

- Intense fear of gaining weight or becoming fat, even though underweight.

- Disturbance in the way in which one's body weight or shape is experienced, undue influence of body weight or shape on self-evaluation, or denial of the seriousness of the current low body weight.

- In postmenarche females, amenorrhea, ie, the absence of at least three consecutive menstrual cycles.

Binge-eating/purging type: The patient regularly engages in binge-eating or purging behavior (ie, self-induced vomiting or the misuse of laxative, diuretics, or enemas).

Restricting type: The patient has not regularly engaged in binge-eating or purging behavior.

TABLE 13-2 Diagnostic Criteria for Bulimia Nervosa

- Recurrent episodes of binge eating (eating in a discrete period of time, eg, within 2 hours, an amount of food that is definitely larger than most people would eat under similar circumstances). During these binges the person feels that the eating is out of control.

- Recurrent inappropriate compensatory behavior in order to prevent weight gain, such as self-induced vomiting; misuse of laxatives, diuretics, enemas, or other medications; fasting; or excessive exercise.*

- The binging and compensatory behaviors both occur, on average, at least twice a week for 3 months.

- Self-evaluation is unduly influenced by body shape and weight.

- The disturbance does not occur exclusively during episodes of AN.

---

*Purging type: The patient regularly engages in self-induced vomiting or the misuse of laxatives, diuretics, or enemas.

Nonpurging type: The patient uses other inappropriate compensatory behaviors, such as fasting or excessive exercise, but has not regularly engaged in self-induced vomiting or the misuse of laxatives, diuretics, or enemas.

characterized by binge eating without the purging aspects of bulimia, is currently under consideration as a distinct diagnosis. Research criteria for BED are shown in Table 13-3. There appears to be a continuum among symptom complexes of self-starvation and the binge-purge cycle. Many patients demonstrate both anorectic and bulimic symptoms or alternate between the two. About half of patients with AN binge eat and purge, and many patients with BN have prior histories of AN.

TABLE 13-3 Research Diagnostic Criteria for Binge Eating Disorder

- Recurrent episodes of binge eating (eating in a discrete period of time, eg, within 2 hours, an amount of food that is definitely larger than what most people would eat under similar circumstances). During these binges the person feels that the eating is out of control.

- The binge eating episodes are associated with three or more of the following:

    Eating much more rapidly than normal

    Eating until feeling uncomfortably full

    Eating large amounts of food when not feeling physically hungry

    Eating alone because of being embarrassed by how much one is eating

    Feeling disgusted with oneself, depressed, or very guilty after overeating

- Marked distress regarding the binge eating present.

- The binge eating occurs, on average, at least 2 days a week for 6 months.

- The binge eating is not associated with the regular use of inappropriate compensatory behaviors (eg, purging, fasting, excessive exercise) and does not occur exclusively during the course of AN or BN.

It is best to ask patients about eating patterns and attitudes directly and sympathetically. The following information should be collected:

- Weight history, including maximum and minimum weights
- Desired weight
- Weight preoccupations
- Body image distortions
- Dieting and fasting behaviors
- Food avoidances and self-defined "allergies" or "sensitivities"
- Binge eating—frequency and quantity
- Purging (vomiting, laxatives, diuretics, emetics)
- Regular and compulsive exercise
- Over-the-counter, prescription, and illicit diet pills
- Unusual beliefs about nutrition
- Menstrual history

Tactful questions to elicit such information include: How much do you weigh, and how much do you really want to weigh? What do you think is really a healthy weight for you—the weight where your menstruation and ovulation are best and where you have the most energy and vigor? To what extent do you find yourself unhappy with the way you look? Do you ever spend time in front of the mirror just looking at your body, or parts of your body, wishing they looked different? What sorts of things have you tried to make sure you don't gain weight?

Anorexia Nervosa

AN appears in restricting and binge eating-purging subtypes, which occasionally alternate in the same patient. Restricters may limit intake to as little as a few hundred kilocalories per day, with narrow food selection, obsessional thoughts, and compulsive behaviors regarding food, eating habits, and exercise. Binge eating-purging subtypes are unable to refrain from these behaviors, although some patients purge without actually binge eating. They are often self-destructive; may have impulsive, dramatic, and emotional personality structures; and sometimes abuse alcohol and drugs. At least 50% of patients with AN develop major depression; at least a third have significant anxiety disorders; and virtually all demonstrate mood lability, irritability, and some degree of social isolation. The lifetime prevalence of obsessive-compulsive disorder is about 25%. Many patients have avoidant, shy, and/or perfectionistic personalities; in chronic cases, many complain of having no real sense of who they are apart from their eating disorder.

Patients with AN present in various stages of malnutrition. Although weight loss leading to a weight that is at least 15% below normal is necessary for the diagnosis, patients often lose considerably more weight than this before presenting for medical attention. Often, family members seek treatment for such patients against their will.

Full recovery occurs in 30% to 50% of patients. The best prognosis is seen in younger-onset patients and restricting subtypes, although full recovery may take 5 to 7 years even in these patients. Death from starvation, cardiac arrhythmias, and suicide occurs in 5% to 10% of patients within 10 years and in nearly 20% within 20 years. The death rate has been estimated to be 12 times higher than comparably aged nonclinical populations and twice that of any other female psychiatric population.

Bulimia Nervosa

BN is manifest by recurrent episodes of binge eating and purging in which patients binge eat large quantities of food in a short, discrete time period. Two subtypes have been defined: the purging type uses self-induced vomiting, laxatives, or diuretics to avoid weight gain, and the nonpurging type uses other inappropriate compensatory behaviors such as excessive exercising or fasting. Patients frequently consume between 2000 and 10,000 kilocalories per binge episode, and binge-purge cycles may occur up to several times per day. Patients feel that their eating is entirely out of control. Many are secretive about this problem due to shame. Most patients with BN are distressed by their condition and want to change. As many as 75% concurrently suffer from major depression or anxiety disorder; patients also show increased rates of alcohol use, substance abuse, and personality disorders.

Binge Eating Disorder

BED is characterized by recurrent binge eating without the inappropriate compensatory behaviors seen in BN. It is more common among females than males, but males constitute 35% of patients, a much higher percentage than in other eating disorders. Quite common among individuals seeking obesity treatment, it is estimated that 70% of participants in Overeaters Anonymous and 25% to 30% of participants in weight loss programs display BED. This disorder is also associated with significant psychiatric comorbidity, particularly mood and anxiety disorders, although comorbid rates are not as high as for other eating disorders.

Associated Medical Findings

Patients with AN and/or BN may have severe medical complications, including sequelae of malnutrition, even if they are of normal weight. These medical complications are summarized in Table 13-4.

Many patients appear superficially healthy, even when seriously underweight, and continue to deny the seriousness of their condition. Accordingly, careful assessment is necessary. The signs and symptoms of starvation often accompany the weight loss and include fat depletion, muscle wasting (in severe cases cardiac muscle involvement), marked orthostatic hypotension, constipation, leukopenia, hypercortisolemia, cold intolerance, hypothermia, gastric motility disturbances, and lanugo (fine babylike hair over the body). Metabolic alterations to conserve energy may result in low T_3, LH, and FSH levels. Cardiac abnormalities range from bradycardia and benign arrhythmias to premature ventricular contractions and consequent sudden death. Toxic myopathies, including cardiomyopathy, are associated with the chronic use of ipecac to induce vomiting.

By definition, all postmenarchal female patients with AN stop menstruating; up to a third stop menstruating prior to losing enough fat reserve to account for the amenorrhea. Prepubertal growth arrest is common, and patients may not grow to their anticipated heights. Amenorrhea that lasts longer than 6 months is associated with potentially irreversible osteopenia and osteoporosis and increased rates of pathologic fractures. AN patients in their mid-20s with prolonged amenorrhea sustain stress fractures at about seven times expected rates. Infertility is common; eating disorders account for about 20% of cases seen in infertility clinics.

TABLE 13-4 Medical Complications of Eating Disorders

Related to Weight Loss

- *Cachexia:* Loss of body fat, muscle mass, reduced metabolism (low T_3 syndrome), cold intolerance, and difficulty maintaining core body temperature

- *Cardiac:* Loss of cardiac muscle, small heart size, cardiac arrhythmias, including atrial and ventricular premature contractions, prolonged Q-T interval, bradycardia, ventricular tachycardia, sudden death

- *Dermatologic:* Lanugo (fine baby-like hair covering body), edema

- *Gastrointestinal:* Delayed gastric emptying, bloating, constipation, abdominal pain

- *Hematologic:* Leukopenia

- *Neuropsychiatric:* Abnormal taste sensation, apathetic depression, mild organic mental symptoms; white and gray matter volume shrinks with malnutrition

- *Renal:* Impaired renal function—decreased glomerular filtration rate

- *Reproductive:* Amenorrhea, low LH and FSH, infertility

- *Skeletal:* Osteopenia and osteoporosis

Related to Purging (vomiting and laxative or diuretic abuse)

- *Metabolic:* Electrolyte abnormalities, particularly hypokalemia, hypochloremic alkalosis, hypomagnesemia

- *Gastrointestinal:* Salivary gland hypertrophy, pancreatic inflammation with increase in serum amylase, esophageal and gastric erosion, dysfunctional bowel with dilatation

- *Dental:* Erosion of dental enamel, particularly affecting front teeth, with corresponding decay

- *Neuropsychiatric:* Seizures, mild neuropathies, fatigue, weakness, mild organic mental symptoms

Common physical findings from binge eating and purging include parotid gland hypertrophy from overstimulation, resulting in "chipmunk cheeks"; dental enamel erosion and decay, especially behind the incisors due to gastric acid wash; and scars on the dorsum of the hand due to recurrent abrasions sustained during self-induced vomiting.

Abnormal laboratory findings may include:

- metabolic abnormalities, particularly hypochloremic, hypokalemic alkalosis, hypomagnesemia, low zinc levels;
- elevated amylase (25% to 40%), cortisol, reverse T_3, carotene, and cholesterol levels;
- abnormal liver function tests;
- occasional hypoglycemia;
- neutropenia with relative lymphocytosis.

Obesity

A full discussion of the medical aspects of obesity is beyond the scope of this chapter. However, assessment and classification of the obese patient is related to the extent to which the individual is overweight, often assessed as body mass index (BMI), calculated as weight in kilograms divided by height in meters squared. Clinical consensus guidelines and standard tables are cited in the list of suggested readings. Briefly, normal BMIs range from 18.5 to 24.9 and mild overweight BMIs range from 25.0 to 29.9. Obesity, diagnosed at BMIs >30.0, is categorized as follows:

- Class I (moderate)   BMI 30.0 to 34.9
- Class II (severe)   BMI 35.0 to 39.9
- Class III (very severe)   BMI >40.0

ETIOLOGY AND PATHOGENESIS

Theories regarding the causes of eating disorders have implicated biological, psychological, family, and sociocultural factors. The common risk factor for all eating disorders is a history of dieting. Additionally, a premorbid tendency toward being overweight or obese may contribute to the risk of BN and BED.

Biological Theories

Primary proximal biologic influences in eating disorders are those related to hunger and starvation. Healthy volunteers who lose 25% of their usual healthy weight through dieting become irritable, moody, depressed, food-obsessed, socially isolated, and apathetic; all of these symptoms are consistent with those found in eating disorders. Furthermore, when food is available, these same volunteers often binge eat and hoard food. Even after regaining their weight, full psychological recovery may take 6 to 12 months. In other words, many of the mood- and food-related psychological and behavioral symptoms seen in AN may result from the severe starvation rather than be causative. Hunger itself is thought to be the primary stimulus for binge eating in low- and normal-weight bulimics because the drive to eat overtakes the patient's desire and ability to restrain eating. Other, still largely speculative, biological theories invoke genetic vulnerability and assorted physiological and neurotransmitter abnormalities at or above the level of the hypothalamus.

Psychological Theories

Eating disorders have been associated with several, not mutually exclusive, pathological psychological processes. Although they have not been established as etiologic, the following models have offered useful psychotherapeutic strategies:

- *Maladaptive learned responses:* These are responses, based on classical or operant conditioning, that reduce anxiety. In AN, food avoidance may reduce anxiety due to food or weight phobias. In contrast, binge eating in BN or BED may initially reduce anxiety. Secondary anxiety resulting from overeating or loss of control may, in turn, be relieved by purging.
- *Cognitive distortions:* These misguided, erroneous, obsessional, self-directed statements confuse self-worth with physical appearance and have a self-reinforcing quality. The distortions may include overgeneralizations, magnification of minor issues, and "all or none" thinking, eg, "If I permit myself one bite of chocolate, I'll turn into a fat pig."
- *Perceptual distortions regarding body size:* Such perceptions are ubiquitous among women, but the extent and degree of such distortions are greater among women with eating disorders.
- *Difficulty identifying inner sensory and emotional states:* Sensory states include hunger and satiety (interocepts) and emotional states include anger or disappointment.

- *A pervasive sense of ineffectiveness and low self-worth:* These perceptions are frequent precursors of eating disorders. These patients may learn to put on a false front of competence and look after their parents' needs but ignore their own. What may develop in appearance-preoccupied families is a pre-anorexic child whose face to the world, which is a "false self," seems like the "best little girl in the world."
- *Conflicts over adolescent development and sexual maturation:* AN results in regression to a largely prepubertal state, both physiologically and psychologically. Thus, AN may serve to put off the developmental tasks of adolescence, including identity formation, emerging sexuality, and separation from the family.

Family Theories

Although dysfunctional family patterns are common in the general population, they are far from ubiquitous and by themselves are neither necessary nor sufficient to cause eating disorders. Nonetheless, families with higher rates of familial depression, eating disorders, and alcoholism seem more likely than others to produce children with eating disorders. Such families may also exhibit destructive patterns of unrelenting criticism toward the patient (negative expressed emotion), enmeshment between parent and child, and a preoccupation with weight and appearance. Patterns of childhood physical, psychological, and sexual abuse and other less overt forms of parental "boundary violations" and overintrusiveness have been cited as contributing factors to BN, in particular. Blaming parents for their child's eating disorder is not therapeutically useful; however, involving parents in recovery is useful.

Sociocultural Theories

The prevalence of eating disorders has paralleled society's attitudes about beauty and fashion, documented by the steadily decreasing weights among fashion models, center-folds, and beauty pageant winners over the past 40 years. Popular views promoting thinness as a way of attaining desirable high status are thought to have contributed to increased rates of these disorders.

Etiology of Obesity

Obesity results from a variety of complicated biological, psychological, and social influences. More than 200 genes related to eating, metabolism, and energy expenditure have been identified that may contribute to individual propensities for obesity. The heritability of obesity is estimated to be at least 50%, with genetic influences greater in severe forms of obesity. Research currently centers on a variety of peptides and their receptors, including leptin, ghrelin, and gastric-inhibitory polypeptide. Other important obesity-related risk factors include food-oriented family environments during early childhood, access to food, cultural attitudes regarding eating and body shape, and demands for physical activity. For most people, excessive intake of calories from readily available highly palatable foods and insufficient physical exercise contribute significantly to high rates of obesity.

TREATMENT OF EATING DISORDERS

Treatment for eating disorders must be based on thorough assessments that attend to physical status, psychological and behavioral features, comorbid psychiatric conditions, and family dynamics. A multidisciplinary team approach (eg, primary care physician, psychiatrist, psychotherapist, dietitian) is usually necessary. Treatment includes weight normalization; symptom reduction through cognitive-behavioral strategies; nutrition counseling; supportive nursing care; individual, family, and sometimes group psychotherapies; and psychopharmacological intervention for appropriate patients. Optimal treatments combine these elements pragmatically and are adjusted in relation to each patient's motivational stage and readiness for change.

Anorexia Nervosa

Low weight. Weight restoration should be the first and central focus of treatment for AN. Weight gain restores physical health and may foster psychological improvements, reducing obsessional thinking and improving mood. Successful outpatient treatment requires a highly motivated patient, cooperative family, and good prognostic features such as younger age and brief duration of symptoms. Most severely emaciated patients, those 25% to 50% below recommended weight, require initial inpatient hospitalization in a psychiatric unit, general hospital, or, preferably, specialized eating disorder unit to ensure medical stability, permit adequate behavioral evaluation and monitoring, and reduce denial.

Programs that combine large meals and snacks, informational feedback regarding weight gain and caloric intake, and behavioral programs that include both positive rewards (such as desired visits) and negative consequences (such as bed rest and activity restrictions) make the greatest impact. Education, individual and family psychotherapy, and sometimes medications are integral aspects of treatment. To obtain therapeutic effects, such programs typically require several weeks to months of inpatient hospitalization or intensive outpatient day programs. Nasogastric tube feedings and total parenteral nutrition, though rarely necessary, are occasionally lifesaving. Rates of weight gain must be carefully monitored to avoid cardiac complications of overfeeding, particularly related to congestive heart failure and arrhythmias, and edema, which may occur during refeeding. Supplemental phosphorus should be administered to avoid hypophosphatemia, common in early stages of vigorous refeeding. Individual psychotherapy may increase the patient's motivation for change, but patients often make best use of psychotherapy after they have regained some weight and are able to think more clearly.

Because malnourished patients may be especially prone to serious medication side effects, medication treatment is often avoided initially. Despite early favorable open trials and collections of small series of patients' cases, recent studies suggest that because of the ceiling effects that result from good nursing care in well-organized eating disorders inpatient programs, selective serotonin reuptake inhibitors (SSRIs) do not increase the rate or amount of weight gain for patients treated in these settings. However, SSRIs are sometimes used for prominent depressive, obsessional, and compulsive symptoms in the still-underweight patient. Low doses of atypical neuroleptics have been used to promote weight gain, but existing studies do not support their general use. After nutritional rehabilitation has been accomplished, fluoxetine hydrochloride (average 40 mg/day) has been shown to sustain weight gain, reduce relapse, and reduce exacerbations of depression. Of note, in a study of adolescent AN patients treated as outpatients, citalopram hydrobromide was associated with weight loss.

Psychological issues. The most effective individual psychotherapies appear to be empathic and reality-based, providing education, effecting behavior changes, and encouraging patients to examine and confront the many distortions and developmental issues described above. Cognitive-behavioral therapy is helpful for weight gain and weight maintenance. Psychotherapy sessions are usually scheduled once or twice weekly. Families can benefit from counseling as soon as an eating disorder is identified, and family therapy following hospital discharge is of proven value for younger patients with AN.

Bulimia Nervosa

Controlled studies have demonstrated the superior efficacy of cognitive-behavioral individual and group psychotherapies. Interpersonal psychotherapy is also effective and psychodynamic psychotherapy may be of value as well. Although no systematic studies exist, many patients find Overeaters Anonymous helpful, partly due to the sense of connectedness and 24-hour-per-day support against cravings offered by this organization. The role of 12-step programs that do not address nutritional counseling and psychological and behavioral deficits remains controversial, especially as sole interventions.

A cognitive-behavioral approach includes several stages, each consisting of several weeks of weekly individual and/or group sessions. Several workbooks are listed in the suggested readings. These stages are described here.

1. The first stage helps establish control over eating through behavioral techniques such as self-monitoring (eg, keeping a detailed symptom-relevant diary), response prevention (eg, eating until satiated without being allowed to vomit), prescribing patterns of regular eating, and stimulus-control measures (eg, avoiding situations most likely to stimulate an eating binge). During this stage, patients are educated about dieting, weight regulation, and the deleterious effects of bulimia.
2. The second stage attempts to restructure unrealistic cognitions (eg, assumptions and expectations) and develop more effective methods of problem solving.
3. The third stage emphasizes maintaining gains and preventing relapse with weekly sessions during the first year when relapse is most likely to occur.

Intensive outpatient day programs featuring specific group programs several hours each day for several weeks have also been used with varying results. For those completing cognitive-behavioral therapy, 50% to 90% attain substantial reductions in binge eating and purging and approximately one third become asymptomatic. However, dropout rates are high. Follow-ups of up to 10 years indicate that many gains are maintained, although some recidivism is seen, particularly at times of severe stress.

Controlled studies show that several classes of antidepressant medications are effective in reducing binge eating and purging in BN. Common obstacles to treatment include medication adherence and maintaining adequate blood levels in the face of persistent vomiting. Fluoxetine hydrochloride (60 mg/day) and the tricyclics (particularly imipramine hydrochloride and desipramine hydrochloride, 150 to 300 mg/day), which are the best studied and most frequently used, are effective in patients with or without comorbid major depression. Results of medication treatment alone are similar to, though more modest than, those with cognitive-behavioral therapy alone. Evidence suggests that best results are obtained from combinations of cognitive-behavioral psychotherapies and psychopharmacological approaches.

Hospitalization is rarely necessary for uncomplicated BN. Indications to hospitalize include failure to respond to adequate outpatient treatment trials, severe medical complications not manageable in outpatient settings, severe mood disorders, and suicidality.

Binge Eating Disorder

Most treatments for BED have been extrapolated from programs designed for BN or obesity. Cognitive-behavioral therapy is the single most effective approach. Most antidepressants that are helpful for BN have also been shown to be effective for binge eating alone. Studies have demonstrated that when added to behavior therapy, fluoxetine hydrochloride (60 mg/day), but not fluvoxamine maleate (100 mg/day), enhanced weight loss for both binge-eating and nonbinge-eating obese subjects. However, all patients rapidly regained weight when medication was stopped. Although the combination of phentermine hydrochloride and fenfluramine hydrochloride was effective for both binge-eating and nonbinge-eating obese individuals, cardiac complications resulted in removal of fenfluramides from the market. Recently, the anticonvulsant medication topiramate has been shown to reduce binge-eating symptoms and produce weight loss, but larger studies are needed to prove its effectiveness and assess reported cognitive side effects (occasional confusion) before it can be generally recommended. Controlled studies of sibutramine hydrochloride monohydrate for BED are in progress.

Obesity

Mild obesity. Patients with mild obesity are 20% to 40% over ideal body weight, with BMIs ranging from 27 to 29.9. There is relatively little increased risk to health, so conservative treatment, consisting of sensible, well-balanced diets and exercise, sometimes with the assistance of self-help programs such as Weight Watchers and Overeaters Anonymous, is recommended.

Moderate obesity. For patients with BMIs ranging from 30 to 34.9 who are 40% to 100% overweight, realistic weight loss goals of 5% to 10% are appropriate, particularly if associated high-risk medical conditions such as hypertension, diabetes mellitus, hyperlipidemia, hypercholesterolemia, and/or smoking are present. Carefully constructed behavioral weight management programs that consist of monitored meals and exercise are used. If these efforts are not successful after 12 weeks, very low-calorie diets and/or medications such as sibutramine hydrochloride monohydrate, 5 to 15 mg/day, or orlistat, 120 mg per fat-containing meal up to three per day, may be of help. However, the effects of these medications are modest and side effects may be considerable. The side effects of sibutramine hydrochloride monohydrate may include increased blood pressure, depression, insomnia, and severe headache. This medication is not recommended for patients with hypertension or histories of cardiac illness or cerebrovascular accidents and should not be used for more than 2 years. For orlistat, which acts by blocking the absorption of fat from the gastrointestinal tract, prominent abdominal and fecal side effects occurred in more than 25% of patients starting treatment, including oily spotting, flatus with discharge, fecal urgency, and fatty-oily stool. Supplements of fat-soluble vitamins are required.

Severe obesity. For patients with BMIs ranging from 35 to 39.9, weight loss goals of more than 10% are appropriate. In addition to the behavioral programs described earlier, very low-calorie diets and medications are usually recommended.

Very severe obesity. Individuals with BMIs of 40 and above are at very high risk of several medical complications, including cardiovascular disease, obstructive sleep apnea, daytime respiratory compromise (Pickwickian syndrome), and a wide range of musculoskeletal problems. In patients who are in their 40s or older, death rates due to cardiovascular disease are about 12 times higher than expected. Suggested weight loss goals are at least 30% to 40%. Gastric surgery is recommended if medical treatment fails. Current procedures include open and laparoscopically conducted adjustable silicone gastric banding, Roux-en-Y gastric bypass, and, for superobese patients, long-limbed Roux-en-Y bypass. Although the ultimate long-term success rates of these procedures may be no more than 50% to 60%, the extremely high death and morbidity rates in untreated patients usually justify these procedures. Prior to surgery, the patient should diet to reach his or her lowest attainable weight to minimize operative risks.

Current research into the basic biology of obesity and the creation of novel anti-obesity agents is extremely active. Many new medications, which are based on recent findings concerning obesity-related genes and their proteins and receptors, are in various phases of clinical development. However, the cautionary medico-legal experiences associated with the so-called phen-fen phenomenon ensure that few anti-obesity drugs are likely to be rushed to market in the near future before being adequately tested for safety. Physicians are advised to caution their patients about the lack of therapeutic efficacy and potential dangers of using over-the-counter agents and "health supplements" such as caffeine or ephedra preparations.

SUMMARY

Eating disorders (AN, BN, and BED) are psychiatric disorders commonly seen in primary care settings, particularly where younger women are treated. These disorders can have substantial medical complications as well as psychiatric comorbidity. Primary care physicians may play a vital role in their recognition, evaluation, and management. Although obesity is not a mental illness, treatment of this extremely prevalent and important condition often requires counseling, behavioral therapy, pharmacotherapy, and sometimes surgical intervention.

ADDITIONAL READINGS

American Psychiatric Association. Practice guideline for the treatment of patients with eating disorders. *Am J Psychiatry*. 2000;Jan:157(1 Suppl):1-39. www.psych.org/clin_res/guide.bk.cfm

Bacaltchuk J, Hay P. Antidepressants versus placebo for people with bulimia nervosa. *Cochrane Database Syst Rev*. 2001;(4):CD003391.

Bacaltchuk J, Hay P, Trefiglio R. Antidepressants versus psychological treatments and their combination for bulimia nervosa. *Cochrane Database Syst Rev*. 2001;(4):CD003385.

Cash TF. *The Body Image Workbook*. New York, NY: Fine Communications; 1998.

Clinical guidelines on the identification, evaluation, and treatment of overweight and obesity in adults. Available at: www.nhlbi.nih.gov/guidelines/obesity/practgde.htm

Executive summary of the clinical guidelines on the identification, evaluation, and treatment of overweight and obesity in adults. *Arch Intern Med*. 1998;158:1855-1867. Available at: www.nhlbi.nih.gov/guidelines/obesity/ob_exsum.htm

Devlin MJ, Yanovski SZ, Wilson GT. Obesity: what mental health professionals need to know. *Am J Psychiatry*. 2000;157:854-866.

Fairburn C. *Overcoming Binge Eating*. New York, NY: Guilford Press; 1995.

Fairburn CG, Cooper Z, Doll HA, Norman P, O'Connor M. The natural course of bulimia nervosa and binge eating disorder in young women. *Arch Gen Psychiatry*. 2000;57:659-665.

Garner D, Garfinkel P, eds. *Handbook of Psychotherapy for Anorexia Nervosa and Bulimia*. 2nd ed. New York, NY: Guilford Press; 1996.

Hay PJ, Bacaltchuk J. Psychotherapy for bulimia nervosa and bingeing. *Cochrane Database Syst Rev*. 2001;(3):CD000562.

Johnson JG, Cohen P, Kasen S, Brook JS. Eating disorders during adolescence and the risk for physical and mental disorders during early adulthood. *Arch Gen Psychiatry*. 2002;59:545-552.

Lyznicki JM, Young DC, Riggs JA, Davis RM. Council on Scientific Affairs, American Medical Association. Obesity: assessment and management in primary care. *Am Fam Physician*. 2001;63:2185-2196.

Villapiano M, Goodman LJ. *Eating Disorders: A Time for Change: Plans, Strategies, and Worksheets*. New York, NY: Brunner-Routledge; 2001 (and companion volume, Goodman LJ, Villapiano M. *Eating Disorders: The Journey to Recovery Workbook*. New York, NY: Brunner-Routledge; 2001).

Wadden TA, Berkowitz RI, Sarwer DB, Prus-Wisniewski R, Steinberg C. Benefits of lifestyle modification in the pharmacologic treatment of obesity: a randomized trial. *Arch Intern Med*. 2001;161:218-227.

Wadden TA, Stunkard AJ. *Handbook of Obesity Treatment*. 3rd ed. New York, NY: Guilford Press; 2002.

Chapter **14**

Psychiatric Aspects of Common Medical Conditions

Bezalel Dantz, MD

Psychiatric disorders are more common in the medically ill than in the general population. Medical disorders can cause psychiatric symptoms directly, as in the case of hyperthyroidism, pancreatic cancer, and multiple sclerosis. Treatment of medical disease can have psychiatric sequelae, such as steroid-induced psychosis or interferon-induced depression. The impact of medical illness on mental health can also be indirect. Pain, loss of independence, fatigue, uncertainty, and shame may lead even the most resilient of medically ill persons into a state of depression or anxiety.

Psychiatric illness can in turn have a direct or an indirect impact on medical disease. Eating disorders and substance abuse are examples of high-risk behaviors that can have dire medical consequences. Treatment of psychiatric illness may also produce medical complications, as is the case with the neuroleptic malignant syndrome. Indirect effects of psychiatric disorders on medical illness have been recognized. Depression is associated with adverse outcomes in diseases as varied as rheumatoid arthritis, cardiovascular disease, and HIV/AIDS.

The co-occurrence of medical illness and psychiatric symptoms poses unique challenges. Clinicians must be able to detect and distinguish between various coping styles, adjustment disorders, and psychiatric syndromes. When the medical illness itself causes anorexia, insomnia, or fatigue, a psychiatric disorder may be obscured. Nonetheless, psychiatric disorders in the medically ill patient can impact both quality and duration of life. These disorders must be identified and treated aggressively. Psychopharmacologic management must take into account drug-drug interactions, side-effect profiles, and the impact of medications on the medical illness.

Some disorders, though controversial, appear at the interface of medicine and psychiatry. Included in this category are irritable bowel syndrome, fibromyalgia, and multiple chemical sensitivities. Patients with these disorders may face skeptical physicians who dismiss their symptoms as psychiatric. Though their etiology is elusive, it should be noted that peptic ulcer disease once was considered a psychosomatic disease. Irritable bowel syndrome may one day, too, be understood in the physiologic terms by which diseases gain legitimacy. In the meantime, we must empathize with our patients' concerns, admit our own limitations, and help patients cope with their distress.

This chapter summarizes key issues in diagnosing and managing psychiatric problems in a variety of common medical and "interface" conditions.

CARDIOVASCULAR DISEASE

William Osler attributed premature heart disease in his physician colleagues to their long hours and stressful occupation. The psychosocial risk factors for developing cardiac disease have intrigued investigators ever since. More recently, the association between type A personality (impatience, competitiveness, excessive commitment to work) and cardiovascular morbidity has been revisited. Hostility has been identified as the core link between the type A personality and premature atherosclerosis. Other psychosocial risk factors are social isolation, hopelessness, low socioeconomic status, anxiety, and chronic and subacute life stress. Among psychiatric disorders, the best available evidence supports an association between depression and ischemic heart disease.

Depression

Case Vignette

Mr Aaron, a 61-year-old man, comes to his physician's office for a routine visit. He has an 8-year history of hypertension, which has been well controlled with enalapril maleate. Mr Aaron smoked one pack of cigarettes per day from the age of 22 until 3 months ago, when he had an anteroseptal myocardial infarction that was complicated by mild congestive heart failure.

After his MI, Mr Aaron lost about 20 pounds and began exercising three times per week. Today he reports that he has not exercised for the past month: "What's the point? It's too much work, I don't have the energy, and I know I'm just going to have another heart attack anyway." His weight is unchanged, "but not because I'm trying; I just don't feel much like eating these days." When asked directly, he admits that his mood has been "kind of blah, mostly lousy." Mr Aaron has been waking up early most mornings unable to return to sleep, and he feels his thinking lately has been "fuzzy." He wants to live, but he is pretty sure he "won't last much longer: My Dad died from a heart attack when he was only 63."

On examination, Mr Aaron is normotensive and shows no evidence of congestive heart failure. Chemistries, blood count, and thyroid studies are all normal. His physician tells him that he has a major depression, which is a fairly common complication of a myocardial infarction and a significant risk for future cardiac events. Mr Aaron agrees to a trial of sertraline and to see a psychotherapist.

Major depression is present in nearly one fifth of patients post-myocardial infarction (MI). Large, long-term studies have demonstrated that depression is a risk factor for cardiac morbidity in patients with and without baseline heart disease. After adjusting for known cardiac risk factors, depressed patients incur adverse outcomes at more than twice the rate of nondepressed patients. In a study of 879 subjects hospitalized with MI, the presence of depression was the best predictor of 5-year cardiac mortality. Depression was a more likely predictor than diabetes, left ventricular ejection fraction, or a history of revascularization. Other studies have shown a dose-dependent relationship between mood and cardiac outcomes, with even minor depression posing significant risk. Among the multiple mechanisms that have been identified are the following:

- Depressed patients are less likely to receive medical and surgical interventions.
- Depressed patients have an increased prevalence of cardiac risk factors such as smoking.
- Depression is associated with lower adherence to diet, exercise, and medications.
- There is increased sympathoadrenal activity in depression.
- Depressed subjects have decreased heart rate variability.
- Depression is associated with increased platelet aggregation.

Evidence for a physiologic basis is convincing. First, depression is associated with heightened hypo-pituitary-adrenal activity, as demonstrated by a paradoxical cortisol response to dexamethasone suppression. Hypercortisolemia leads to premature atherosclerosis. Second, depressed patients display an increased resting heart rate and decreased heart rate variability, both of which are associated with poor outcomes following MI. Finally, studies of platelet activation show increased amplitude and velocity of platelet aggregation in depressed patients. This may be mediated by the increased density of 5HT-2 receptors in the platelets of patients with untreated depression.

Although the link between depression and heart disease is well established, the outcome following treatment of depression is not known. Retrospective case-control studies suggest an increased risk of MI in patients taking tricyclic antidepressants. Other studies show a favorable effect in patients taking selective serotonin reuptake inhibitors (SSRIs). In preliminary studies of patients post-MI, psychosocial interventions have led to decreased cardiac morbidity. Two randomized controlled trials, one studying the impact of sertraline and the other of cognitive-behavioral therapy in post-MI depressed patients, yielded disappointing results. Although both are successful in treating depression, neither treatment proved to be superior to a placebo in improving cardiac outcomes. The sertraline trial was not powered to detect these differences; however, the group randomized to the active drug showed a trend toward improved cardiac outcomes.

SSRIs seem to be safe and effective in post-MI patients. Short-term studies have shown no increase in the incidence of arrhythmias, ischemia, or cardiac conduction delay. Case-control analyses reveal no excess in cardiac mortality. SSRIs may cause a relative bradycardia (their sympatholytic properties have rendered SSRIs, in addition to beta-blockers, the treatment of choice for vasovagal syncope). However, caution should be practiced when prescribing these agents in conjunction with cardiac medications. Warfarin may be displaced from protein-binding sites, leading to increased prothrombin times. Certain SSRIs are potent inhibitors of the cytochrome P450 enzymes and may increase the plasma concentration of beta-blockers, calcium channel blockers, statins, and antiarrhythmics. Sertraline and citalopram hydrobromide are least likely to cause an interaction.

Tricyclic antidepressants are no longer recommended for patients with heart disease. Tricyclics, which have properties similar to class I antiarrhythmics, can cause orthostatic hypotension, tachycardia, prolongation in cardiac conduction intervals, and decreased heart rate variability. They are deadly in overdose. Of greatest concern is the finding that class I antiarrhythmics increase mortality in patients following MI. Although no study has linked therapeutic doses directly to cardiac mortality (retrospective case-control studies have obvious flaws), the availability of alternative antidepressants has rendered tricyclics as second-line agents in this population. Tricyclics also should be avoided with patients who have bundle branch block or prolonged QTc intervals. Lower doses (such as those used to treat neuropathy and chronic pain) may carry a more favorable risk:benefit ratio.

Although bupropion hydrochloride and venlafaxine hydrochloride seem to be safe for this population, both medications (in particular, venlafaxine hydrochloride) may cause hypertension in a dose-dependent fashion. Limited data are available to comment on the safety of nefazodone hydrochloride or mirtazapine. The former has been associated with a low risk of fulminant hepatic failure; the latter is associated with weight gain and hyperlipidemia. Nefazodone hydrochloride inhibits the metabolism of digoxin, statins, and calcium channel blockers, causing a rise in serum levels. Monoamine oxidase inhibitors (MAOIs) have demonstrated safety in patients with heart disease, but their use is limited by dietary restrictions and the risk of hypertensive (tyramine-induced) crises.

Other somatic treatments include the use of psychostimulants and electroconvulsive therapy (ECT). Low doses of methylphenidate (eg, 2.5 to 5 mg bid) are associated with a modest rise in pulse and blood pressure; they are considered safe in patients with stable coronary disease. Pemoline has minimal sympathomimetic activity; however, its use is associated with a 2% risk of hepatotoxicity. In patients with ischemic heart disease and good functional capacity, ECT is associated with a low risk of cardiac complications.

Cardiac rehabilitation is an underused, yet extremely important, component of post-MI care. In addition to improving cardiac performance, rehabilitation may enhance self-esteem and restore well-being. Some individuals, particularly those with type A personalities, benefit from stress-reduction treatments. Cognitive-behavioral therapy is a proven, nonpharmacologic alternative for patients with post-MI depression.

Controversy continues with respect to the role of beta-blockers in precipitating or aggravating a depressive episode. Reviews of controlled studies have failed to show a relationship. In cases where a beta-blocker is suspected to cause depression, switching to a nonlipophilic beta-blocker (eg, atenolol) or lowering its dosage is an alternative.

Anxiety

Panic attack is the most common diagnosis in patients under age 40 presenting to the emergency room with chest pain. Yet, cardiac risk factors are absent in 50% of patients with myocardial infarction, and it is estimated that more than half of ischemic events are precipitated by acute psychological stress. Clinicians are faced with a dilemma whenever a patient presents with atypical symptoms. An extensive workup is often unnecessary to rule out cardiac, pulmonary, or gastrointestinal (GI) causes. A panic attack is the likely etiology for chest pain when most of the following factors are present:

- Atypical symptoms and absence of traditional risk factors
- Improvement with ambulation
- Rapid onset and complete resolution of symptoms within 20 minutes
- Recent (not necessarily acute) psychosocial stressor
- Improvement in symptoms with benzodiazepines
- History of panic disorder or alcohol abuse
- Strong family history of psychiatric illness

It is unusual (though not impossible) for patients older than age 50 to present with a first-time panic attack. In many cases, a remote history of panic attacks or other psychiatric symptoms can be elicited. A diagnostic maneuver is the reproducibility of symptoms with electrocardiogram (ECG)-monitored hyperventilation. Mitral valve prolapse, detected in 10% to 25% of patients, is neither a sensitive nor a specific marker of a panic attack. Treatment of panic disorder is discussed in Chapter 8. Most patients who present with their first or second panic attack do not require long-term treatment; reassurance is usually sufficient.

"Atypical chest pain" is an unknown cause of recurrent chest pain that lacks features of panic disorder. Many of these cases are found in young and middle-aged women and may be associated with vasospasm of the microvasculature (syndrome X). Even in the absence of a psychiatric disorder, antidepressants are useful in treating atypical chest pain. Placebo-controlled trials have demonstrated that both imipramine and sertraline are efficacious when organic etiologies have been ruled out.

Many patients report anxiety symptoms following MI. Supportive, interpersonal, cognitive-behavioral, and psychodynamic therapies are the preferred modalities in patients with mild to moderate symptoms. The pharmacologic treatment of anxiety disorders in patients with cardiovascular disease is outlined in Table 14-1.

TABLE 14-1 Agents Recommended for Comorbid Psychiatric Illness and Cardiovascular Disease

Class	Recommended	Alternates	Not Recommended
Antidepressants	sertraline citalopram hydrobromide[b] bupropion hydrochloride	fluoxetine hydrochloride[a] paroxetine hydrochloride[a] venlafaxine hydrochloride[c] mirtazapine[d] nefazodone hydrochloride[a]	tricyclics
Anxiolytics	sertraline citalopram hydrobromide[b] beta-blockers buspirone hydrochloride	fluoxetine hydrochloride[a] paroxetine hydrochloride[a] venlafaxine hydrochloride[c] mirtazapine[d] nefazodone hydrochloride[a] benzodiazepines gabapentin	tricyclics
Hypnotics	Zolpidem tartrate Zaleplon	benzodiazepines mirtazapine[d] nefazodone hydrochloride[a] gabapentin trazodone hydrochloride[e]	tricyclics
Antimanic agents	Valproic acid	lithium[f] olanzapine[g] risperidone	carbamazepine
Antipsychotics	Risperidone quetiapine	olanzapine[g] haloperidol[i] aripiprazole[j]	ziprasidone hydrochloride[h]
Psychostimulants	Pemoline	methylphenidate hydrochloride[k] dextroamphetamine[k]	
Treatment of alcohol dependence	Naltrexone hydrochloride		disulfiram

[a] These agents are considered alternate choices because of their potential for drug-drug interactions.
[b] Includes the enantiomer s-citalopram hydrobromide.
[c] May cause or exacerbate hypertension.
[d] Associated with weight gain and hyperlipidemia.
[e] Associated with priapism in approximately 1 in 10,000 patients.
[f] Associated with sick sinus syndrome; toxic levels can induce nonspecific T-wave abnormalities.
[g] Associated with weight gain, hyperglycemia, and hyperlipidemia.
[h] Associated with prolonged QTc intervals.
[i] May cause QTc prolongation; reports of torsades with high parenteral doses.
[j] Though this agent has a desirable profile on lipids and weight, data are limited.
[k] Modest rises in pulse and blood pressure at low doses (eg, 2.5 to 5 mg bid); generally safe in patients with stable disease.

PULMONARY DISEASE

Chronic obstructive lung disease (COPD) is the fourth leading cause of death in the United States. Asthma affects approximately 5% of the US population. The incidence and morbidity associated with these diseases are rising. The following section explores the treatment of psychiatric illness in the setting of lung disease. Functional pulmonary syndromes are also briefly considered.

Anxiety

Whereas depression is the most common psychiatric illness affecting cardiac patients, anxiety disorders are prominent in patients with respiratory disease. One in 10 asthma patients develops panic disorder (the respiratory illness usually comes first). Stress is associated with clinically significant bronchoconstriction in 20% to 40% of asthma patients. When the dyspneic patient becomes anxious, it triggers a vicious cycle: Anxiety exacerbates shortness of breath, leading to even greater anxiety. Fear of leaving home, overuse of medications, and excessive visits to emergency rooms may indicate an uncontrolled pulmonary condition, anxiety disorder, or both. In patients with compromised pulmonary function, hyperventilation may decrease efficiency of breathing and cause respiratory decompensation. Behavioral strategies such as diaphragmatic breathing, meditation, and relaxation training can help avert an attack.

Medications used to treat pulmonary disease can cause or exacerbate anxiety. These medications include decongestants, antihistamines, beta-agonist inhalers, theophylline, and systemic steroids. The primary care physician can limit the patient's use of decongestants by prescribing nasal steroids and noncentrally acting antihistamines. Long-acting beta-agonist inhalers, such as salmeterol xinafoate, are preferred over shorter-acting agents. Inhaled corticosteroids have little systemic absorption and thus pose a low risk of psychiatric side effects. Anticholinergic inhalers, leukotriene antagonists, and mast cell stabilizers are relatively free of psychiatric side effects. The management of steroid-induced psychiatric symptoms is discussed in the section on rheumatology.

Most psychotropics can be used safely by patients with pulmonary disease. SSRIs do not affect ventilatory drive and are effective in treating a broad range of disorders, including generalized anxiety, panic disorder, posttraumatic stress disorder, social phobia, obsessive-compulsive disorder, and depression. However, the therapeutic effects of SSRIs do not appear for several weeks, and they may be anxiogenic in the short term.

Tricyclic antidepressants can be useful because they possess rapid hypnotic and anxiolytic effects. They are effective in treating most anxiety disorders as well as depression. Their anticholinergic properties may dry bronchial secretions and promote bronchodilation. Antihistaminic effects can reduce the need for supplementary antihistamines and decongestants. The secondary amine tricyclics, nortriptyline hydrochloride and desipramine hydrochloride, are preferred because of their improved tolerability. Tertiary agents, such as amitriptyline and imipramine, have more potent antihistaminic and anticholinergic effects. Nortriptyline hydrochloride is an effective treatment for nicotine dependence. Caution is advised in using any tricyclic medication with patients who have underlying cardiovascular or cardiac-conduction disease. A baseline ECG is warranted in at-risk patients.

Benzodiazepines decrease the sensation of dyspnea but suppress respiratory drive, particularly while sleeping. For this reason, they are contraindicated for patients with sleep apnea and should be used with caution in patients with congestive heart failure (CHF) or chronic obstructive pulmonary disease (COPD). Benzodiazepines are relatively safe for patients with asthma but should be avoided in patients with a history of alcohol or drug dependence. The use of hypnotic agents with patients who have respiratory disease is discussed below.

In animal and human studies, buspirone hydrochloride has been shown to stimulate respiratory drive and thus may be a good option for patients with COPD or sleep apnea who have comorbid anxiety. The effects of buspirone hydrochloride do not appear for several weeks, and it is effective only for generalized anxiety. An alternative is gabapentin, an anticonvulsant that has been used with some success in treating certain patients who have generalized anxiety and panic disorders.

Depression

Psychotherapy, including cognitive-behavioral and interpersonal therapy, has long-term efficacy and should be considered first-line in the motivated patient with mild to moderate depression. In addition, exercise conditioning has a salutary effect on mood and should be recommended to all patients with COPD.

The tricyclic antidepressants and the SSRIs are both effective in treating depression in patients with respiratory illness. Bupropion hydrochloride has no adverse cardiac or pulmonary effects and is approved for treating both depression and nicotine dependence. However, bupropion hydrochloride does not have anxiolytic properties and is the most stimulating of all available antidepressants. Therefore, its use should be reserved for depressed patients in whom anxiety is not prominent. It is contraindicated for patients with eating disorders and those at risk for seizures.

Few studies have been done on the effects of newer antidepressants in treating patients with respiratory illness. Venlafaxine hydrochloride, nefazodone hydrochloride, and mirtazapine all have little effect on respiratory drive and have been used safely in patients with pulmonary disease. These antidepressants are effective in treating depression and most anxiety disorders. The antihistaminic properties of mirtazapine may be helpful in patients with insomnia and/or allergies. The propensity of this agent to produce weight gain, however, should be considered. MAOIs also are safe and effective with this population, but their use is limited by dietary restrictions and drug-drug interactions.

Insomnia

Chapter 11 covers the differential diagnosis of, and general treatment approaches to, insomnia in considerable detail. For patients with known pulmonary illness, the principles of using psychopharmacologic agents include a number of options:

- Benzodiazepines, which are respiratory depressants, must be used with caution. Zolpidem tartrate, a benzodiazepines receptor agonist, does not impact respiratory drive and therefore is an acceptable alternative. Both zolpidem tartrate and zaleplon can be associated with physiologic tolerance, withdrawal, and dependence. Continuous use of these agents is not recommended for more than 2 consecutive weeks.

- Antihistamines are sedating and do not cause respiratory suppression, although patients may complain of a hangover or anticholinergic side effects.

- Other options include low-dose tricyclic antidepressants, trazodone hydrochloride, mirtazapine, and anticonvulsants (eg, gabapentin, tiagabine hydrochloride).
- Low doses of atypical antipsychotics also may be used.

Recommended sleeping agents and dosages are listed in Table 14-2.

Functional Pulmonary Syndromes

Hyperventilation syndrome. Hyperventilation syndrome is diagnosed in patients who present with shortness of breath and lack the history, physical findings, and laboratory evidence consistent with pulmonary disease. In addition to dyspnea, patients experience light-headedness, paresthesias, diaphoresis, and rapid heart rate. Arterial blood gases reveal low pressures of carbon dioxide.

The benign nature of this syndrome can be illustrated to patients in the office by reproducing the symptoms through hyperventilation. Breathing into a paper bag and diaphragmatic breathing can help abort an attack. It is ideally treated with cognitive-behavioral therapy. Pharmacologic options include SSRIs, benzodiazepines, and tricyclic antidepressants.

Vocal cord dysfunction. Another disorder that presents as respiratory distress is vocal cord dysfunction. Found mostly in young women, this disease is caused by the unconscious, paradoxical motion of vocal cords during breathing. Patients frequently are misdiagnosed with asthma, prescribed multiple medications, and treated inappropriately with steroids. When patients present in acute distress, they may get intubated.

TABLE 14-2 Recommended Sleeping Agents in Patients With Respiratory Disease	
Class	**Example**
Antihistamines*	Hydroxyzine[†], 25 to 50 mg Diphenhydramine hydrochloride[†], 25 to 50 mg
Tricyclic antidepressants	Amitriptyline[†], 10 to 50 mg Doxepin[†], 10 to 50 mg
Other antidepressants	Trazodone hydrochloride[á], 25 to 150 mg Mirtazapine, 7.5 to 15 mg
Selective benzodiazepine receptor agonist*	Zolpidem tartrate, 5 to 10 mg
Anticonvulsants	Gabapentin, 300 to 1800 mg Tiagabine, 2 to 16 mg
Antipsychotics	Quetiapine fumarate, 25 to 300 mg Olanzapine, 2.5 to 5 mg Risperidone, 0.25 to 1 mg Haloperidol, 0.5 to 1 mg

*Tolerance is common.

† Anticholinergic effects may cause confusion in elderly and demented patients.

á Associated with priapism in 1 in 10,000 patients.

Clues to vocal cord dysfunction include upper-airway wheezing on auscultation, the absence of hyperinflated lungs on chest x-ray, and normal findings on pulmonary-function tests. When intubated, wheezing disappears and the patient's respiratory distress dramatically reverses. Diagnosis is definitively made through direct visualization of vocal cords during breathing. Treatments include psychotherapy and speech therapy.

Multiple environmental allergies. Multiple environmental allergies, also known as multiple chemical sensitivities, is a controversial illness as there are no reliable laboratory abnormalities associated with this syndrome. Patients develop multiple symptoms when exposed to such agents as fabrics, cosmetics, smoke, disinfectants, foods, and other substances. Symptoms include burning eyes, rhinorrhea, nasal congestion, tinnitus, shortness of breath, pruritis, myalgias, fatigue, irritability, headaches, dizziness, and neurocognitive dysfunction. Onset of illness may be tied to an inciting event, such as installation of new carpeting or exposure to a spilled chemical. The "allergic" response becomes generalized to multiple agents, even when present in minute concentrations (a phenomenon known as *kindling*). Eventually patients learn to avoid exposure to the offending agents and may develop severe phobias, environmental restrictions, and obsessive cleaning rituals. Results from allergy testing are equivocal. Many patients have preexisting psychiatric illness.

Spurned by traditional physicians, patients seek the care of clinical ecologists who perform assays of various chemicals in such specimens as blood, fat, urine, and hair. Levels of serum immunoglobulins, complement, and quantitative counts of lymphocyte subsets are analyzed. Some patients are diagnosed with systemic candidiasis and are treated with long-term antifungal therapy. Patients may provide their primary care physician with a staggering amount of data and a long list of attempted remedies. The skeptical physician should not confront such patients. Rather, a therapeutic alliance should be formed, benign treatments offered (see discussion on chronic fatigue syndrome), and comorbid psychiatric illness addressed.

The greatest quandary is posed by patients with documented airway disease and psychophysiologic illnesses such as hyperventilation syndrome, vocal cord dysfunction, or multiple chemical sensitivities. A collaborative approach with a psychiatrist is necessary with these patients. The risk of iatrogenic harm (eg, unnecessary treatment with steroids and intubation) is great enough to warrant mandatory psychiatric evaluation. Reluctant patients should be told that further treatment is contingent on psychiatric assessment.

GASTROENTEROLOGY

With over 100 million neuronal cell bodies embedded in the gastrointestinal tract, the enteric nervous system has been called the "brain of the gut." The enteric and central nervous systems share the same neurotransmitters and are interconnected. Ninety-five percent of the serotonin produced in the body resides in the enterochromaffin cells of the gastrointestinal tract. It comes as no surprise, then, that the gastrointestinal system is affected by most psychiatric illnesses. In this section, we explore the functional gastrointestinal disorders as well as psychotropic considerations in the patient with liver disease.

Functional Gastrointestinal Syndromes

It has been estimated that up to 60% of gastroenterology practice is devoted to psychosomatic complaints. These disorders include globus, esophageal dysfunction, functional dyspepsia, pseudo food allergies, psychogenic vomiting, and irritable bowel syndrome. Common to all these disorders is visceral hypersensitivity. Functional GI syndromes are common in patients with psychiatric illness, including those with eating disorders, substance abuse, psychosis, anxiety disorders, trauma, and depression. Patients with personality disorders can have particularly refractory symptoms. When patients present with significant weight loss (ie, more than 5% of initial body weight), an organic cause should be sought, regardless of preexisting psychiatric or psychosomatic disease. The most common of the functional GI disorders are briefly considered here.

Globus. Globus is defined as a persistent or intermittent sensation of a lump in the throat. The sensation occurs between meals and must not be accompanied by difficult or painful swallowing. Nearly 50% of the population has experienced globus at least once, and it usually resolves on its own. Precipitated by an emotional event, globus is more common in women than men. Some specialists recommend that patients receive an upper GI series to rule out achalasia. Most patients with globus will respond to reassurance alone. In others, psychiatric treatment may be warranted. Interventions such as biofeedback, relaxation therapy, supportive counseling, and other behavioral therapies have been used. Pharmacologic options include benzodiazepines, buspirone hydrochloride, and SSRIs. One study showed the tricyclic antidepressant imipramine to be more effective than placebo.

Functional dyspepsia. A common presenting complaint in primary care is functional dyspepsia, defined as 3 or more months of pain or discomfort in the upper abdomen in the absence of known organic disease. Patients complain of a variety of symptoms, including early satiety, recurrent retching or vomiting, and bloating. Though chronicity of symptoms suggests a benign cause, no historical elements are available to rule out organic disease. In addition to a careful history and physical exam, the workup should include tests of liver function, electrolytes, lipase and amylase, upper endoscopy, abdominal ultrasound, and, if necessary, computerized tomography (CT) imaging. Treatment for *Helicobacter pylori* for patients with non-ulcer dyspepsia is controversial.

Benign treatments, such as dietary modification, antacids, and H_2 blockers, can be used. Cimetidine hydrochloride and omeprazole interact with many psychotropics, causing enzymatic inhibition and induction, respectively. Metoclopramide hydrochloride, used in cases of delayed gastric emptying, may cause acute dystonia or extrapyramidal symptoms. Opioids should be avoided, given their risks for physiologic tolerance and dependence. Unfortunately, the use of psychotropic agents is limited by their GI side effects. SSRIs may cause nausea, bloating, constipation, and diarrhea. These side effects can be limited by using lower than usual doses and titrating slowly. Tricyclics may exacerbate reflux. Benzodiazepines and mirtazapine are relatively free of GI side effects.

Food allergies. The complaint of food allergies is common, and patients may inappropriately restrict their dietary intake. The consequences are as varied as osteopenia, weight loss, and anemia. True allergies are more common in children and infants. Typical are allergies to eggs, peanuts, cow's milk, wheat, mustard, seafood, and soy products. Additives such as yellow dye number 5, monosodium glutamate, and sulfites may cause allergic reactions. Because of cross-reactivity, people with ragweed allergies may become allergic to melons. Individuals typically outgrow sensitivities to most offenders but not to nuts, fish, or eggs. The only true food allergies that may present in adulthood are allergies to shellfish.

Mast cell degranulation occurs in the nasopharynx, bronchi, GI tract, vascular system, and skin and is responsible for the varied symptomatic presentation of food allergies. The most common manifestation of food allergies is urticaria; the most dangerous are angioedema and anaphylaxis. Most allergic reactions to food occur within minutes to an hour after ingestion. GI symptoms are present in only 30% of patients with food allergies and include abdominal pain, vomiting, or diarrhea. If specific foods are suspected to cause GI symptoms, a food diary can be helpful.

Though not true allergies, idiosyncratic reactions to some foods are common. Lactase and sucrase deficiency, cholelithiasis, gastroesophageal reflux, peptic ulcer disease, celiac sprue, and caffeine or monosodium glutamate intolerance should be considered. Diagnostic tests include scratch skin testing and serologic tests for food-specific IgE. These tests are diagnostic only in the setting of a convincing history.

There is no evidence that specific foods cause psychiatric symptoms. A primary psychiatric disorder should be suspected in any patient who complains of vague somatic and psychological reactions to food or a history of other somatoform illness. Management involves establishing a therapeutic alliance, avoiding harmful treatments, discouraging visits to noncertified health care providers, promoting a balanced diet, and treating comorbid psychiatric illness.

Case Vignette

Mrs Mind, a 32-year-old woman previously in good health, presents to her physician's office with complaints of abdominal pain of 8 months' duration. The pain is described as periumbilical and crampy and it usually is relieved by defecation. Mrs Mind previously moved her bowels daily but now does so about every third day, and the cramping resumes about a day after each bowel movement, increasing in intensity until she next defecates. Her stools contain no mucus or blood, nor have they changed color. Her appetite has been normal, and her weight has been unchanged.

Mrs Mind has been very worried that her symptoms might represent a colon cancer, even though there is no family history of malignancy. She has been taking lorazepam several times per week for a vague "nervous condition." Physical examination reveals an afebrile, anxious woman with normal bowel sounds and no organomegaly. Her abdomen is soft and minimally tender, although some tenderness can be induced by palpating deeply along the left lateral abdominal wall. The rectal examination is normal, and the stool sample is negative for occult blood. The complete blood count (CBC), comprehensive metabolic panel, and thyroid-stimulating hormone (TSH) test are all normal. Irritable bowel syndrome is diagnosed, and treatment with bulk-forming agents is initiated.

Irritable bowel syndrome. Roughly one quarter of the ambulatory cases seen by gastroenterologists are for irritable bowel syndrome (IBS), defined as 12 or more weeks of abdominal discomfort associated with altered bowel habits, in the absence of warning signs. Features not consistent with a diagnosis of IBS include weight loss, anemia, fever, symptoms during sleep, blood in the stools, severe chronic diarrhea, and a rapid onset of symptoms. A family history of GI malignancy should prompt further investigation.

A 2002 consensus statement by the American College of Gastroenterology recommends against laboratory testing in patients without alarm symptoms or signs, with the possible exception of serologies to exclude celiac sprue. Patients with IBS have an approximately 5% risk of having celiac sprue, compared to a prevalence of 1% in the general population. Nonetheless, a few simple tests can be reassuring to both the clinician and the patient. A CBC, comprehensive metabolic panel, TSH, erythrocyte sedimentation rate (ESR), stool studies, and testing for antiendomysial antibodies should be sufficient to exclude organic disease when the pretest probability is low. All patients deserve a trial of abstinence from dairy products. In the absence of alarm symptoms, endoscopic evaluation is not necessary. Routine colon cancer screening is recommended for all patients older than 50 years of age, regardless of symptoms.

IBS can be classified as diarrhea-predominant, constipation-predominant, or mixed. Though roughly 15% of the US population has symptoms of IBS, only a fraction of affected persons seek medical care. Studies have shown that patients with IBS have higher psychological morbidity than nonpatients who meet the criteria for IBS. Psychiatric illness often precedes the development of GI symptoms. A history of childhood sexual or physical abuse is common. Like other psychosomatic illnesses, patients with IBS have a high incidence of comorbid somatoform disorders, including hypochondriasis, multiple chemical sensitivities, chronic fatigue syndrome, chronic tension headaches, and fibromyalgia. Despite its benign nature, psychological distress is more common in patients with IBS than in those with inflammatory bowel disease.

Treatment of IBS involves several principles. Patients must be educated that this is a chronic disease with a relapsing and remitting course, which can be exacerbated by stress. IBS does not affect life expectancy or predict future disease. It can be managed effectively but not cured. The mainstays of treatment include a balanced diet, exercise, stress management, proper sleep hygiene, and avoidance of noxious substances (eg, caffeine, gas-producing legumes, alcohol, and tobacco). Cognitive-behavioral therapy can help patients adapt to unpredictable symptoms, identify and manage stressful situations, and avoid catastrophic thought patterns. Hypnotherapy is also an effective intervention.

Medical management can be effective. Though controlled studies are lacking, patients with primarily abdominal pain can be treated with antispasmodics such as hyoscyamine or dicyclomine. A low-dose tricyclic (eg, desipramine hydrochloride, 10 to 25 mg qhs) may also be helpful. Benzodiazepines are successful in some cases, particularly when combined with antispasmodics (eg, commercially available Librax).

Individuals with prominent diarrhea may benefit from prn loperamide hydrochloride or a low-dose tricyclic antidepressant such as nortriptyline hydrochloride or amitriptyline. Therapeutic doses of tricyclics should be used with patients who have comorbid depression or anxiety. If an SSRI is chosen, paroxetine hydrochloride is the preferred choice because it is the most anticholinergic of available agents. Alosteron, a 5HT-3 receptor antagonist, has had a profound benefit in some patients with severe diarrhea-predominant IBS. After cases of ischemic colitis were reported, it was temporarily withdrawn from the US market. Practitioners must now be certified in its use.

Patients with constipation-predominant IBS should be treated initially by increasing fiber intake. Osmotic agents (eg, polyethylene glycol) are preferred over irritant laxatives because the latter may induce gut immotility. The only treatment with proven efficacy in constipation-predominant IBS is the 5HT-4 receptor agonist tegaserod maleate. Despite the widespread use of SSRIs, there are no published data of SSRIs in treating any form of

IBS. In patients with comorbid anxiety or depression, remission of the psychiatric illness often leads to reduction in GI distress. Prognosis in IBS is best for males, those with a brief history of symptoms, those with constipation-predominance, and those reporting an acute illness at the onset of GI upset.

Liver Disease

Patients with liver disease have many psychological symptoms, including fatigue, depression, anxiety, delirium, insomnia, and sexual dysfunction. Portal hypertension poses the risk of encephalopathy, which can present with subtle findings, including cognitive disturbance, affective lability, irritability, and sleep disturbance. Hepatic encephalopathy is particularly common in patients who have received a portocaval shunt. It may be precipitated by infection, GI bleeding, dehydration, increased dietary protein intake, electrolyte abnormalities, and medications. Neurologic examination may reveal tremor, asterixis, and poor coordination. Frank delirium occurs only in advanced stages of encephalopathy; therefore, a high level of suspicion is warranted for subtler cases. An electroencephalogram (EEG) is highly sensitive (but not specific), showing diffuse slowing and triphasic waves. Serum ammonia levels are increased in 90% of patients with hepatic encephalopathy, but ammonia levels and severity of encephalopathy are not correlated.

Treatments include low-protein diets and clearing the intestines of ammonia-producing bacteria. Lactulose, metronidazole, oral vancomycin hydrochloride, and neomycin have been used. Low-dose antipsychotics can be helpful in controlling agitation and psychotic symptoms.

Medications used in liver disease can cause significant psychiatric sequelae. Spironolactone, used to treat ascites, is an androgen-antagonist that may exacerbate preexisting hypogonadism in the patient with liver failure. In men with liver disease who complain of sexual dysfunction, free-testosterone levels, taken in the morning, should be measured. If low, hormone replacement should be considered. Topical and intramuscular testosterone preparations are preferred. Alpha interferon is another medication with psychiatric side effects, most frequently depression. Suicidality and psychosis may be precipitated by interferon and can occur in patients with no prior psychiatric history. For this reason, patients receiving interferon must be monitored closely for development of psychiatric symptoms.

In one small placebo-controlled study, prophylactic treatment with paroxetine hydrochloride was effective in reducing the incidence of depression while patients were receiving high-dose interferon. Patients with psychiatric complaints should be aggressively treated prior to initiating interferon. Patients with prior episodes of depression should be considered for prophylactic antidepressants.

The use of psychotropic agents in patients with hepatic disease follows several principles. Low doses should be used, and they should be titrated slowly. Medications with shorter half-lives, limited hepatic metabolism, and inactive metabolites are preferred. Agents with idiosyncratic or dose-dependent hepatotoxicity should be avoided if possible. Tests of liver function should be assessed before and during the addition of any new agent, and withdrawal of the suspected medication should be attempted if liver function worsens. Whenever possible, serum levels (eg, tricyclic antidepressants) should be monitored. Table 14-3 lists the recommended agents in treating patients with hepatic disease.

TABLE 14-3 Recommended Agents, With Starting Doses, in Patients With Advanced Liver Disease

Class	Recommended	Alternates	Not Recommended
Antidepressants	Sertraline, 12.5 mg Citalopram hydrobromide, 5 mg Venlafaxine hydrochloride, 18.75 mg Nortriptyline hydrochloride*, 10 mg Desipramine hydrochloride *, 10 mg	Mirtazapine, 7.5 mg Paroxetine hydrochloride, 5 mg	Nefazodone hydrochloride Bupropion hydrochloride[†]
Anxiolytics	Same as above Gabapentin, 100 mg Buspirone hydrochloride, 7.5 mg Also see antipsychotics	Mirtazapine, 7.5 mg Lorazepam[‡], 0.5 mg Oxazepam[‡], 10 mg	Most benzodiazepines
Hypnotics	Hydroxyzine, 25 mg Doxepin hydrochloride, 10 mg Gabapentin, 100 mg Olanzapine, 2.5 mg	Trazodone hydrochloride[‡], 25 mg Temazepam[§], 5 mg	Most benzodiazepines
Antimanics	Lithium, 150 mg Olanzapine, 2.5 mg	Risperidone, 0.25 mg Quetiapine, 25 mg	Valproic acid Carbamazepine
Antipsychotics	Olanzapine, 2.5 mg Haloperidol, 0.5 mg	Risperidone, 0.25 mg Quetiapine, 25 mg	Chlorpromazine hydrochloride Thioridazine hydrochloride
Stimulants	Methylphenidate, 2.5 mg	Dextroam-phetamine, 2.5 mg	Pemoline

---

* These tricyclics have known therapeutic concentrations; dosages should be titrated according to blood level.

[†] Bupropion hydrochloride may accumulate in patients with advanced hepatic disease and thereby increase the risk of seizures.

[‡] Associated with priapism in approximately 1 in 10,000 patients.

[§] These benzodiazepines are metabolized by conjugation and have inactive metabolites.

RHEUMATOLOGY

Depression is common in patients with rheumatologic disease, occurring in 20% of patients with rheumatoid arthritis. Pain, disfigurement, restricted mobility, and fears of dependence can cause significant distress. This is particularly so in rheumatologic diseases, to which young and middle-aged women have a predilection. If the afflicted person is a working mother, the impact extends to the marriage, the children, and the financial well-being of the family. Even after controlling for severity of disease, individuals with both rheumatoid arthritis and depression demonstrate poorer functional status, more pain, increased use of health care, and higher levels of unemployment. Studies suggest that depression lowers the threshold for perception of pain.

Medications used to treat rheumatologic diseases may cause or contribute to psychiatric illness. Nonsteroidal antiinflammatory drugs (NSAIDs) are a frequently overlooked cause of psychiatric morbidity. NSAIDs are associated with cognitive changes and sleep disturbance, as well as affective and psychotic symptoms. Other agents that can cause psychiatric symptoms include tramadol hydrochloride, corticosteroids, antimalarial agents, and methotrexate sodium. Tramadol hydrochloride has been associated with abuse and dependence.

Rheumatoid Arthritis

Cognitive-behavioral therapy is effective in treating depression and anxiety related to rheumatoid arthritis and has been shown to reduce both pain behaviors and perception of pain. Patients cite stress as the chief precipitant of disease flares. Physicians caring for these patients should emphasize the importance of social support, active problem solving, and finding meaning in the experience of illness. Catastrophic thinking should be challenged. Feelings of helplessness are countered through assertiveness training and encouraging self-help abilities. Families may benefit from family counseling. Maintaining hope is of critical importance in coping with any chronic disease.

Pharmacologic management is the same as with the general patient, paying close attention to the side effects of the chosen agent. Tricyclic antidepressants have mild antiinflammatory effects independent of their antidepressant activity. Because of their anticholinergic properties, however, they should be avoided in patients with sicca. SSRIs inhibit the metabolism of several opiates, increasing the action of hydrocodone while paradoxically decreasing the analgesic effects of tramadol hydrochloride and codeine. Serotonin syndrome in combination with tramadol hydrochloride is rare. Fatigue, common in patients with rheumatologic and connective tissue disease, can be treated with dopaminergic agents (eg, psychostimulants or bupropion hydrochloride).

Systemic Lupus Erythematosis

Although involvement of the central nervous system (CNS) is rare in rheumatoid arthritis, it is common in patients who have systemic lupus erythematosis (SLE). Neuropsychiatric manifestations of lupus occur in nearly 50% of cases. Features suggesting an organic etiology include symptoms in a patient with no prior psychiatric history, evidence of systemic or neurologic disease activity, recent change in steroid dosage, and the presence of cognitive impairment. A careful review of medications, cognitive exam, neurological evaluation, and metabolic workup are warranted. Antibodies to ribosomal P proteins are common in SLE-induced psychiatric illness.

When CNS lupus is suspected, treatment of psychiatric symptoms should be directed toward treatment of SLE. Otherwise, treatment of psychiatric illness in lupus patients should proceed as described for rheumatoid arthritis. Steroid-associated syndromes are discussed below.

The Patient on Steroids

The psychiatric sequelae of systemic steroids are variable, idiosyncratic, and dose-dependent; they may appear during therapy or its withdrawal. These symptoms may include depression, anxiety, agitation, insomnia, fatigue, mania, and psychosis. Women are more susceptible than men. The onset of psychiatric symptoms is usually within the first 2 weeks after initiating treatment. When a brief period of treatment is required, low-dose psychotropics can be added to target specific symptoms (see Table 14-4). Patients on long-term steroids who develop psychiatric symptoms should receive the same treatment as any other patient. Nefazodone hydrochloride, fluvoxamine maleate, and fluoxetine hydrochloride inhibit the metabolism of all steroids.

Although psychosis occurs in 1% of patients receiving 40 mg or less of prednisone daily, it occurs in 28% of patients receiving 80 mg or more daily. Patients with SLE and pemphigus are at highest risk. Episodes begin with mood lability, dysphoria, and hyperarousal and evolve rapidly into florid psychosis. In most cases, psychiatric symptoms resolve rapidly after medication has been discontinued; rarely do the symptoms persist for weeks. Antipsychotics will hasten recovery. Contrary to popular belief, neither a previous nor a current psychiatric disorder predicts the psychiatric response to steroids. Patients with a prior history of steroid psychosis may tolerate future treatment uneventfully. Nonetheless, most clinicians should proceed with caution when prescribing steroids to these patients. Alternate day-dosing and divided daily doses may lower the risk. If patients with a history of steroid psychosis are reluctant to undergo a future course, they can be offered prophylactic antipsychotic medication.

TABLE 14-4 Psychopharmacologic Management of Acute Steroid-Related Symptoms	
Symptom	**Recommended Agents**
Depression or fatigue	Methylphenidate, 2.5 to 10 mg bid
	Modafinil, 100 to 200 mg qd bid
	Amantadine hydrochloride, 100 mg tid
Insomnia	Hydroxyzine, 25 to 50 mg qhs
	Doxepin, 10 to 25 mg qhs
	Zolpidem tartrate, 5 to 10 mg qhs
	Trazodone hydrochloride, 25 to 150 mg qhs
Anxiety	Lorazepam, 0.5 to 1 mg tid
	Clonazepam, 0.5 to 2 mg bid
	Gabapentin, 300 mg tid
	Antipsychotics (see below)
Mania or psychosis	Risperidone, 0.25 to 1 mg qhs or bid
	Olanzapine, 2.5 to 10 mg qhs or bid
	Haloperidol, 0.5 to 2 mg bid

Psychiatric symptoms, most commonly depression, also may arise when withdrawing from steroids. Slowing the reduction in dosage (eg, by 2.5 mg every week) may minimize symptoms. Adrenocortical deficiency must be ruled out in any patient being tapered from chronic steroids who complains of depressive symptoms. Patients who become psychologically dependent on steroids warrant psychiatric consultation.

Chronic Fatigue Syndrome

Chronic fatigue syndrome (CFS) is a disorder characterized by the symptoms listed in Table 14-5. Patients may also complain of low-grade fevers, night sweats, orthostasis, environmental allergies, and abdominal cramps. The diagnosis is one of exclusion. The criteria exclude patients with a history of melancholic depression, psychosis, eating disorders, dementia, morbid obesity, and those who have abused substances within 2 years prior to the onset of fatigue. A complete history and physical examination should be performed.

Appropriate laboratory studies include a CBC; electrolyte panel; urinalysis; liver function tests; total protein; ESR; C-reactive protein (CRP); and TSH. Abnormal laboratory findings should prompt an investigation for alternative diagnoses. When lightheadedness is a prominent complaint, a corticotropin stimulation test and/or tilt table test may be considered. The differential diagnosis of chronic fatigue is included in Table 14-6.

Though complaints of fatigue are ubiquitous, only 0.4% of the population qualifies for a diagnosis of CFS. The CFS patient is typically white, above the age of 30, and female. Symptoms are of sudden onset, usually precipitated by a viral illness or after

---

TABLE 14-5 Chronic Fatigue Syndrome Diagnostic Criteria (CDC)

Six or more months of persistent or relapsing fatigue that:

1. Is of new or definitive onset

2. Has remained unexplained after clinical evaluation

3. Is not the result of ongoing exertion

4. Is not relieved by rest

5. Produces significant reduction in previous level of activities

6. Concurrently, patients must have at least four of the following symptoms:

    a. Impairment in short-term memory and concentration

    b. Sore throat

    c. Tender cervical or axillary lymphadenopathy

    d. Muscle pain

    e. Arthralgias

    f. Headaches of a new type, pattern, and severity

    g. Unrefreshing sleep

    h. Postexertional malaise lasting more than 24 hours

TABLE 14-6 Differential Diagnosis of Chronic Fatigue

Type of Condition	Specific Diagnosis
Infections	Tuberculosis, subacute bacterial endocarditis, HIV, Lyme disease, hepatitis, parasitic disease, post-viral syndrome
Endocrine disorders	Hypothyroidism/hyperthyroidism, diabetes, adrenal insufficiency, Cushing syndrome, hypoparathyroidism/hyperparathyroidism, menopause, pregnancy
Metabolic disorders	Kidney and liver disease, hypocalcemia/hypercalcemia, hypophosphatemia, hyponatremia/hypernatremia, hypokalemia, hypomagnesemia, vitamin deficiencies
Cardiopulmonary disease	CHF, COPD, obstructive sleep apnea, chronic sinusitis
Neurologic disease	Head trauma, multiple sclerosis, myasthenia gravis, dementia, poststroke, Parkinson disease
Rheumatologic disorders	SLE, rheumatoid arthritis, polymyalgia rheumatica, vasculitis, polymyositis, dermatomyositis, myopathies
Hematologic disorders	Anemia
Sleep disorders	Narcolepsy, restless legs, nocturnal myoclonus, sleep apnea, circadian rhythm disturbance
Cancer	Pancreatic, multiple myeloma, lymphoma, paraneoplastic syndromes, others
Medications	Psychotropics, NSAIDs, beta-blockers, antihistamines, others
Psychiatric disorders	Depression, anxiety disorders, eating disorders, substance abuse
Social disorders	Domestic violence, shift work
Other	Amyloidosis, sarcoidosis, deconditioning, malnutrition

suffering minor head trauma. They are worsened by emotional stress and overexertion. More than half of the patients have mild to moderate depression, which may precede the diagnosis of CFS.

A high proportion of patients have irritable bowel syndrome, fibromyalgia, tension headaches, and multiple chemical sensitivities. There is no evidence of a viral etiology. Studies linking Epstein-Barr virus, herpesvirus-6, and other viral agents to CFS have failed under scrutiny. Cortisol dysregulation, alterations in cellular and humoral markers of immunity, and autonomic dysfunction have been found in subjects with CFS. These findings are inconsistent across studies, have low sensitivity and specificity, and do not correlate with severity of disease. Thus, a pathophysiologic explanation for CFS remains elusive.

In a frustrated search for an explanation and a cure, patients may seek consultations with rheumatologists, infectious-disease specialists, allergists, and clinical ecologists.

Patients may present to homeopaths, acupuncturists, body workers, and other alternative providers. Herbal treatments may include SAM-e (S-adenosylmethionine), nicotinamide adenine dinucleotide (NADH), coenzyme Q, malic acid with magnesium, and carnitine. Among the more noxious treatments are intravenous immunoglobulin, long-term antibiotics, megadose vitamins, and antiviral and antifungal agents. None of these treatments has demonstrated efficacy in placebo-controlled trials. Ultimately, patients may become angry, isolated, and depressed.

The cornerstone of treatment is the patient-physician relationship. The physician must take the illness seriously and perform a complete and thorough evaluation. The impact of the illness on the patient's family, occupation, social activities, and emotional well-being must be explored. The patient should be informed of the diagnosis, its relapsing and remitting course, and its exacerbation by stress. As with irritable bowel syndrome, patients need reassurance that the illness is benign and is associated with a normal life expectancy. It is important to convey confidence in the diagnosis and optimism about the possibility for improvement. Although consultation with alternative healers may be unavoidable, the patient should be warned about unscrupulous practitioners and unproved remedies. A timetable for consultations and the type of remedies sought should be negotiated. Periodic reassessment for possible underlying illness is important, as is evaluation of any new symptoms, without preconceptions.

Only cognitive-behavioral therapy and graded exercise programs have demonstrated efficacy in randomized trials. Lifestyle recommendations include avoidance of caffeine, alcohol, and illicit drugs; maintenance of regular sleep and dietary habits; prevention of overexertion; and avoidance of prolonged rest. Permanent disability status should be discouraged as it predicts a poor prognosis. Patients can be told that unemployment leads to deconditioning, poor self-esteem, increased symptoms, and social isolation. Continued employment thus can be parlayed into a prescription for symptomatic relief.

The goals of cognitive therapy include acceptance of chronic illness, respecting one's limits, choosing among competing priorities, and managing interpersonal conflict. Cognitive distortions (eg, "my life has been ruined") are confronted. A carefully graded exercise program has been proved to decrease symptoms and improve exercise tolerance.

In addition to psychological treatment and lifestyle changes, the physician may offer symptom-targeted therapies. When comorbid psychiatric illness is present, its treatment will result in significant reduction in CFS symptoms. Even in the absence of psychiatric morbidity, modest doses of antidepressants (including SSRIs and tricyclic antidepressants [TCAs]) may be helpful. Low-dose tricyclic antidepressants (eg, nortriptyline hydrochloride or amitriptyline, 10 to 50 mg qhs) are effective in improving the quality of sleep. When lightheadedness is a major complaint, alpha agonists (eg, midodrine hydrochloride, 5 to 10 mg tid) or mineralocorticoid replacement (fludrocortisone acetate, 0.1 to 0.3 mg qd) can be attempted. A positive tilt table test suggests vasovagal reactivity; beta-blockers and SSRIs may then be considered. Dopamine agonists (eg, modafinil, 100 to 400 mg qd) can alleviate fatigue. Though pharmacologic approaches have been disappointing in randomized trials, individual patients may benefit from one or more of these agents. Dosing always should start low, given these patients' sensitivity to medication.

A minority of patients recover fully. Among poor prognostic indicators are longer duration of symptoms, rejection of a psychological component to the illness, comorbid somatization disorder, and lifelong dysthymia.

Fibromyalgia

Fibromyalgia is a related syndrome that has a high concurrence with CFS, IBS, chronic headaches, multiple chemical sensitivities, depression, and anxiety disorders. Fatigue and sleep disturbance are common. Fibromalgia is distinguished by pain of longer than 3 months' duration in 11 of 18 tender point sites on digital palpation. Pain must be present in the axial skeleton, on both sides of the body, and above and below the waist.

Fibromyalgia affects approximately 5% of the population, occurring mostly in women between the ages of 20 and 50. As with CFS, half of the patients recall a precipitating trigger such as a viral illness or trauma. Nonpharmacologic treatments include supportive and cognitive psychotherapies, biofeedback, hypnotherapy, and a graduated exercise program. Among drug treatments are bedtime doses of tricyclic antidepressants, cyclobenzaprine, NSAIDs, tramadol hydrochloride, trazodone hydrochloride, anticonvulsants (eg, gabapentin), mexiletine hydrochloride, SSRIs, and trigger point injections. Opioids should be avoided if possible.

ENDOCRINE DISORDERS

Perturbations in the endocrine system are common during mental crises. Studies of depressed patients reveal a blunted TSH response to TRH (thyrotropin-releasing hormone) and nonsuppression of cortisol following a dexamethasone challenge. Investigators have found higher bone turnover and lower bone mineral density in women with depression. Reproductive hormones are particularly sensitive to psychological stress. The menstrual cycle may be disturbed even in women who do not meet the criteria for adjustment disorders.

Endocrine disorders are among the reversible causes of psychiatric illness and should be considered whenever patients present with an atypical history (eg, older age of onset, absence of external stressors) or with constitutional symptoms. In addition, many psychotropics have idiosyncratic or direct endocrinologic effects. This section focuses on psychiatric syndromes in two of the most common endocrinologic disorders: diabetes and thyroid disease. Two syndromes that may be caused by psychotropic medications—syndrome of inappropriate secretion of antidiuretic hormone (SIADH) and hyperprolactinemia—are also considered. See Table 14-7 for a list of psychotropic-induced endocrinopathies. For a discussion of steroid-induced psychiatric illness, see the section on rheumatology.

Obesity, Diabetes, and the Insulin-Resistance Syndrome

The prevalence of depression in patients with diabetes is noted to be as high as 20%. Depressed diabetics have lower adherence to medication, are less likely to follow a diabetic diet, and have poorer glycemic control than nondepressed diabetics. Medications used to treat diabetes can cause hypoglycemia, which may manifest as anxiety or irritability. Diabetics who develop panic attacks or intermittent explosive behaviors should be carefully evaluated for hypoglycemia.

Cognitive-behavioral therapy improves glycemic control in depressed diabetic patients and should be considered first-line treatment in patients with mild to moderate depressive symptoms. Individual controlled trials have demonstrated neutral or favorable changes in glycosolated hemoglobin in patients randomized to cognitive therapy,

TABLE 14-7 Psychotropics and Endocrinologic Disease

Agent	Effect
Antipsychotics and SSRIs*	Hyperprolactinemia
Atypical antipsychotics†	Weight gain, hyperlipidemia, diabetes
Lithium	Hypothyroidism
Lithium	Nephrogenic diabetes insipidus
Lithium and anticonvulsants	Osteoporosis
Lithium	Hyperparathyroidism
Mirtazapine	Weight gain and hyperlipidemia
SSRIs, carbamazepine, and TCAs	SIADH
Tricyclics	Weight gain and impaired glycemic control
Valproic acid	Polycystic ovarian disease

*Of the atypical antipsychotics, risperidone is the agent most commonly associated with hyperprolactinemia. Psychotropic-induced elevated prolactin levels rarely exceed 100 mg/dL.

† Clozapine and olanzapine have been conclusively linked with medication-induced diabetes and hyperlipidemia. Two newer agents, ziprasidone hydrochloride and aripiprazole, appear to be weight-neutral and unlikely to dysregulate glucose or lipid metabolism.

sertraline, and benzodiazepines. Other psychotropic medications may aggravate diabetic control through weight gain or via direct metabolic effects. SSRIs (and, to a lesser extent, TCAs) can exacerbate sexual dysfunction. Conversely, some agents, including the tricyclic antidepressants and some anticonvulsants, may be particularly helpful for patients with neuropathy. Table 14-8 addresses adverse effects of psychotropics that are of particular concern.

Obesity has grown to epidemic proportions in the United States, with 25% of the population maintaining a body mass index greater than 30 kg/m^2. This has been accompanied by a corresponding increase in the prevalence of the insulin-resistance syndrome, a disorder characterized by abdominal obesity, glucose intolerance, hypertension, and dyslipidemia. Obese patients may have low self-esteem, depression, and anxiety.

The choice of psychotropic agent with this population depends on its effect on the patient's weight. With some medications (eg, SSRIs), the effect on body weight is idiosyncratic. When the psychiatric illness itself causes a weight disturbance, the priority should be to use the most effective agent available. Table 14-9 lists recommended psychotropics when weight gain is an important issue. In cases in which iatrogenic weight gain is unavoidable, exercise and diet alterations should be discussed. Pharmacologic antidotes include histamine-2 receptor blockers, metformin hydrochloride, amantadine hydrochloride, and topiramate. Successful use of these antidotes has not been demonstrated in randomized controlled trials.

Thyroid Disease

Though psychiatric symptoms are common in patients with overt thyroid disease, less is known about the relationship between subclinical hypothyroidism and psychiatric illness.

TABLE 14-8 Psychotropic Considerations in the Diabetic Patient

Agent	Effect
Tricyclics	Weight gain, impaired glycemic control, worsened gastroparesis or neurogenic bladder; effective for peripheral neuropathy
SSRIs	Sexual dysfunction
Bupropion hydrochloride	Low risk of weight gain or sexual dysfunction
Mirtazapine	Weight gain and hyperlipidemia
Venlafaxine hydrochloride	Hypertension
Gabapentin	Effective for peripheral neuropathy
Lithium and valproic acid	Weight gain
Topiramate	Possible weight loss
Atypical antipsychotics*	Weight gain, worsened diabetic control, hyperlipidemia

*Note that several newer atypical antipsychotics, including ziprasidone hydrochloride and aripiprazole, may have favorable effects on weight, glucose metabolism, and lipids.

In one population of elderly depressed patients, only 0.7% of subjects were found to have TSH of 10 µIU/L or greater, suggesting that the risk of hypothyroidism is no higher in depressed patients than in the general population. Other studies suggest that subclinical hypothyroidism doubles the lifetime prevalence of major depression. Though common practice, the routine testing of thyroid function in depressed patients is supported by little data. Women older than age 35 are at particular risk for subclinical hypothyroidism; the American Thyroid Association recommends testing these patients regardless of symptoms. When thyroid screening is performed, TSH should be assessed, given the prevalence of the sick euthyroid syndrome (isolated low free T4) in the psychiatric population.

Few guidelines are available on how to treat psychiatric syndromes in patients who have active thyroid disease. Occasionally, psychiatric symptoms may persist several months (or permanently) after thyroid function has been corrected. More commonly, psychiatric symptoms resolve once thyroid status has been stabilized. Hyperthyroid patients with anxiety can be treated successfully with beta-blockers while they are undergoing definitive therapy. Mania can be stabilized with benzodiazepines or atypical antipsychotics.

Patients with hypothyroidism and depression should be treated with thyroid replacement first, typically levothyroxine sodium (T4). Because hypothyroidism is associated with sleep apnea, benzodiazepines should be avoided. In cases of subclinical hypothyroidism, depression may be coincidental. Treatment should be based on the severity of the depression and the presence of predisposing risk factors, such as a personal or family history of psychiatric illness. Generally, thyroid replacement is attempted first; if symptoms persist, psychotropic agents are added.

Thyroid replacement therapy in patients with subclinical hypothyroidism should be initiated in the presence of: (1) depression or cognitive deficits; (2) positive antithyroid antibodies; (3) women older than age 50; (4) hypercholesterolemia; (5) goiter; and

TABLE 14-9 Weight Gain Associated With Psychotropics		
Class	**Less Weight Gain**	**Most Weight Gain**
SSRIs	Fluoxetine hydrochloride (0/+) Sertraline (0/+)	Paroxetine hydrochloride (+/++)
TCAs	Desipramine hydrochloride (+)	Amitriptyline hydrochloride (+++) Imipramine hydrochloride (+++)
Other antidepressants	Bupropion hydrochloride (-/0) Nefazodone hydrochloride (0) Venlafaxine hydrochloride (0/+)	Mirtazapine (+++)
Anxiolytics	Buspirone hydrochloride (0) Benzodiazepines (0/+)	Gabapentin (+)
Mood stabilizers	Carbamazepine (0/+) Oxcarbazepine (0/+) Lamotrigine (0) Topiramate (—/-)	Lithium (+++) Valproic acid (+++)
Antipsychotics	Ziprasidone hydrochloride (0) Aripiprazole (0) Molindone hydrochloride (0) Haloperidol (+)	Olanzapine (++++) Quetiapine (+++) Risperidone (+++)

Agents are scored from — to ++++ based on likelihood of weight gain.

Note that some individuals may gain or lose weight with any of the above agents. It is recommended to document weight before and after treatment with any psychotropic.

(6) patients on lithium. Patients with independent psychiatric illness and concomitant thyroid disease should receive the same considerations as patients without a thyroid disorder.

Patients receiving lithium should have TSH measured every 3 months for the first 2 years and annually thereafter; those who develop hypothyroidism should be managed according to TSH levels.

Syndrome of Inappropriate Antidiuretic Hormone Secretion

Patients who develop confusion, fatigue, or somnolence while taking antidepressants should have their serum sodium levels evaluated. The syndrome of inappropriate antidiuretic hormone secretion (SIADH) has been increasingly recognized as a side effect of psychotropics, occurring most commonly in patients older than age 65. Among 53 elderly patients taking SSRIs, approximately 25% had below-normal sodium levels.

Hyponatremia is typically mild, begins within 1 month of starting an antidepressant, is transient, and resolves within 2 weeks after discontinuation of the offending agent. In a minority of cases, hyponatremia becomes severe and symptomatic. If patients are rechallenged, two thirds will have a recurrence. Patients who develop asymptomatic hyponatremia while they are on psychotropics should be monitored closely. Antidepressants should be discontinued if sodium levels drop below 129 mEq/L or if the patient becomes symptomatic; an antidepressant from a different class should be substituted.

Hyperprolactinemia

Elevated prolactin levels are a common side effect of antidepressants and many antipsychotics (among the atypicals, risperidone is the most common offender). A quandary is posed when a female patient has responded well to a specific agent but develops a menstrual disturbance. At abnormal values below 50 ng/dL (the upper limit of normal in most laboratories is 15 to 20 ng/dL), production of progesterone is impaired, resulting in an abbreviated luteal phase of the menstrual cycle. Galactorrhea is common. Oligomenorrhea and amenorrhea are rare at prolactin levels below 50 ng/dL, so other causes of menstrual disturbance should be sought. Infertility may occur even in the absence of changes in menstruation.

When prolactin levels exceed 50 ng/dL, oligomenorrhea, amenorrhea, infertility, sexual dysfunction (in men and women alike), and accelerated bone metabolism may occur. Values above 100 ng/dL are rarely associated with psychotropic medications; at these levels, a prolactinoma should be ruled out.

When iatrogenic hyperprolactinemia is suspected, discontinuation of the offending agent should result in a prompt (ie, within 2 weeks) normalization of prolactin levels. In the case of fluoxetine hydrochloride, normalization may require a longer period given its prolonged half-life (up to 2 weeks for fluoxetine hydrochloride and its active metabolite, norfluoxetine).

RENAL DISEASE

Patients with renal disease are at risk for sexual dysfunction, depression, and cognitive impairment. Pruritis, joint pain, dyspnea, and restless leg syndrome may interfere with sleep. Delirium is most predicted by the rate of increase (rather than the absolute value) of the blood urea nitrogen (BUN) concentration.

Multiple studies have shown decreased medical adherence in depressed patients on dialysis. Patients with an external locus of control, lack of family support, and low frustration tolerance are at high risk for dietary noncompliance. Psychiatric hospitalization in dialysis patients occurs at nearly twice the rate of patients with other chronic diseases. Studies suggest a higher prevalence of suicide in these patients compared to the general population. Even after accounting for increased rates of suicide, survival may be lower in dialysis patients with depression. A psychosocial assessment on all patients with end-stage renal disease should be performed, and those at risk should be considered for medication or referral for counseling.

When prescribing psychoactive medications to patients with kidney disease, the recommendation is to use between one half and two thirds of the usual starting dose. Dialysis does not clear most psychotropics. Agents with established therapeutic blood levels (eg, nortriptyline hydrochloride, desipramine hydrochloride, valproic acid, and carbamazepine) can be dosed accordingly (a morning level should be drawn 7 to 10 days after the last dose adjustment). SSRIs with shorter half-lives (eg, paroxetine hydrochloride and citalopram hydrobromide) are preferred. Dosages should be initiated at low levels (eg, 5 to 10 mg) and increased slowly (every 2 to 3 weeks) as tolerated. Bupropion hydrochloride may accumulate in the patient with end-stage renal disease, lowering the seizure threshold. The tendency of venlafaxine hydrochloride to raise diastolic blood pressure renders this medication a poor choice in patients who have poorly controlled hypertension.

Benzodiazepines with inactive metabolites (eg, lorazepam and oxazepam) are preferred; even so, the half-life of these agents is dramatically extended, rendering a single daily dose sufficient in most patients with end-stage renal disease. The half-life of the sedative hypnotic zolpidem tartrate is unchanged in renal failure, although patients may be more sensitive to its cognitive effects. Both typical and atypical antipsychotics are effective treatments for anxiety, psychosis, and agitation. Low doses are used (eg, risperidone, 0.25 to 0.5 mg bid; olanzapine, 2.5 mg qhs or bid). Gabapentin is excreted renally; once-daily dosing is recommended in patients with creatinine clearance less than 30 cc/min (in dialysis patients, administer dose after each dialysis session). Lithium should be avoided except with patients receiving long-term hemodialysis. Because it is completely dialyzed, lithium can be given in a single dose after each dialysis session. With these caveats, psychoactive medications can be used safely with most patients.

HIV/AIDS

The advent of highly active antiretroviral therapy (HAART) has changed the course of HIV infection from that of terminal illness to one of chronic disease. In addition to the struggles that patients with chronic illness face, individuals with HIV disease must adapt to these unique challenges:

- Belonging to groups sidelined by mainstream society (gay men, racial and ethnic minorities, substance users, the homeless and the poor)
- Facing the stigma of HIV illness and coping with reactions from family, friends, and colleagues
- Managing rigid dosing schedules and long-term medication side effects that can be disabling (eg, chronic diarrhea, fatigue, neuropathy) and alter one's appearance (lipodystrophy)
- Negotiating the terms of sexual intimacy with non-HIV-infected partners
- Mourning the loss of close friends and intimates victimized by AIDS

Psychiatric issues may arise from several sources: problems adapting to these challenges, preexisting mental illness including substance-use disorders, HIV-related neuropsychiatric effects, and iatrogenic psychiatric complications. Before discussing the treatment of HIV-related mental illness, a few general points must be considered: HIV-infected patients respond to the same psychotropic medications that are used to treat psychiatric disorders in non-HIV-infected individuals. These patients are extremely susceptible to psychotropic side effects; thus, geriatric dosing should be used. Finally, because of the common enzymatic pathways involved in the metabolism of antiretroviral and psychiatric medication, drug-drug interactions must be considered whenever psychiatric medications are prescribed.

The prevalence of HIV-associated dementia (HAD) increases from 5% in patients with asymptomatic infection to nearly 60% of patients with advanced HIV disease. HAD is considered to be a subcortical dementia affecting frontostriatal pathways. Symptoms include cognitive, neurologic, and behavioral manifestations. Cognitive deficits include impairment in attention and concentration, short-term memory, processing speed, visuospatial skills, abstraction, and language. Motor symptoms include gait disturbances, slowing of movements, clumsiness, and changes in handwriting. Among psychiatric complications are apathy, irritability, emotional lability, and behavioral disinhibition. Of these, apathy and inertia are the most common behavioral manifestations of HIV-associated dementia.

The differential diagnosis includes opportunistic infections, CNS neoplasms, metabolic abnormalities, endocrinopathies, anemia, and drug effects. Assessment should encompass a complete neurologic and mental status exam; review of medications; CBC; comprehensive metabolic panel; measurements of TSH, B_{12}, VDRL, and testosterone levels; an adrenocorticotropic hormone (ACTH) stimulation test; neuroimaging; and a lumbar puncture. Bacterial, fungal, and viral cultures and serum antibody and antigen tests are used to rule out infection. An EEG is rarely helpful.

In addition to HAART (preferably a regimen that includes azidothymidine [AZT]), treatment of HAD with psychostimulants may enhance cognitive function and improve motivation. Methylphenidate (2.5 to 20 mg on awakening and at noon) has been studied extensively in this population. For patients with HAD and significant mood lability, irritability, or psychotic features, treatment with a low-potency atypical antipsychotic is recommended. Risperidone (0.25 to 1 mg bid), olanzapine (2.5 to 5 mg bid), or quetiapine fumarate (25 to 100 mg bid) are typically used. Because individuals with HIV are extremely sensitive to extrapyramidal effects of traditional neuroleptics, these agents should be avoided whenever possible. When parenteral tranquilization is necessary (as with agitated and uncooperative patients), low-dose intramuscular haloperidol (0.5 to 2 mg) or intramuscular ziprasidone hydrochloride (10 to 20 mg) may be used. Benzodiazepines may contribute to confusion and lead to paradoxical increases in agitation.

Among other psychiatric illnesses common in the HIV population are depression, anxiety disorders, mania, and substance-use disorders. Once reversible causes are addressed (see discussion of HIV-associated dementia), geriatric (low) doses of standard psychiatric medications (such as those used in patients without HIV disease) are used to target specific psychiatric syndromes. TCAs may be useful with patients who have concomitant neuropathy or refractory diarrhea. SSRIs are well tolerated and efficacious for depressive and anxiety disorders alike. Bupropion hydrochloride may be well suited for patients with lethargy and low motivation but should be avoided with patients at risk for seizures. Gabapentin has anxiolytic properties in addition to treating neuropathic pain. Benzodiazepines should be prescribed with caution for patients who have underlying cognitive dysfunction or are active substance abusers. Divalproex sodium is the treatment of choice for HIV patients with bipolar disorder.

Cognitive-behavioral therapy is a nonpharmacologic alternative that has proven efficacy in treating depressive and anxiety disorders in patients with HIV. In one study, cognitive-behavioral therapy resulted in improved markers of immunity at 1-year follow-up, even in patients without psychiatric illness.

Patients with substance-use disorders must be strongly encouraged to engage in substance-abuse treatment, in many cases before HAART is instituted. Poor compliance with HAART is common in this population and may lead to treatment resistance. Heroin-using patients should be urged to enroll in methadone-maintenance programs; these programs improve adherence to medication and have been shown to lower HIV-associated morbidity. As with all patients on multiple medications, drug-drug interactions should be considered whenever psychotropic agents are prescribed.

The development of depression in patients with HIV warrants special attention. Adrenal insufficiency should be considered in patients with CD4 counts under 100; hypogonadism is common in patients with higher CD4 counts. To diagnose the latter, morning free-testosterone levels should be measured. Men with low or low-normal levels are candidates for androgen-replacement therapy. Testosterone replacement has been shown to improve mood, libido, muscle mass, and overall quality of life in HIV-infected male patients with hypogonadism. Recommended options include intramuscular (eg, testosterone cypionate, 50 to 300 mg q 1 to 3 weeks), and transdermal (eg, Androgel, 1% 5 to 10 g patch daily) administration.

In addition to clinical response, morning free-testosterone levels should be measured once a steady state is achieved (midway between the third and fourth injections for intramuscular preparations, a month after dosing of transdermal formulations). The goal is to achieve morning free-testosterone levels in the middle range of normal. Testosterone replacement therapy is not recommended for patients with normal gonadal function and has not been studied in females.

A study of HIV-infected women with baseline depression found lower CD4 counts and decreased survival 5 years later. Suicide occurs at increased rates in HIV-infected individuals compared to age-matched controls. Risk factors include depression, social isolation, substance abuse, other psychiatric illness, occupational and financial problems, unrelieved physical pain, and delirium. At every visit, patients with these risk factors should be questioned about suicidal ideation, and aggressive reduction of modifiable risk factors should be undertaken.

CANCER

Despite widespread belief, most patients with cancer do not have psychiatric problems. Of those who develop symptoms, most are diagnosed with adjustment disorders. The remainder of patients suffer from major depression, an organic mental disorder, a personality disorder, or an anxiety disorder.

Cancer patients at high risk for depression include those with:

- poor physical condition,
- poorly controlled pain,
- advanced illness,
- family or personal history of depression,
- pancreatic, lung, head, and neck cancers,
- other life stressors or losses, or
- treatment with drugs known to cause depression.

Depression may be particularly difficult to distinguish from the somatic manifestations of cancer because sleep impairment, loss of appetite, and low energy are common to both. Nevertheless, the cognitive and affective symptoms of depression can be distinguished from those of cancer and its treatments (Table 14-10). Suicidal ideation by itself does not indicate the presence of depression. In some cancer patients the option of sui-

TABLE 14-10 Symptoms That Distinguish Depression From Somatic Manifestations of Cancer	
Present in Both Depression and Cancer	**Present in Depression Only**
Low energy	Persistent sadness
Loss of appetite	Anhedonia
Sleep disturbance	Hopelessness
Impaired concentration	Low self-esteem
	Feelings of guilt and worthlessness

cide provides a sense of control. Thus, the stockpiling of medication or the presence of a weapon at home should give pause.

The first line of defense should be the aggressive management of pain, insomnia, nausea, fatigue, and anxiety. Patients fear the 6 Ds: disability, disfigurement, discomfort, dependency, disruption of interpersonal relationships, and death. Eliciting these fears will offer insight into the patient's priorities and strengthen the therapeutic relationship. Bad news should be "dosed" according to the patient's needs, always with an offer of hope. Hope may mean the opportunity to reach one more birthday or it may mean the possibility of a cure.

While encouraging realistic plans, the physician should acknowledge that patients can outlive even the most dire predictions. Patients may need to hear explicitly that they will not be abandoned, even as they undergo treatment by other specialists. Those who fear pain, nausea, or fatigue will require reassurance that all symptoms will be aggressively managed and controlled. Discussion of past coping mechanisms may be helpful. Religious, social, and family supports should be mobilized. Although support groups may offer solace, a large multicentered study has failed to confirm previous reports of increased survival in breast cancer patients randomized to support groups.

Treatment with antidepressant medication is as effective in cancer patients as in the general population. Nonetheless, a response may not be apparent for several weeks, and fewer than three quarters of patients respond. Faster-acting agents may be warranted. The use of psychostimulants with the medically ill has been well established; therapeutic effects can be seen within 48 hours. Psychostimulants result in increased appetite, enhanced concentration, and improved energy and mood. Stimulants may counter opioid-induced sedation and are synergistic when prescribed with analgesics. Among other treatments for fatigue are amantadine hydrochloride and bupropion hydrochloride.

Anxiolytics and hypnotics have a rapid onset of action. Benzodiazepines and the traditional antipsychotics have intrinsic antiemetic effects. Benzodiazepines should be used cautiously with patients who have advanced lung or heart disease. For patients with liver cancer or metastases, lorazepam and oxazepam are preferred. In elderly and demented patients, atypical antipsychotics may control anxiety, agitation, or insomnia without impairing cognition.

Dronabinol, an oral cannabinoid, is commonly used as an antiemetic and appetite-stimulant. It also has anxiolytic and mood-enhancing properties. Studies have demonstrated synergistic analgesic effects when combined with opiates. Dronabinol also may enhance sexual response. Side effects include hallucinations and delirium. Among other antiemetics are antihistamines, phenothiazines, 5HT-3 receptor antagonists, steroids, and metoclopramide hydrochloride. Appetite stimulants include dronabinol, megestrol acetate, and the psychostimulants.

Specific agents can be chosen based on their side-effect profiles. SSRIs are the most commonly prescribed, with supporting data for their efficacy with this population. SSRIs inhibit the metabolism of several opiates, increasing the action of hydrocodone, while paradoxically decreasing the analgesic effects of tramadol hydrochloride and codeine. Mirtazapine, a selective serotonin and norepinephrine receptor agonist, possesses 5-HT$_3$ antagonism and thus is an excellent choice for patients with anorexia and nausea. Its sedating properties and lack of sexual side effects may be suitable for specific patient concerns.

Tricyclics are effective treatments for depression and most anxiety disorders. Their use is recommended for patients with comorbid pain and insomnia, but they should be avoided in patients at risk for cardiac arrhythmia. Gabapentin is a good anxiolytic, hypnotic, and treatment for chronic pain. Its therapeutic effects are achieved more rapidly than those of SSRIs. Of the antidepressants, bupropion hydrochloride is the most stimulating and thus is an appropriate choice for patients with lethargy. Further, it carries little risk of sexual dysfunction. Bupropion hydrochloride, however, should not be used with patients at high risk for seizures, such as those who have cerebral metastases or metabolic derangement.

Hot flashes caused by anti-estrogen therapies can be controlled with SSRIs or venlafaxine hydrochloride. Paroxetine hydrochloride prophylaxis has been used successfully to decrease the incidence of depression with patients on high-dose interferon. Low doses of atypical antipsychotics may be used to mitigate agitation or delirium with patients on steroids or other drugs.

NEUROLOGIC DISORDERS

Central nervous system (CNS) disorders represent the group of medical diseases most commonly mistaken for psychiatric disturbance. Therefore, clinicians must consider a CNS etiology in the differential of any psychiatric complaint.

Clues to the presence of a neurologic cause include the following elements:

- Focal neurologic deficits
- Headaches, vomiting, or changes in mental status
- Family history of neurologic disease
- History of head trauma
- Onset of symptoms after the age of 50 (after 30 for psychosis)
- Risk factors for HIV
- Abrupt onset of symptoms and rapid deterioration
- Absence of psychosocial stressor
- Atypical presentation
- Refractory to standard psychiatric treatment

Studies that may be performed in suspicious cases include neuroimaging with head CT scan or brain magnetic resonance imaging (MRI), single photon emission computed tomography (SPECT) scan, lumbar puncture, and EEG. These studies, although highly sensitive for CNS pathology, may yield normal findings in some disorders such as the early stages of dementia, paraneoplastic syndromes, and seizure disorders.

Seizure Disorders

The diagnosis of a seizure disorder in patients presenting with psychiatric symptoms requires a high degree of suspicion. The sensitivity of a single EEG is 50% and increases with subsequent EEGs, reaching a sensitivity of up to 90% with four EEGs. Sleep deprivation, caffeine, photic stimulation, and recording during sleep may increase sensitivity. With temporal lobe seizures, nasopharyngeal or sphenoidal leads improve detection. Nonetheless, patients with true seizures may have entirely normal EEGs.

Simple partial seizures (those restricted to a specific area of the brain) and complex partial seizures (those that spread to the opposite hemisphere) can present solely with psychological symptoms. Symptoms may arise during any or all of three phases: the aura (lasting seconds), ictal (also seconds), and post-ictal periods (minutes to hours). Symptoms include cognitive (depersonalization, déjà vu, forced thinking), affective (anxiety, depression, anger, pleasure), perceptual (gustatory, olfactory, visual, auditory, sensory), and behavioral (automatisms, aggression, staring) features. In addition to the clues listed above, the following should raise suspicion of a nonconvulsive seizure:

- The presence of risk factors, even if remote (eg, stroke, head trauma, cancer)
- Family history of seizures
- Episodic, brief, or phasic course of symptoms
- Identical symptoms during each episode
- Unprovoked symptoms
- The occurrence of automatisms
- Amnesia or partial amnesia during events

Patients with seizure disorders have an increased prevalence of psychopathology. Depression occurs in up to one third of patients with epilepsy, and psychotic disorders occur in 10%. The use of psychotropic agents with this population poses the hazard of decreasing the seizure threshold. Patients at risk for iatrogenic seizures include those with a history of seizures (including febrile convulsions), head trauma, cerebrovascular and other neurologic disease, and a family history of epilepsy. Medical risk factors include active eating disorders, alcohol and cocaine abuse, end-stage renal disease, hepatic dysfunction, and uncontrolled hypertension.

Current data on choice of agents are hampered by the lack of controlled data, diverse populations studied, and reliance on animal studies. SSRIs, venlafaxine hydrochloride, and MAOIs are less likely than tricyclics to induce seizures. The antipsychotics of choice are molindone hydrochloride and risperidone. Bupropion hydrochloride, maprotiline hydrochloride, clomipramine hydrochloride, chlorpromazine hydrochloride, clozapine, and lithium should be avoided.

Traumatic Brain Injury

With an incidence of 3 million head injuries each year in the United States, the postconcussive syndrome is a common condition faced by primary care physicians. The single greatest risk factor is alcohol and drug abuse. Most of these injuries are mild to moderate.

The postconcussive syndrome occurs in roughly 50% of patients with mild head trauma and may develop several weeks after the event. Loss of consciousness is not necessary to produce symptoms; nor is degree of injury correlated with severity of postconcussive complaints.

A noncontrast head CT is recommended for patients older than age 65 and those with severe or progressive symptoms. Subdural hematoma can produce symptoms months after a head injury. In patients with the postconcussive syndrome, full recovery is anticipated by 3 months; however, 20% of patients have persistent complaints after 2 years. Neuropsychological assessment will detect malingering, diagnose a psychiatric disorder, and reveal specific deficits that may be addressed through rehabilitation. Curiously, resolution of a compensation case or a lawsuit does not translate into symptomatic improvement.

Pharmacotherapy should be guided by the following principles: Use geriatric dosing, avoid benzodiazepines and medications that lower the seizure threshold (see above), and titrate doses slowly. Psychostimulants (including modafinil) and the dopaminergic agent amantadine hydrochloride may be helpful to counter fatigue and/or deficits in attention. Most medications will require up to 2 months before the patient achieves a full response.

Parkinson Disease

Parkinson disease is characterized by cogwheel rigidity, bradykinesia, stooped posture, shuffling gait, micrographia, and masked facies. Because of the apparent psychomotor retardation and bland (seemingly emotionless) facial expression, this disorder is often mistaken for depression. Parkinson disease is distinguished by the presence of extrapyramidal signs. Psychiatric complications include dementia (20% to 60%) and depression (20% to 60%). Treatment with dopamine agonists may cause psychosis in up to 15% of patients. Other disorders with parkinsonian symptoms have distinctive psychiatric presentations. Lewy body dementia presents with visual hallucinations early in its course. Progressive supranuclear palsy is a rapidly progressive movement disorder associated with vertical-gaze impairment. These patients often exhibit emotional incontinence (pathological crying or laughing). Another rapidly progressive parkinsonian syndrome is multisystems atrophy, in which autonomic insufficiency accompanies parkinsonian symptoms.

Several options are available in the psychopharmacologic management of patients with Parkinson disease. The dopaminergic agonist pramipexole dihydrochloride and the MAO type B inhibitor selegiline hydrochloride may have antidepressant properties. SSRIs are often used to treat depression and anxiety disorders in this population but may be associated with worsening of extrapyramidal symptoms. TCAs also are effective but are associated with orthostatic hypotension. Anticholinergic effects can be helpful in the early stage of the disease. Although little data exist on the use of bupropion hydrochloride in patients with Parkinson disease, its dopaminergic activity renders it a useful alternative; agitation and insomnia are common side effects. ECT has been used effectively and may improve motor symptoms. Antipsychotics of choice are quetiapine and clozapine because these agents are the least likely to exacerbate extrapyramidal symptoms.

Stroke

Poststroke depression occurs in approximately one third to one half of patients, most commonly in infarctions of the left frontal lobe. Depression typically lasts 9 months and is associated with slower functional recovery. As in patients with ischemic heart disease, stroke patients with depression have higher mortality rates than their nondepressed counterparts. Only nortriptyline hydrochloride and citalopram hydrobromide have been studied in placebo-controlled trials of poststroke depression; both agents are more effective than placebo.

Multiple Sclerosis

Patients with multiple sclerosis (MS) may present with vague neurologic symptoms. Many have a strange affect that leads the clinician to dismiss their symptoms as hysterical. Psychiatric presentations include depression (50%), bipolar disorder (13%), cognitive deficits (50%), and emotional incontinence (pathologic crying or laughing). Fatigue is a common complaint.

Treatment with corticosteroids is ineffective when psychiatric disturbance is the sole manifestation of MS. Tricyclics are effective in patients with pathological crying and laughing, bladder incontinence, and depression. Nonetheless, SSRIs are associated with fewer side effects and thus should be considered first-line treatment. Patients with bipolar I disorder have responded well to lithium and atypical antipsychotics. Fatigue may be treated with psychostimulants or amantadine hydrochloride.

Headache

Migraine and tension headaches are commonly seen in primary care. Both are associated with behavioral disturbances that may increase the frequency of headaches and/or lead to functional disability. The comorbidity of psychiatric disorders in chronic headache sufferers is among the highest of any medical disorder. The largest studies show up to a threefold increase in mood disorders and a fivefold increase in anxiety disorders as compared to the general population. The relationship between psychiatric disorders and headache may be bidirectional. A prospective, 3.5-year study of young adults found that baseline depression increased the risk for later development of migraine and vice versa.

The traditional vascular hypothesis of migraine pathogenesis has been challenged. A comprehensive neurovascular model suggests that foci within the brainstem incite spreading neuronal dysfunction and secondary vascular changes that are responsible for aura and headache. The most common triggers for migraine are stress, fatigue, and sleep disturbance. Other triggers are skipping meals, consuming alcohol, eating certain foods, hormonal changes, bright lights, loud noises, noxious odors, overexertion, and changes in weather. Less appreciated is the contribution of analgesic overuse (notoriously Fiorinal, but also over-the-counter medications), which may be responsible for the conversion of episodic migraine to chronic headaches. Many of these triggers are modifiable, and a migraine diary will permit identification of specific targets for intervention. Relaxation therapy (eg, progressive muscle relaxation, meditation, and imagery exercises), thermal (hand warming) biofeedback, electromyogram (EMG) biofeedback, and cognitive-behavioral therapy all have limited empirical support in the treatment of migraine headache. Studies of these interventions have been criticized for their small sample sizes and the absence of control groups.

Pharmacologic treatments have become the mainstay of treatment, and a "stratified care" approach now is preferred over the "step-up approach," in which all migraine sufferers initially receive over-the-counter analgesics. The frequency and severity of headache should guide initial treatment. Patients who have two or more headaches a week and those with headaches refractory to abortive treatments should be considered for prophylactic therapy. Beta-blockers, TCAs, and anticonvulsants have received the most empirical support for prophylactic treatment. Though amitriptyline is the tricyclic with the most supporting data, equal efficacy (and fewer side effects) can be achieved with its metabolite, nortriptyline hydrochloride. When depression is comorbid with headache, therapeutic doses of a tricyclic (eg, 50 to 150 mg of nortriptyline hydrochloride) should be used; lower doses (eg, 25 to 50 mg of nortriptyline hydrochloride) are used for headache prophylaxis alone. The use of SSRIs in the absence of psychiatric indications has not been sufficiently evaluated.

Formerly attributed to muscle tension, current theory posits that the primary cause of chronic tension headaches is CNS sensitization to pain. Behavioral therapy for tension headache has stronger research support than that for migraine headache. Indeed, a large, randomized controlled trial demonstrated equal efficacy of cognitive-behavioral therapy and TCAs in treating chronic tension headache. Both treatments yielded better responses than placebo, and combining the two treatments was even more effective. Limited data exist on the efficacy of biofeedback, relaxation therapy, or hypnosis.

Current recommendations are to treat episodic and chronic tension headaches with cognitive-behavioral therapy, tricyclic antidepressants, or both. As is the case with migraine headaches, analgesic overuse may lead to rebound headaches and therefore should be limited to no more than two times per week.

DERMATOLOGY

The prevalence of psychopathology in dermatologic practice is estimated at 25%. These disorders can be divided into several categories:

1. *Primary dermatologic disorders that are exacerbated by psychiatric illness.* Stressful events provoke flares of atopic dermatitis, psoriasis, herpes simplex, and urticaria, among other skin conditions.
2. *Primary dermatologic disorders that lead to psychiatric complaints.* Acne, rosacea, alopecia, and vitiligo can cause considerable depression and social anxiety. The association of isotretinoin (Accutane) with suicide may be related to the severity of acne in patients treated with the drug rather than a direct pharmacologic action.
3. *Primary psychiatric disorders that lead to skin disease.* Patients who engage in excessive handwashing, alcohol or drug abuse, and eating disorders may present with skin complaints without acknowledging the causative behaviors. Patients also may complain of hyperhidrosis as a side effect of antidepressant therapy.
4. *Primary psychiatric disorders that masquerade as skin disease.* These include body dysmorphic disorder, pathological skin-picking, trichotillomania, and delusions of parasitosis or body odor.
5. *Dermatologic complaints without physiologic explanation,* including psychogenic pruritis, vulvodynia, and glossodynia. They may be considered the irritable bowel syndrome of dermatology.

Patients struggling with chronic skin disease may benefit from cognitive-behavioral therapy to reduce stress and enhance self-esteem. When pruritis is associated with an

TABLE 14-11 The Psychodermatoses: Pharmacotherapy			
Disorder	**Phenotype**	**Drug Class**	**Example**
Obsessions	Body dysmorphic disorder	SSRI	Citalopram hydrobromide, 10 to 80 mg
Compulsions	Skin-picking Hair-pulling	SSRI	Fluoxetine hydrochloride, 10 to 80 mg
Delusions	Parasitosis Body odor	Antipsychotic	Risperidone, 0.5 to 6 mg
Somatic	Pruritis Vulvodynia	TCA	Doxepin, 10 to 150 mg

anxiety or depressive disorder, the tricyclic antidepressants are the treatment of choice (see Table 14-11).

Behavior therapy can be useful in treating patients with pathological skin-picking or trichotillomania; however, many of these patients require adjunctive pharmacotherapy. At high doses, SSRIs are effective.

Another disorder with characteristics of obsessive-compulsive disorder is body dysmorphic disorder (BDD). Patients with BDD are obsessed with an exaggerated defect in appearance. They, too, may benefit from high doses of SSRIs. When the obsessions reach delusional proportions, an atypical antipsychotic should be added.

Because patients with delusions of parasitosis do not respond to reality testing, it is best to express interest in the patient's complaints while performing a complete physical exam. Exploration of the patient's psychological state should be limited to inquiries about how the disorder is affecting his or her life. Benign tests and treatments (eg, use of a topical emollient) can be prescribed while engendering the patient's trust. A psychosocial history is obtained gradually through subsequent visits. Eventually, the clinician can point to difficulties with sleep or anxiety as interfering with the patient's quality of life. While empathizing with the frustration over the mysterious ailment, the physician can turn his or her attention toward the patient's associated distress, then prescribe a "tranquilizer" in the form of an antipsychotic.

SUMMARY

Many general medical and psychiatric disorders are linked. At times the medical condition or its treatment can cause psychiatric symptoms through physiological means, while at other times it is the emotional impact of the medical condition that leads to psychiatric morbidity. Conversely, psychiatric disorders can have important effects on the course of co-occurring medical conditions, particularly through their impact on self-care and adherence to medical regimens. In some conditions (such as in functional disorders), psychiatric illness is associated with visceral hypersensitivity and a lower threshold for pain perception. Other physiologic mechanisms may be responsible for the adverse cardiac outcomes of patients with cardiovascular disease and depression.

ADDITIONAL READINGS

Carney C. Diabetes mellitus and major depressive disorder: an overview of prevalence, complications, and treatment. *Depression and Anxiety*. 1998;7:149-157.

Gupta MA, Gupta AK. Psychodermatology: an update. *J Am Acad Dermatol*. 1996;34:1030-1046.

Jackson JL, O'Malley PG, Tomkins G, Balden E, Santoro J, Kroenke K. Treatment of functional gastrointestinal disorders with antidepressant medications: a meta-analysis. *Am J Med*. 2000;108:65-72.

Kiecolt-Glaser JK, McGuire L, Robles TF, Glaser R. Emotions, morbidity and mortality: new perspectives from psychoneuroimmunology. *Annu Rev Psychol*. 2002;53:83-107.

Kroenke K, Laine C, eds. Investigating symptoms: frontiers in primary care research. *Ann Intern Med*. 2001;134(9):801-930.

Malhotra S, McElory SL. Medical management of obesity associated with mental disorders. *J Clin Psychiatry*. 2002;63(suppl 4):24-32.

Masand PS, Tesar GE. Use of stimulants in the medically ill. *Psychiatr Clin North Am*. 1996;19(3):515-547.

Roszanski A, Blumenthal JA, et al. Impact of psychological factors on the pathogenesis of cardiovascular disease and implications for therapy. *Circ*. 1999;16:2192-2217.

Smith TW, Kendall PC, Keefe FJ, eds. Behavioral medicine and clinical health psychology: special issue. *J Consult Clin Psychol*. 2002;70(3):459-856.

Stoudemire A, Fogel BS, Greenberg DB, eds. *Psychiatric Care of the Medical Patient*. New York, NY: Oxford University Press; 2000:871-887.

Whiting P, Bagnall A, Sowden AJ, Cornell JF, Mulrow CD, Ramirez G. Interventions for the treatment and management of chronic fatigue syndrome. *JAMA*. 2001;286:1360-1368.

Wise MG, Rundell JR, eds. *Textbook of Consultation Liaison Psychiatry*. Washington, DC: American Psychiatric Publishing Inc; 2002:557-562.

Chapter 15

Somatoform and

Related Disorders

Charles V. Ford, MD
Clifton K. Meador, MD
Larry S. Goldman, MD

A significant proportion of patients present to primary care physicians with medically unexplained symptoms. Although some of these patients may have unrecognized underlying physical disease, many, if not most, have "somatized" their psychosocial distress. Research has demonstrated that at least 10% of physically symptomatic patients have no evidence of physical disease and that about 25% of patients in primary care practices have some degree of somatization. Further, it has been repetitively demonstrated that a small proportion of patients uses a disproportionately large percentage of medical care services. Although some of these individuals have serious or significantly severe chronic disease, many have abnormal illness behavior that is remarkably stable year to year, yet they consume a significant proportion of medical care costs.

Primary care remains the de facto major mental health care delivery system. Patients in primary care settings, however, infrequently identify themselves as in need of mental health care services; instead they use a physical symptom as a "ticket of admission" to the physician's office. Katon and colleagues (1984) have labeled this form of somatization as the culturally sanctioned idiom of psychosocial distress. The physician's failure to recognize somatization results in inappropriate and ineffective treatment of the underlying psychosocial problems, as well as the ordering of expensive diagnostic procedures or even unnecessary surgical interventions.

This chapter reviews some of the process, psychological, and referral issues pertaining to somatoform disorders in general. Each specific condition (conversion, somatization disorder, hypochondriasis, body dysmorphic disorder, pain disorder) within this category of illnesses is then examined. Factitious illness and malingering, although they are not strictly somatoform disorders, are also covered because of their phenomenological similarities. For each disorder, diagnostic and management issues are stressed.

SOMATIZATION AS A PROCESS

A patient may preferentially interpret psychosocial distress in terms of physical symptoms (Table 15-1) for many reasons. Further, more than one reason may coexist in any one patient; in fact, multiple processes are probably the norm. These processes include the following:

- The medical care system functions as an auxiliary social support system for persons who are socially isolated or particularly unskilled.

TABLE 15-1 Some Reasons That Patients Somatize

• Obtain social support	• Rationalize life failures
• Manipulate others	• Request assistance (cry for help)
• Misinterpret symptoms	• Reduce stigma from mental illness
• Amplify body sensations	• Obtain secondary gain
• Predisposition from childhood trauma	• Learned behavior

- Physical illness can be used as a socially accepted rationalization for occupational, social, or sexual failures.
- Illness can be used as a means to manipulate others.
- Somatic symptoms can be a "cry for help."
- Physiological concomitants of certain psychiatric illnesses (eg, major depression or panic disorder) may be misinterpreted as evidence of physical disease.
- Physical illness is less stigmatizing than mental illness.
- Some individuals amplify normal bodily sensations and interpret them as physical disease.
- The sick role can provide secondary gains such as gaining disability payments or avoiding social responsibilities.
- Physical or sexual trauma during childhood appears to predispose a person to using somatic symptoms for communication.
- Developing physical symptoms may be a behavior learned in childhood to obtain wanted nurturance from parents and other caregivers.
- Physicians trained with a too-exclusive emphasis on "physical" disease may attend only to physical symptoms and ignore psychosocial information from the patient.

PSYCHIATRIC REFERRAL

Somatizing patients regard themselves as physically, not psychiatrically, ill. Frequently, conferring a psychogenic etiology on medically unexplained complaints or suggesting psychiatric referral leads to resentment and discomfort in the patient-physician relationship. Thus, despite the need of these patients to address their psychosocial distress, management of these patients defaults to the primary care physician.

One potential resource is informal consultation with the primary care physician in the form of advice on how to manage severe personality disorders or psychopharmacologic information. Larger HMO clinics may find that providing such a resource is cost effective. Solo and small-group practitioners may contact a psychiatric colleague for some assistance.

Although overall management of somatization is best handled by the primary care physician, psychiatric referral is necessary at times. These situations include assessment of the patient who expresses suicidal ideation and management of treatment-resistant depressed patients, some patients with body dysmorphic disorder (because of severe and pervasive psychiatric comorbidity), highly self-injurious patients with factitious illness, and patients whose symptoms reflect the need for marital or family therapy.

A psychiatric referral is best made after rapport has been established and in association with a promise for ongoing treatment so the patient does not regard the referral as a rejection. Before making a referral, it is helpful to discuss the following with patients:

- The relationship between their symptoms and an underlying mental health disorder or stressful situation
- Assurance that the primary care physician believes these symptoms are real and not imagined and that the patient is not crazy or a failure
- Mental health care as part of an overall approach to the problem, which also includes ongoing monitoring and, when appropriate, specific treatment by the primary care physician

Shortly after making a referral for mental health care, it is important to schedule a follow-up primary care visit to verify that the patient is not being abandoned and to make sure the patient actually saw the specialist. At times, such as with manipulative, drug-seeking patients, accepting a psychiatric referral may be a condition of continuing involvement with the primary care physician.

SPECIFIC SOMATIZING SYNDROMES

The syndromes shown in Table 15-2 are defined in the *Diagnostic and Statistical Manual of Mental Disorders*, fourth edition (DSM-IV), as psychiatric disorders with specific diagnostic criteria. These textbook classifications, however, are deceptive in that few patients neatly fit into one of these categories. Rather, the various syndromes demonstrate inconsistent boundaries and fluidity of symptoms such that a patient may be described as meeting criteria for one diagnosis at one time and for another diagnosis at a later time. Further, most of these disorders have a dimensional rather than a categorical quality.

TABLE 15-2 Somatoform and Related Disorders

- Somatoform disorders:

    Conversion disorder

    Somatization disorder

    Undifferentiated somatization disorder

    Hypochondriasis

    Body dysmorphic disorder

    Pain disorder

    Somatoform disorder not otherwise specified

- Factitious illness
- Malingering

Conversion Disorder

Conversion symptoms were originally described in Egypt almost 4000 years ago. They were discussed in the *Corpus Hippocraticum* and, more recently, were a major focus of late-19th century neurologists including Charcot, Reynolds, and Freud. Despite occasionally mistaken statements that they belong to the past, conversion symptoms continue to be seen in a wide variety of medical settings.

Case Vignette

Mr Ramos is a 34-year-old single man with a grade school education who had emigrated from Mexico to be able to send money home to his family, in particular to help pay his beloved mother's mounting medical bills. He was successful at first, but after the first year Mr Ramos's homesickness mounted, he began to drink heavily, and his income stream became more erratic.

His mother died, but Mr Ramos was too broke and befuddled by alcohol to be able to arrange to go home for the funeral. Three days after the funeral, while watching a television program about happy mothers and sons, he suddenly became blind. A neighbor brought him to the hospital, and Mr Ramos was admitted for neurologic and ophthalmologic evaluation. The examinations were normal, and conversion disorder was suspected. The consultant psychiatrist found that Mr Ramos felt very guilty about his failure to attend his mother's funeral, and he was also highly suggestible.

Mr Ramos was hypnotized and given a posthypnotic suggestion that his vision would return after he emerged from the hypnotic state. His vision was restored a few minutes later, and he then was referred for brief outpatient grief counseling and alcohol treatment.

Diagnosis. Conversion disorder (as defined by the DSM–IV) consists of one or more symptoms suggesting a neurologic or general medical condition affecting voluntary motor or sensory function. The symptom is, however, medically unexplained, and psychologic factors are judged to be associated with its initiation or exacerbation. The symptom is not intentionally produced or feigned.

Features such as symbolism (ie, the notion that the symptom is metaphoric, such as blindness when the patient was exposed to something he or she did not want to see) and *la belle indifference* (lack of emotional concern about the symptom) may be seen in conversion disorder. Contrary to earlier opinions, though, these factors are not useful in determining the presence of conversion. Factors that do have some diagnostic utility include a prior history of somatization, a precipitating stressor, a human model for the symptom (knowing someone with a similar symptom), and symptoms that are clearly nonphysiologic (eg, total blindness with intact pupillary responses to light or sensory loss in a nonanatomic distribution).

Conversion occurs in persons of all ages. It is more common in adult women than adult men. As a general rule, any factor that reduces a person's ability to articulate distress may predispose to conversion, which then is used to communicate distress. These factors include lower intelligence, deprived economic or cultural background, poor education, highly limited health and medical knowledge, and any type of brain dysfunction. Conversion and neurologic disease are frequently comorbid, presumably because the neurologic disease provides a "model" for symptoms and/or interferes with verbal articulation. For example, up to one third of patients with epilepsy may also demonstrate pseudo-seizures.

The primary care physician must recognize that acute conversion usually represents an effort to communicate distress, suggesting more subtle underlying physical disease or psychiatric disorder. The patient may feel overwhelmed or may have sexual conflicts or abuse issues, eg, and be unable to talk about the distress. In some cases, patients may articulate their distress more clearly (and may even lose their physical symptoms) under hypnosis or during an Amytal (amobarbital sodium) interview, but these should be performed only by those who are experienced in these techniques.

Comorbidity. Persons with conversion disorder are so frequently comorbid for another psychiatric disorder, physical disease (often neurologic), or concurrent stressor in their lives that conversion should be viewed as a symptom rather than a diagnosis. Conversion is often associated with depression or concurrent neurologic disease including recent head trauma. Persons with recurrent conversion symptoms may better fit the diagnostic category of somatization disorder, described in the next section.

Prognosis. Most conversion symptoms are transient and remit either spontaneously or with suggestive therapies, often within hours or days. A few symptoms will persist and become problematic. If the conversion symptom remains untreated, physical complications may develop (eg, contractures from conversion paralysis). Over a period of several years, about 25% of patients will have a recurrence of conversion symptoms and/or the emergence of neurologic disease that explains the original symptom.

Treatment principles. Each person with conversion disorder should be evaluated from the perspective of the three Ps:

- **P**redisposition
- **P**recipitating stressor(s)
- **P**erpetuating factors

The treatment plan will be guided, to a large extent, by this information. Predisposing factors include issues such as a low level of psychological sophistication, prior somatization, and a model for the symptom (eg, prior history of genuine epileptic fits). Precipitating factors may be current sexual or physical abuse, eg, or a feeling of being overwhelmed with demands of housework, children, and employment. Perpetuating factors (present in more chronic symptoms) may include attention from previously uninvolved relatives, disability payments, relief from usual and onerous responsibilities, or other secondary gains.

Each patient with conversion symptoms (even if transient) should receive a careful physical and neurologic evaluation, including a search for comorbid psychiatric diagnoses and, when present, treatment. External stressors (eg, physical abuse) must be identified and addressed as indicated. Symptoms that are persistently disabling require careful assessment of reinforcers in the environment that perpetuate the sick role. Hospitalization, either psychiatric or in a rehabilitation unit, may be necessary to institute behavior-modification techniques to extinguish sick role behaviors. These techniques often can be combined with physical therapy, providing the patient with a face-saving mechanism to discard his or her symptoms.

Psychotherapy, either individual or family-oriented, may be useful to help resolve the conflicts underlying the need for conversion as a means of communication. Insight psychotherapy focusing on a search for symbolizing has not proved, as a general rule, to be efficacious for those patients who are not psychologically minded. Because much of the treatment is driven by more formal psychotherapeutic methods, the primary care physician can play an important role in reinforcing, to the patient and the family, the need for such care, and to avoid additional fruitless searches for medical "zebras" once the diagnosis of conversion has been made.

Somatization Disorder and Undifferentiated Somatization Disorder

A pattern of medically unexplained physical complaints was first studied systematically by Pierre Briquet in the mid-19th century. More recent research in the mid-20th century by Guze and colleagues at Washington University has led to the current phenomenologic and descriptive knowledge of what is a relatively common disorder in primary care. Diagnostic criteria have evolved from original descriptions of hysteria to that which was termed *Briquet's syndrome*. The DSM–III term *somatization disorder* (SD), incorporating prior concepts of hysteria, was introduced in 1980.

Case Vignette

Ms Margie, a 34-year-old, twice-divorced mother of three, sought care from Dr Morales because as she noted, "I've had it with all of those other doctors. Everyone tells me you're the best primary care doctor in town. You'll get all my problems straightened out." She said she had been somewhat "sickly" ever since she had "abdominal lymphadenitis" at age 13, although she denied any current complaints at the time except "migraine headaches, but they are part of my environmental allergies."

The physical examination was remarkable only for an old cholecystectomy scar and three different breast biopsy scars. Two days later the pharmacy called, asking for authorization to renew Ms Margie's Fiorinal and alprazolam prescriptions. Later that week Ms Margie's old medical records from the clinic were delivered. Dr Morales reviewed them: 3 years at the clinic, 14 pounds of records, 12 physicians (5 of them primary care), 22 items on the problem list, 4 surgeries, 4 biopsies, 17 different medications.

Later that day Ms Margie called, urgently asking for an appointment because she was having "another one of my kidney infections." She commented on how much she had liked Dr Morales' tie and his aftershave the last time she had seen him.

Diagnosis. The DSM–IV criteria for somatization disorder (SD) specify that the disorder begins before age 30 and must include at least eight unexplained medical symptoms, four pain symptoms, two nonpain gastrointestinal (GI) symptoms, one sexual symptom, and at least one pseudoneurologic symptom (see Table 15-3). Undifferentiated somatization disorder is defined by one or more medically unexplained symptoms and a duration of at least 6 months.

From a phenomenologic viewpoint, somatization disorder and undifferentiated somatization disorder seemed to be dimensional differences of the same process on a continuum. Undifferentiated somatization disorder (eg, a history of one to seven unexplained medical symptoms) has many of the same phenomenologic findings as somatization disorder, only to a lesser degree. Thus, it is a subsyndromal variant of somatization disorder. The following discussion focuses on somatization disorder. The reader must keep in mind that the same general principles regarding care are applicable to undifferentiated somatization disorder.

Persons with SD are most frequently of lower socioeconomic status and often of minority groups. Women, particularly unmarried mothers, comprise the large majority of patients, although men with the disorder have been reported. Persons with SD frequently come from chaotic childhood homes in which divorce, substance abuse, and/or sexual or physical abuse are common. There is an increased incidence of SD in female relatives and of alcoholism and/or antisocial personality disorder among male relatives. Women who later develop SD often have ventured prematurely into sexual behavior, they often marry early, and they may have alcoholic and/or abusive sexual partners. They themselves frequently have problems with alcohol or other drugs of abuse, including prescribed medications. Persons with SD tend to live disorganized chaotic lives, and their somatization can be conceptualized as an attempted coping mechanism. Some exhibit incongruent smiling or affect as if in a shell with their "serious medical problems."

Comorbidity. Essentially all patients with SD are comorbid for at least one axis I diagnosis (particularly major depression and substance-use disorders) and one or more axis

---

TABLE 15-3 Summary of DSM-IV Diagnostic Criteria for Somatization Disorder

- History of many physical complaints beginning at less than 30 years of age, occurs over several years, and results in treatment being sought or significant impairment in functioning.

- Each of the following:

  Four pain symptoms: eg, head, abdomen, back, joints, extremities, chest, rectum, during menstruation, during sexual intercourse, or during urination

  Two nonpain GI symptoms: eg, nausea, bloating, vomiting other than during pregnancy, diarrhea, or intolerance of several different foods

  One nonpain sexual or reproductive symptom: sexual indifference, erectile or ejaculatory dysfunction, irregular menses, excessive menstrual bleeding, vomiting throughout pregnancy

  One pseudoneurological symptom: impaired coordination or balance, paralysis or localized weakness, difficulty swallowing or lump in throat, aphonia, urinary retention, hallucinations, loss of touch or pain sensation, double vision, blindness, deafness, seizures; dissociative symptoms such as amnesia; or loss of consciousness other than fainting

- Each symptom cannot be fully explained by a known general medical condition or the direct effects of a substance, or the complaints or resulting impairment are in excess of what would be expected.

- Symptoms are not intentionally feigned or produced.

Adapted with permission from the *Diagnostic and Statistical Manual of Mental Disorders*. 4th ed, Text Revision. Copyright 2000. American Psychiatric Association.

II personality disorders (most frequently histrionic, borderline, and dependent). Persons with SD frequently have a history of psychiatric treatment in addition to their complex medical histories. Women with SD typically see multiple medical specialists concurrently. Histories of multiple surgical procedures are common. Substance abuse (including that of iatrogenic origin) and suicidal gestures are seen frequently, and these risks have complications for treatment and management (see below).

SD patients frequently carry the label of one or more chronic diseases, often poorly substantiated, such as lupus erythematosus and irritable bowel syndrome. They also are likely to be labeled with fashionable diagnoses such as fibromyalgia, chronic fatigue syndrome, multiple chemical sensitivities, or dysautonomia. Frequently they are taking multiple prescribed (and over-the-counter) drugs, which may be producing side effects—a situation that can further complicate the task of reaching an accurate diagnosis.

Prognosis. In its full-blown form, SD is a chronic, undulating disorder with relapses occurring at times of personal stress. Patients are at risk for complications of substance abuse, partner abuse, and, most important, iatrogenic disease. Despite these patients' perceiving themselves as "sicker than the sickest," they do not have a shortened life span and their symptoms frequently continue into old age.

The major serious complications of SD seem to be iatrogenic. Unwise decisions about invasive testing or therapeutics may leave patients with chronic complications (eg, adhesions) that increase patient distress and further complicate subsequent symptom evaluation.

Management principles. Patients with SD almost always have multiple problems—social, medical, and psychiatric. They rarely are psychologically minded, and they are poor candidates for traditional forms of psychotherapy. Their management generally falls to the primary care physician.

Several general treatment principles have been demonstrated to reduce excessive medical use. Sometimes the goals are as basic as preventing unnecessary visits to emergency departments or unneeded surgeries. The overall strategy must be to contain symptoms and prevent iatrogenic complications rather than to effect a "cure." As with many chronic illnesses, SD should be approached with an eye toward optimizing function rather than eradicating symptoms, as noted here:

- One primary care physician should manage medical care (and prescriptions). Consultants are used for advice rather than to shift responsibility for medical care. Consultants should be asked to communicate their findings and suggestions to the primary care physician only. This policy should be explained in advance to the patient as necessary to prevent confusion and miscommunication.
- The etiology of symptoms should be explained to patients rather than their being blamed for a psychogenic etiology, eg, "You seem to have an exacerbation of your pelvic pain when you're under stress," rather than, "Your pain is all in your head."
- Decisions about invasive diagnostic and therapeutic procedures should be based on objective findings, not on subjective complaints alone.
- Patients should be seen on a regularly scheduled basis (eg, every 2 to 4 weeks), not dependent on the development of new symptoms (ie, prn). This type of predictable support significantly reduces emergency-room visits and other unnecessary emergent medical interventions.
- Habituating or addictive medications must be used sparingly and only when necessary for objective indications. Caution must be used in the quantity of medications prescribed. These patients are prone to develop home pharmacies and also are at risk for suicidal gestures via overdoses.
- Co-occurring psychiatric disorders (eg, depression, anxiety, substance abuse, sexual dysfunction) should be sought, diagnosed, and treated appropriately.
- Group therapy, particularly therapy with an education and/or cognitive-behavioral therapeutic approach, has been shown to reduce medical utilization significantly. This service may be offered by HMOs, large group practices, or governmentally supported medical care (eg, military medical clinics).
- For patients who have prominent pain complaints, many of the management suggestions indicated below in the section on pain disorder may be helpful.

Hypochondriasis

Hypochondriasis is a long-recognized condition that some have believed in the past, inaccurately, to be the male equivalent of hysteria. The term literally means "below the cartilage," reflecting observations that these patients frequently complain of abdominal symptoms.

Diagnosis. Hypochondriasis is defined as the preoccupation with, fears of, or conviction that one has a serious disease. Symptoms must last at least 6 months, persist despite adequate medical evaluation and reassurance, and cause significant distress or social or occupational impairment. Exclusionary factors include somatic delusions, such as those that occur with psychotic depression.

Hypochondriasis, which affects 4% to 6% of all patients, is commonly seen in primary care. It often starts in adolescence or young adulthood and is seen in persons from childhood to old age. The male:female ratio is approximately equal and, contrary to popular belief, it is not more prevalent among elderly persons. Although hypochondriasis (and its associated comorbid disorders) tends to run in families, there is no specific evidence of a genetic etiology.

The most frequently presented symptoms include those reflecting the musculoskeletal system, GI tract, and cardiopulmonary function. Symptoms, however, can include a wide breadth of complaints such as tinnitus, headaches, vision complaints, and so forth. Symptoms are not generally presented in a dramatic fashion with an urgency for action (as with conversion or somatization disorder) but, rather, in a worried, obsessive manner. Symptoms reflecting normal body functions or minor illnesses may be misinterpreted as evidence of catastrophic disease.

Many hypochondriacal patients seem to thrive on the suffering that their symptoms cause and thus be reluctant to hear any "good news." They greet physician reassurances with disbelief, requests for further diagnostic assessment, or even disparagement of the physician's skills or knowledge. Despite the often obvious psychological nature of the illness to the physician, hypochondriacal patients themselves usually are quite focused on physical symptoms and are reluctant to entertain the idea that emotional factors could be involved. They may become quite angry if the physician suggests this possibility. Recommendations for psychiatric evaluation or care—unless handled deftly in the context of a solid patient-physician alliance—may rupture the relationship.

By contrast, transient hypochondriasis following serious illness, such as after cancer surgery, is common and normal and should be differentiated from primary hypochondriasis. These transient patients frequently scan their bodies and regard any mild symptoms as a potential sign that the disease is recurring.

Comorbid disorders. Comorbidity in hypochondriasis is so common that some investigators have questioned whether it should be regarded as a distinct entity or as a common final symptomatic pathway for a number of disorders. The most common comorbid disorders are major depression, dysthymia, panic disorder, generalized anxiety disorder, and obsessive-compulsive disorder. Patients also frequently have symptoms reflecting irritable bowel syndrome, which are misinterpreted as a sign of more serious illness. It also has been proposed that hypochondriacs may differentially attend to symptoms. For example, they might have an irrational fear that the tachycardia or dizziness accompanying a psychiatric illness (such as panic disorder) is indicative of a disease process.

Prognosis. Hypochondriasis tends to be a chronic disorder that fluctuates in severity of symptoms. Paradoxically, many patients respond best to the physician's limited expectations for improvement. Some patients deteriorate and become disabled by their preoccupations with disease, perhaps reflecting severe forms of depression or obsessive-compulsive disorder.

Transient hypochondriasis, by definition, generally remits after several months if the patient's disease process is stable (eg, postcancer surgery or postmyocardial infarction).

Management. Treatment of the hypochondriac is a long-term process that should be tempered with modest expectations for improvement. Each new complaint should be evaluated by obtaining an appropriate history of the symptom in association with at least a limited physical examination. Invasive diagnostic and therapeutic procedures should be based on objective findings rather than subjective complaints. With negative findings (the usual situation) the patient should be reassured that there is no evidence of any serious disease, and a follow-up visit (generally for about 1 month) should be scheduled. The overall goal for hypochondriasis is optimization of functioning, which largely means preventing the patient's health concerns and help-seeking from becoming too large a part of his or her life.

The physician's demeanor should be warm and concerned but not condescending. Patients who are observed to respond to reassurance with an increase in complaints may require a different approach; they may do better with no reassurance but, rather, praise for their bearing up so well under such a burden. It is important to gradually obtain personal information about the patient and to establish rapport and a working relationship. With time, the primary care physician may be able to help the patient associate the emergence of certain symptoms with life stressors or with specific emotional states. It also is helpful for the physician to identify the patient's explanatory model of his or her illness (if there is one) and to address issues raised by that model. Finally, the physician should offer patients specific suggestions about signs for which they can look that indicate a need for further medical investigations or treatments.

Treatment of comorbid disorders is important but may have to be delayed until the patient has developed sufficient rapport with the physician so that he or she will accept treatment. Premature efforts to prescribe medication for depression or panic disorder may meet with resistance, disabling side effects, or the patient's change of physicians. When prescribing medications, the physician must take into account the hypervigilance to bodily symptoms that these patients manifest and must keep in mind that they are inclined to report a number of side effects from the medication. In fact, many hypochondriacs own a copy of the *Physicians Desk Reference*. It is prudent for the physician to explain to the patient that he or she understands the sensitivity to medication, to start with a low dosage, and to increase it slowly until therapeutic levels are achieved.

Many hypochondriacal patients have reduced symptoms following the prescription of one of the selective serotonin reuptake inhibitors (SSRIs), such as fluoxetine or sertraline hydrochloride. This is because of the relationship between hypochondriasis and obsessive-compulsive disorder (OCD); hypochondriasis may represent a subtype of OCD in which the obsession is a preoccupation with somatic symptoms.

Cognitive-behavioral therapy has been demonstrated to be helpful in hypochondriasis. Through this treatment the patient learns that the somatic preoccupations and fears are cognitive distortions and is taught methods by which to redirect thinking. Because of time constraints, providing cognitive-behavioral therapy would be difficult for most primary care physicians, but larger medical groups and HMOs may be able to provide some adjunctive psychological services.

Body Dysmorphic Disorder

Body dysmorphic disorder (BDD) is a relatively new diagnosis introduced in DSM-III to clarify the prior unsatisfactory vague terms of dysmorphophobia and monosymptomatic hypochondriasis. Although persons with BDD may be seen in a primary care setting, they most frequently seek consultations from dermatologists and plastic surgeons.

Case Vignette

Mr Paul, a 25-year-old single postal worker, presents to his new primary care physician, Dr Dahl, requesting a referral to a plastic surgeon. He feels that his nose was misshapen, and he believes that his impoverished social life and low self-esteem would improve if he were to have his nose reshaped. The nose does not appear deformed to Dr Dahl, but he authorizes a consultation with Dr Blair, a plastic surgeon. Dr Blair agrees that surgery is not necessary.

Two months later Mr Paul returns to Dr Dahl, requesting another referral for the same problem. He seems more pressured about the surgery, and he tells Dr Dahl that he switched to the night shift at work because he could not bear to be seen by so many people at work and in public when going to and from work.

After further questioning, Dr Dahl discovers that Mr Paul almost never leaves his home during the weekend and that he has no social contacts other than his family. Dr Dahl offers Mr Paul a prescription for fluoxetine, 20 mg q AM. Paul seems puzzled about how this could help his nose, but he agrees to a trial.

Over the next 3 months the dose is increased gradually to 60 mg/day, and Mr Paul reports less preoccupation with his nose, more comfort in social situations, and a return to day-shift work. The medication is continued, and 3 months later Mr Paul goes out on his first date.

Diagnosis. Body dysmorphic disorder consists of an overvalued belief (sometimes of a delusional magnitude) that something about one's body is deformed, unattractive, or inadequate. The defect, which must be a major preoccupation of the sufferer of the syndrome, is nonexistent or is perceived by others as essentially insignificant. This disorder has been aptly called "the pain of imagined ugliness." Examples include preoccupation over the size or shape of one's nose, lips, or other facial features, and preoccupation with the size or shape of one's breasts or penis.

Distortions of body image such as those associated with anorexia nervosa are better described by an eating disorder diagnosis. Patients with primary psychotic disorders (eg, schizophrenia) may describe bizarre symptoms, whereas those with BDD tend to describe those that are at least plausible, even if unlikely.

The incidence of BDD is unknown. There seems to be a continuum of severity, with persons who have milder cases typically seen in late adolescence. Persons with more severe and clinically significant symptoms are most frequently young adults, equally distributed between men and women. These persons may be completely disabled from work and spend much of their waking time examining themselves, looking at themselves in reflecting surfaces, and being intensely preoccupied with their appearance. They may be reluctant to leave their place of residence for fear of humiliation because of the perceived deformities.

Comorbidity. BDD frequently is comorbid with obsessive-compulsive disorder. In fact, some investigators believe that BDD is a form of OCD with an obsessional focus on a body part. Other frequent comorbid disorders include major depression, dysthymia, and social phobia. Some of the more severe BDD patients evoke consideration of a psychotic process such as delusional disorder or schizophrenia. In this regard, BDD seems to have some relationship with the monosymptomatic hypochondriacal syndromes of delusions of bromosis (the belief that one is emitting an odor) and delusions of parasitosis (the mistaken, and generally unshakable, belief that one is infected by parasites).

Prognosis. The prognosis for BDD is unknown. Follow-up studies have suggested that persons with monosymptomatic hypochondriasis are at high risk for developing psychosis or for suicide. Fortunately, with the advent of more effective pharmacologic treatment, the prognosis for these unhappy people will be more favorable.

Treatment. Treatment of BDD prior to the introduction of SSRIs was largely limited to treatment of comorbid conditions. Some success using pimozide for the monosymptomatic hypochondriacal states was reported but was never replicated in large-scale studies. Psychotherapy, despite the intriguing promise of some relationship to apparent psychodynamic issues, has never been shown to be consistently useful for BDD patients.

The SSRIs have proved to be highly efficacious for BDD. Patients treated with these medications may experience a significant reduction in the intensity of their symptoms, even when the symptom is of psychotic proportion. This specific response to treatment, in association with some other phenomenologic features, is what has led some clinicians to conclude that BDD and OCD are closely related, possibly variations of the same disorder. Treatment of BDD also must include consideration of the frequent comorbid disorders, including severe depression and social phobia, and the fact that these persons are at high risk for suicide.

Pain Disorder

Pain disorder is the latest of the various terms used over the years in an attempt to categorize and explain chronic unexplained physical pain. Previous terms, such as *chronic pain*, *psychogenic pain*, and *somatoform pain disorder*, were not well accepted; and they failed to assist in systematic research for this disorder, which is known to all clinicians, yet is elusive to define and quantitate. Patients with chronic pain are among the most commonly seen in primary care, and their treatment and concurrent disability result in the spending of billions of dollars annually for medical costs and payments for disability. These are among the most vexing of all patients. There are a multitude of pain syndromes, but in the interest of brevity, the following comments are limited to general concepts and common phenomenologic observations. Pain, however, is of heterogeneous etiologies, and the following descriptions do not fit all patients.

Diagnosis. The DSM-IV diagnostic criteria for pain disorder require that pain in one or more body sites be the predominant focus of the clinical presentation. The pain must be of sufficient severity to cause significant distress or impairment of function. Psychological factors are regarded as important in the initiation, perception, or perpetuation of the pain. Pain is classified as chronic if it persists longer than 6 months.

The new diagnostic criteria allow for further categorization as to whether the pain is associated with primarily psychological factors, primarily psychological factors and a general medical condition, or primarily resulting from a general medical condition. This classification attempts to avoid the previous dualism of psychologic vs the physiologic etiology of pain and takes into account the fact that most patients with pain may have an organic nidus for pain perceptions but react with exaggeration or elaboration.

Phenomenology. Pain is a ubiquitous symptom, and pain syndromes occur in all ages and in both sexes. Among the various manifestations are chronic low-back pain, temporomandibular joint pain, atypical facial pain, chronic pelvic pain, and phantom pain. Pain disorder frequently is described as the "disorder of the Ds":

- **D**isability
- **D**rugs
- **D**epression
- **D**octor-shopping
- **D**ependency

The pain-disorder patient is generally nonpsychologically minded and attributes all depressive feelings and interpersonal problems as secondary to the pain. In contrast to overt statements as to what an independent person he or she is, the pain disorder patient repetitively behaves in a dependent manner and, despite a lack of objective findings to substantiate disability, resists all efforts to return him or her to work. A frequent underlying factor in disability is anger at a supervisor at the place of employment.

Prognosis. Pain patients often are remarkably refractory to any therapeutic intervention. Outcome studies are complicated by their tendency to "doctor-shop," and they frequently are lost to follow-up. They often deteriorate, with increasing disability and social withdrawal. The physician must show patience with the anticipation of a chronic and lengthy illness. Unfortunately, many patients are self-defeating, so they sabotage improvement in pain and function, leading to a relapse.

Management. As with other somatoform disorders, a major goal in managing the pain disorder patient is to avoid iatrogenic complications. These patients are at risk for habituation of anxiolytics and analgesics, and they often accept, or even seek out, surgical procedures that in retrospect have little indication. For example, patients with facial pain frequently have a history of multiple surgical and dental procedures with no lasting relief from pain.

Established principles and techniques in managing pain disorder patients include:

- Setting goals that emphasize rehabilitation rather than pain relief, helping the patient learn to function despite pain rather than focus on pain relief, and on decreasing the risk of addiction
- Acknowledging the reality of the patient's pain while also making the link to psychosocial factors (ie, the relationship between mood and pain, and stressors and pain)
- An approach emphasizing that the patient take responsibility for his or her behavior and discard magical expectations that the right physician, drug, or surgical procedure will relieve his or her discomfort
- Avoiding unnecessary habituating drugs; if they worked, the patient wouldn't continue to have pain
- When opiate-type or other analgesics are objectively indicated (eg, postoperatively), prescribe them on a scheduled basis rather than an as-needed basis (this reduces the patient's need to engage in pain behaviors to seek medications and reduces tension between the patient and health care staff)
- Treating comorbid disorders, particularly depression (even for nondepressed patients, low-dose tricyclics, such as amitriptyline hydrochloride, often are beneficial)
- Communicating to the patient that complete pain relief is improbable and that, as in the National Football League, one must learn how to "play hurt"

Pain patients are difficult to manage, and treatment often must include family members because they frequently reinforce pain behaviors, knowingly or unwittingly. Some patients require treatment at a behaviorally oriented, multidisciplinary pain clinic or program because of the need to address multiple issues in a comprehensive fashion.

Factitious Illness

Factitious disorders (FD), originally described by the Roman physician Galen, present an intriguing paradox: Patients seek treatment for diseases that they surreptitiously produce in themselves. Although the extreme forms of factitious illness (eg, Munchausen syndrome) are relatively rare, an estimated one in five somatizing patients engages in factitious behavior on at least one occasion.

Case Vignette

Mr Terry, a 30-year-old unmarried emergency medical technician, presents to Dr Judd requesting further care for his stage IV lymphoma. He had been diagnosed a month earlier at Sloan Kettering Hospital in New York and had completed the induction phase of a four-drug chemotherapy protocol there. Then he returned to the Midwest to be with his family. When his wallet was stolen at the airport, he lost his chemotherapy prescriptions, but a neighborhood pharmacist who knew his mother gave him a 3-week supply.

On examination, Mr Terry has a temperature of 101.5°, pallor, petechiae, pharyngeal injection, and evidence of consolidation in his left lung. Stat labs reveal pancytopenia. Mr Terry is admitted to the hospital. A call to Sloan Kettering reveals that the hospital has never heard of the patient.

Mr Terry proceeds to have a stormy hospital course, spending 6 weeks in the intensive care unit with a variety of infections and their sequelae. After stabilization and confrontation about the information from Sloan Kettering, Mr Terry admits that he has never been diagnosed with a lymphoma and that he played on the pharmacist's sympathies, knowing that the pharmacist would never believe that anyone would take medications such as these without medical supervision.

Mr Terry becomes indignant and signs out of the hospital against medical advice when Dr Judd proposes a psychiatric consultation to understand what made Mr Terry do such a thing. Later that day, Mr Terry's mother, who is aware of the deception, calls to complain to Dr Judd about his "outrageous care" of her son in proposing a psychiatric evaluation.

Diagnosis. Factitious disorders consist of consciously motivated surreptitious production or simulation of physical or psychological symptoms. They differ from malingering (see below) in that there is no determinable benefit other than seeking the sick role. Persons with factitious behavior have simulated essentially all common, and some rare, physical diseases. Among the most common simulations are anemia (self-phlebotomy), kidney stones (finger pricked to create hematuria), and hypoglycemia (surreptitious self-administration of insulin). Psychological symptoms include feigned bereavement, pseudodementia, and factitious posttraumatic stress disorder.

There are three primary factitious disorder syndromes:

- Patients with *simple factitious disorder* tend to have one symptom (eg, anemia), do not use aliases, and seek medical care in their own locales. They may or may not demonstrate pseudologia fantastica (a form of pathological lying that includes untruthful information unrelated to the medical situation), but they frequently are skillful liars. Most commonly, they are unmarried women 20 to 40 years of age, usually work in a health-related field such as nursing, come from dysfunctional families, and meet diagnostic criteria for histrionic or borderline personality disorder.

- The *Munchausen syndrome* consists of multiple hospital admissions, often with the use of aliases, traveling from city to city, and associated pseudologia fantastica. Persons with this syndrome typically are middle-aged men estranged from their families. They have complex psychiatric and/or legal histories and often fit the criteria for antisocial personality disorder. Substance abuse is a common finding in these patients. Many seek opiates during their medical encounters.

- The *factitious illness by proxy syndrome* (sometimes referred to as *Munchausen by proxy syndrome*) consists of one person surreptitiously inducing illness in another person. Most frequently this person is a mother inducing an illness or misrepresenting symptoms in one or more of her preverbal children. Presumably the mother gains attention from her dramatic role of mother of a sick child and vicariously reaps the benefits of a sick role "by proxy." Common presentations are apnea (prolonged smothering of the child by the mother), false reports of seizures, and the consequences of repeated administration of a toxic substance. The perpetrators, even when apprehended in the act, rarely admit to their behaviors, and the diagnosis must be established by covert surveillance, finding the presence of a toxic substance or nonprescribed medication, or by circumstantial evidence (eg, the child recovers or has no symptoms when kept away from the perpetrator). This is a particularly covert form of child abuse, and cases should be reported to local child protective services.

Comorbidity. Essentially all persons who engage in factitial disease-inducing behavior have a personality disorder, most frequently borderline, histrionic, narcissistic, or antisocial. A small minority of factitious disorder patients has some significant depression or psychosis. Many, if not most, of the perpetrators of Munchausen by proxy syndrome have no overt psychopathology but have underlying narcissistic pathology (ie, an inability to distinguish their own needs and wishes from the interests of others).

Prognosis. The lack of good follow-up studies limits our knowledge of the fate of most FD patients. Patients do suffer irreparable iatrogenic injuries (eg, unnecessary amputations, removal of internal organs, and so forth) and also may misjudge their disease-producing behaviors and accidentally die from complications. Persons with full-blown Munchausen syndrome seem to have an intractable illness. Persons with simple FD often appear to discard their illness-producing behavior spontaneously as they grow older, perhaps to be replaced by other forms of somatization. The mortality rate for the childhood victim of Munchausen by proxy syndrome is approximately 10%, and there are long-term psychological and developmental problems resulting from this form of victimization. One such effect is to engage in FD behavior or somatization as an adult. Thus, FD becomes a multigenerational problem.

Management. The primary goal in managing FD is to prevent further extension of physical damage self-inflicted by patients and to avoid iatrogenic complications caused by invasive diagnostic or therapeutic procedures. Patients with FD present a variety of complex management problems, summarized below. Medico-legal and ethical issues frequently emerge with the FD patient, and it is recommended that the primary care physician seek early consultation for help in anticipating and making contingency plans to deal with complications in management. General principles for management include these:

- Good communication among staff members on the treatment team is essential because FD patients usually are comorbid for personality disorders and they tend to play medical care staff off against each other, creating considerable dissension among their caretakers.
- The FD patient should be confronted in a manner that conveys a continuing concern for the patient and redefines the patient's illness as reflecting psychosocial distress rather than physical disease. Even if confrontation is done well, most FD patients will leave a physician who tells them the truth.
- If the physician strongly suspects FD but lacks enough evidence for a direct confrontation, use of the subjunctive may be helpful: "One of the things that would explain your illness is that you have done this to yourself, and *if this were to be the case*, it would mean that you were so upset about matters in your life that it led you to do something this extreme."
- Medico-legal and ethical principles require adherence to the usual rules for patient consent, privacy, and confidentiality. Deviating from these principles must clearly be for reasons to protect the patient or others from harm. Medical records should reflect consideration of FD as soon as it is suspected; these patients do sue. When Munchausen by proxy syndrome is suspected, it must be reported to the appropriate protective services agency because it is a form of child abuse.
- An ongoing supportive relationship with the primary care physician and frequent office visits may provide sufficient attention and the desired nurturance to significantly reduce the patient's FD behavior. Most primary care physicians feel more comfortable in offering support if they have concurrent consultation assistance from a psychiatrist.

Malingering

Malingering, by definition, is less a medical diagnosis than a legal or social accusation. It is not regarded as a mental disorder in the DSM-IV, largely because malingering may be adaptive under certain circumstances (eg, feigning illness in a POW camp to get better rations or less harsh treatment). The malingerer produces, simulates, or exaggerates physical illness for an external gain such as disability payments, a settlement from an insurance company, avoidance of military conscription, or the obtaining of controlled substances. Table 15-4 highlights the differences between malingering, factitious illness, and conversion.

TABLE 15-4 Conversion, Factitious Illness, and Malingering		
Disorder	**Intentional Symptom Production?**	**Patient Aware of His or Her Motivations?**
Conversion disorder	no	no
Factitious illness	yes	no
Malingering	yes	yes

Although thought to be most common in institutional settings (prisons, the armed forces), malingering, unfortunately, is seen elsewhere, and the primary care physician must neither try to play the role of detective nor be an unwitting accomplice to nefarious behavior. Malingering must be a part of the differential diagnosis when there is a discrepancy between objective findings and subjective complaints and a discernible potential benefit to illness. The physician is advised to carefully document both the presence and the absence of objective findings and make decisions for therapeutic interventions based on objective evidence.

SOMATIZATION AND POSTTRAUMATIC STRESS DISORDERS

Research interest in posttraumatic stress disorder (PTSD) has been increasing during the past decade. PTSD has been shown to cause a variety of physiological dysfunctions, including anatomic brain changes, and is associated with significant psychiatric and medical surgical comorbidities. Medical use markedly increases for persons with PTSD, and much of this is related to medically unexplained symptoms (eg, somatization).

Conversion disorder, somatization disorder, and pain syndromes are associated with PTSD at rates considerably higher than that in the general population. Patients with one of these somatoform disorders, which are comorbid for PTSD, often present with physical complaints rather than characteristic symptoms of PTSD, such as autonomic arousal, increased startle reaction, reexperiencing phenomenon, and phobias. It is important to establish the correct underlying diagnosis of PTSD so effective treatment can be initiated (see Chapter 8). The somatizing patient's first presentation is usually to the primary care physician. Thus, a part of the initial evaluation is to inquire about the possibility of past trauma, including sexual and physical abuse, as well as the presence of typical PTSD symptoms.

SOMATIZATION IN CHILDREN AND ADOLESCENTS

Transient somatization is common in children and generally can be managed using a commonsense approach. What child has not on at least one occasion developed a stomachache, or the equivalent, to avoid an unpleasant task or test? Persistent or recurrent somatization, however, is another matter. Accurate assessment of these situations is crucial in that the symptom(s) may be a cry for help from someone who is dealing with family or environmental issues (eg, abuse issues), a means to perpetrate school refusal, the symptomatic presentation of an anxiety or mood disorder, or undiagnosed physical disease.

Treatment interventions for the somatizing child necessarily depend on identification of the various etiologies that drive the symptoms. Techniques often must include an investigation of the family dynamics (and active intervention if conditions such as sexual or physical abuse are present), as well as communication and consultation with school personnel including teachers, counselors, and the school nurse. Consolidation and coordination of medical care by the primary care physician are desirable to reduce "doctor-shopping" and "doctor-splitting" behaviors. Further, all medications preferably should be prescribed by one physician to minimize drug interactions and the potential for abuse.

SUMMARY

Somatizing patients are common in primary care settings. Early identification results in lower medical care costs, less iatrogenic morbidity, and more effective therapeutic interventions. Management of these patients defaults to the primary care physician, and psychiatric referral is generally limited to specific indications. Principles of management include frequent, regularly scheduled office appointments that are not contingent on the development of new symptoms; avoidance of invasive diagnostic and therapeutic procedures except for *objective* indications; limited use of habituating analgesic and anxiolytic medications; treatment of comorbid psychiatric disorders such as panic disorder and depression; and avoidance of statements (eg, "It's all in your head") that inhibit rapport. Somatizers tend to be long-term chronic patients, and the goal must be "care" rather than "cure."

ADDITIONAL READINGS

Barsky AJ. Hidden reasons some patients visit doctors. *Ann Internal Med.* 1981;94:492-498.

Barsky AJ, Borus JF. Somatization and medicalization in the era of managed care. *JAMA.* 1995;274:1931-1934.

Blackwell B, DeMorgan NP. The primary care of patients who have bodily concerns. *Arch Fam Med.* 1996;5:457-463.

Campo JV, Fritz G. A management model for pediatric somatization. *Psychosomatics.* 2001;42:467-476.

Fink P, Rosendal M, Toft T. Assessment and treatment of functional disorders in general practice. *Psychosomatics.* 2002;43:93-131.

Ford CV. *Lies! Lies!! Lies!!!: The Psychology of Deceit.* Washington, DC: American Psychiatric Press Inc; 1996.

Ford CV. Somatic symptoms, somatizations and traumatic stress: an overview. *Nord J Psychiatry.* 1997;51:5-13.

Ford CV. Somatization and fashionable diagnoses: illness as a way of life. *Scand J Work Environ Health.* 1997;23(suppl 3):7-16.

Goldberg RJ, Novack DH, Gask L. The recognition and management of somatization. *Psychosomatics.* 1992;33:55-61.

Katon W, Ries RK, Kleinman A. Part II: A prospective DSM-III study of 100 consecutive somatization patients. *Compre Psychiatr.* 1984;25:305-314.

Koenig TW, Clark MR. Advances in comprehensive pain management. *Psychiatric Clin North Am.* 1996;19:589-612.

Smith GR, Monson RA, Ray DC. Psychiatric consultation in somatization disorder: a randomized, controlled study. *N Engl J Med.* 1986;314:1407-1413.

Smith RC. A clinical approach to the somatizing patient. *J Fam Pract.* 1985;21:294-301.

Chapter **16**

Difficult Patient Situations

Larry S. Goldman, MD
Steven R. Hahn, MD

Although practicing medicine has many rewards, even generally satisfied physicians find that certain clinical situations are particularly difficult or frustrating. Some situations have to do with unpleasant duties, such as breaking bad news or seeing patients suffer, but with experience most physicians find these situations manageable. Yet, even seasoned clinicians frequently report that certain types of patients invariably manage to "get under their skin." The temptation may be strong to label these patients "difficult" or "personality-disordered" and to think of ways to unload them, but there are other ways to conceptualize such situations and physicians can find effective ways to work with difficult patients.

This chapter provides a review of frameworks by which to understand difficult patient-physician situations and types of patients who commonly cause physicians distress. This group includes patients who are nonadherent, hostile or angry, demanding or entitled, dependent or clinging, and seductive. Somatizing patients are covered more fully in Chapter 15.

What constitutes a difficult patient situation? For the purposes of this chapter, this situation represents an *interpersonal* dissonance between physician and patient that leaves the physician feeling dysphoric in encounters with the patient. The dysphoria may take the form of anger or rage, a feeling of powerlessness, guilt, embarrassment, feeling duped, or other negative emotional states. The physician may or may not be aware of these feelings, but he or she is generally aware of dreading calls or visits from these patients and may contemplate ways to avoid the patients or transfer their care elsewhere.

UNDERSTANDING DIFFICULTY IN THE PATIENT-PHYSICIAN RELATIONSHIP

Empirical research has shown that physicians perceive about 15% of patients in primary care settings to be "difficult." Most of these patients are characterized by clinical syndromes (ie, *Diagnostic and Statistical Manual of Mental Disorders,* fourth edition [DSM-IV], axis I disorders), especially major depression, dysthymic disorder, panic disorder, generalized anxiety disorder, alcohol abuse; an abrasive personality style; and/or multiple physical symptoms. The latter group is generally seen as difficult because of disparities between the patient and the physician in expectations regarding care. The Difficult Doctor-Patient Relationship Questionnaire (DDPRQ; see Hahn, 2001) is a research instrument that has been used to identify difficult patients.

Nevertheless, the view that difficulty in the patient-physician relationship can be understood exclusively in terms of the patient's psychopathology is too limiting. The physician and the patient together form an interpersonal system, and that dyadic unit, too, is embedded in a broader sociocultural system. Changes in any of these three components can affect the patient-physician relationship and thus determine whether the patient situation is indeed "difficult."

Transference and Physicians' Emotional Reactions to Patients

Although the term *transference* was developed for the psychoanalytic situation, it has been found to be a useful construct in thinking about many interpersonal relationships.

Transference is the process by which an individual colors or distorts his or her experience of a current relationship because of experiences in earlier relationships, usually in childhood. Transference is not limited to patient-physician relationships, nor does it occur exclusively in people with psychiatric illnesses. It is found to varying degrees in all relationships.

Why, then, does it seem that there are so many problematic transferences in patient-physician relations? First, numerous aspects of the healing relationship are akin to features of childhood relationships. These factors include being cared for, being touched, being fed (in actuality or symbolically), being hurt, and being told what to do, among others. The physician's role, thus, frequently resembles a parental one, and this may trigger in the patient complementary childlike behavior. Second, stress and illness often induce a childlike dependence in patients, accompanied by psychological regression that fosters transference of old, childhood emotional experiences onto the parentlike physician. Being sick almost invariably causes regression. Not surprisingly, then, some adult patients who were oppositional, needy, or demanding as children will return to these patterns when they are under the pull of regression caused by an illness.

The physician's emotional responses to patients can be shaped by a similar process, sometimes called true counter-transference. In this process the patient's behavior triggers old emotional responses that color or distort the physician's experience of the present patient-physician relationship. True counter-transferential reactions should be suspected when other physicians do not seem to share the negative emotional response. This is a relatively uncommon source of problems in the patient-physician relationship. The more common causes of difficulty are the universal reactions provoked in most physicians by the emotionally charged life events, fears, anxieties, and frustrations intrinsic to the challenge of caring for people who are ill or are experiencing life stress or interpersonal conflict.

A central feature of the patient-physician relationship, essential to understanding this difficulty, is that the physician *always* has *some* reaction to the patient. Most of the time the patient simply stirs mild feelings in the physician and the reaction is easily overlooked. When the reaction is more intense, though, there may be difficulties. Certain types of patients provoke strong negative feelings in nearly all of the physicians they encounter. These almost universal emotional responses (sometimes called generalized counter-transference) characterize the patient-physician relationship with difficult patients. An example of a patient care situation likely to universally provoke a strong negative reaction is shown in the following vignette.

Case Vignette

Mr Henry, a 55-year-old businessman, has hypertension and diverticular bowel disease. He has fired six physicians over the past 10 years for "incompetence and borderline malpractice." He typically schedules "urgent" appointments on short notice, berates the office staff for making him wait, and prolongs his visits with his current physician, Dr Carlson. He relates circumstantial descriptions of his symptoms, hints that Dr Carlson will never help him anyway, and tells of his ruthless business successes and reckless extramarital affairs. He rarely follows through with Dr Carlson's suggestions about diet, exercise, safe sex, or use of medications. Mr Henry is only too happy to discuss his childhood of poverty, repeated physical abuse, and belittling at the hands of his father and how he overcame it all by becoming a self-made millionaire.

Dr Carlson gets a sinking feeling when he sees Mr Henry's name on his schedule for the day. Dr Carlson is comforted only slightly by having discussed Mr Henry with three of Mr Henry's previous physicians, all of whom Mr Henry treated similarly and who loathed Mr Henry as much as Dr Carlson does. Dr Carlson can appreciate that Mr Henry's interpersonal style is a maladaptive way of dealing with his childhood deprivation and abuse, primarily by identifying with Mr Henry's sadistic father. Dr Carlson understands that he feels as powerless, demeaned, and paralyzed as he supposes that Mr Henry did when he was growing up, but this insight alone does not lead to a way out of the impasse.

A Sociocultural Role Framework

Roles, expectations, and cultural beliefs also influence the patient-physician relationship. Talcott Parsons, a medical sociologist, described the "sick role" as a social construct of expected behaviors on the part of both patient and physician. In brief, the patient seeks medical care because of symptoms that are causing distress. There is to be an exchange of information with the physician, a wish to find relief from one's suffering and become well, acknowledgment that being sick is undesirable, and deference to the physician's expert opinions and advice. In exchange for playing this role, patients are allowed some exemption from other roles they normally play vis-à-vis work, within their family system, and behaviorally in terms of display of emotions and expressions of distress.

The specifics of each component of the sick role are influenced by ethnic and cultural factors. For example, complaining about pain is considered far more acceptable by Americans of Italian or Jewish ancestry than by New England Yankees.

The physician has a defined role as well. Most important, he or she is the authority who legitimizes (or fails to legitimize) the sick role for the patient. How physicians perceive the patient and illness and whether they confer such a role will be influenced by their own background, which in turn shapes their concepts of disease and the appropriate expression of disease. This is a powerful role and, therefore, at times invites coercion or manipulation by patients who are eager to adopt the sick role to meet their financial or psychological needs.

Thus, both partners in this dyadic relationship—the patient and the physician—are sizing up one another's performances of their respective roles. For the dyad to work, the roles must complement one another sufficiently. If the role expectations are too divergent, a difficult patient-physician situation is likely to develop. Note that the role expectation approach, like the transference model, emphasizes the interaction and reciprocity between the patient and the physician. Neither approach seeks blame or unilateral pathology as an explanation when difficulties arise in the relationship.

The four most common ways in which role expectations may diverge and cause problems are discussed below.

Disagreement about explanatory model of the disease. In this disagreement the physician typically adheres to a traditional biomedical explanation of disease while the patient understands the illness differently. The difference could stem from an alternative biological explanation, a faulty understanding of the illness, or a cultural or folk interpretation of etiology or treatment. Thus, a physician who insists on pharmacologic management of hypertension might be at odds with a patient who believes that dietary manipulations or a less stressful work or home life would be preferable.

Differing perspective for evaluating health status (disease vs illness). Arthur Kleinman noted that patients and physicians typically view health status from different perspectives. Physicians interpret symptoms and laboratory data in terms of their implications for the pathophysiological status of the disease, while patients focus on the subjective experience of the illness, including unpleasant symptoms, damaged self-esteem, the burden of treatment, and impaired function. For example, in the management of hypertension, patients typically are concerned more with the side effects, expense, and inconvenience of medication, and physicians focus on blood pressure and laboratory measures of end-organ damage. As another example, a patient with HIV is distressed by debilitating night sweats and diarrhea, but the physician is satisfied because the patient's weight is stable, the viral load is satisfactory, and stool cultures are negative.

Power imbalance between patient and physician. The socially defined roles of physician and patient give substantial power to the physician. He or she has more control over the agenda and the content and tone of the patient-physician interaction. When accepted uncritically, this imbalance can interfere with every stage of the health care process, from negotiating an agenda, to gathering information, to developing a therapeutic alliance, to educating the patient about proposed treatment. Evidence of this imbalance may be seen when friends and family who have just seen their own physicians ask us questions they were obviously inhibited about asking, reveal requests and concerns they were afraid to bring up, or admit to leaving the office without even learning what their physician thought about their problem. (It is the nature of this problem that if our own patients are experiencing these difficulties, we will not know it ourselves!)

Unless physicians recognize the intrinsic power gradient in the patient-physician relationship and take steps to adjust it, patients are afraid to share their model of the disease for fear of being seen as foolish or ignorant. They may simply not take their medications rather than complain about side effects, and they may leave with important concerns unmentioned. Many of them leave the clinical encounter dissatisfied if the physician does not empower them to take a more active role. Patients who feel powerless to negotiate with their physicians may refuse evaluation or treatment of a problem or they may choose not to keep an appointment. They are afraid that if they agree to any part of the process, they will be unable to influence the physician's actions when it comes to specific interventions.

Some patients, because of their personalities, have especially strong reactions to the imbalance of power and react with demanding or defiant postures. Many patients who are experiencing pain have learned to anticipate power struggles with clinicians over getting adequate pain medication. They often become preemptively demanding of larger and more frequent doses when clinicians have the power to control the supply. These same patients, however, may be satisfied with much smaller doses when they control administration using patient-regulated infusions. Contrariwise, difficulties may arise when the patient wants the physician to make more decisions than the physician feels comfortable making or when the patient insists on a certain treatment that the physician thinks is inappropriate or unwise (eg, futile end-of-life care or unnecessary aesthetic surgery).

Use of the health care process to solve nonmedical problems. In one sense, this disagreement can be thought of as patient and physician disagreeing about health status. Sometimes patients want to be considered sicker than the physician regards them, as in a request for disability documentation or in the examples below. At other times the patient wants to be seen as less sick, either because the illness threatens the patient's internal sense of himself or herself or because of concerns about the impact of the illness label on his or her social system.

Because the sick role can significantly alter patients' interactions with persons in their social system, it creates an interface between the health care process and other aspects of patients' lives that otherwise might be unrelated to their medical problems. Dramatic examples are patients with factitious illness who inappropriately seek the sick role for financial gain, entitlements, or dispensation from work responsibilities. A subtler, more common, and frequently equally disturbing form of this process involves using the sick role to cope with dysfunction in the patient's family system (see Chapter 1). Examples include:

- a family in which an elderly man amplifies his medical complaints in a way that leaves his young adult daughter uncomfortable about leaving home;
- a young adult woman, anxious about leaving home, who fosters her elderly mother's illness-related dependency, thereby providing an emotionally acceptable rationale for avoiding the anxiety of leaving home and becoming more independent herself;
- a young mother of three preschool-age children who "finally" gets some attention and assistance from her husband and extended family only after presenting with symptoms of chest pain and panic attacks that precipitate an admission to "rule out a myocardial infarction."

The physician does not easily tolerate this process, sometimes called a compensatory alliance, because patients engage the physician in an alliance that compensates for the dysfunction and deficit in the family system. It appears to the physician that the patient is inappropriately seeking the sick role, does not wish to get well, and is subverting the health care process for so-called secondary gain.

An alternative view is that the patient and the entire family system, having limited resources and alternatives, are using the sick role in an effort to cope with overwhelming problems and dysfunction. According to this view, the physician's role is to reframe the patient's (and family's) attention away from the putative reason for adopting the sick role and toward the family's underlying psychosocial problems in an effort to find a better, less self-destructive, and more growth-promoting coping strategy.

Case Vignette (continued)

Mr Henry and Dr Carlson can be thought of as diverging in two ways in the model above. First, they have different frameworks for evaluating health and preventing disease. Mr Henry isn't troubled by his hypertension, so he takes his medication erratically; he also does not accept Dr Carlson's suggestions to help his cardiovascular status and to prevent sexually transmitted diseases. A power imbalance also is present, although in this less typical case, the patient may be said to be bullying the physician. Mr Henry sees the physician's role as that of obedient service provider, while Dr Carlson would prefer to be seen as an autonomous professional.

GENERAL APPROACHES TO EVALUATION AND INTERVENTION

Difficult patient care situations often are overwhelming and baffling and initially seem too complex to understand. The first step in dealing with these situations is to break down the experience into more manageable and understandable components. Among the many components of the difficult patient care situation are seven elements that usually should be explored and examined. They are:

Characteristics of the Patient

- Axis I psychopathology
- A somatoform disorder or pattern of somatization
- Challenging personality traits or a frank personality disorder

The Physician's Contribution

- The physician's subjective emotional response to the patient (universal emotional response, as well as any true counter-transference)
- The behavior of the physician provoked by the subjective emotional response to the patient

The Context and Process of Care

- The patient's family and interpersonal system and its effects on health care–seeking behavior
- Conflicts between the physician's and the patient's explanatory models, disparities in concern over disease vs illness, power balance, and the effect of the interpersonal system on the process of care

Evaluation requires appreciating both these elements and their impact on the physician and the delivery of care. Similarly, interventions can be directed at managing the element itself and/or managing the emotional reactions created by the element. It is normal and to be expected that physicians will have difficulty relating to or working with certain types of patients, and these feelings or difficulties may increase when there is the added burden of guilt for having the feelings.

Axis I Psychopathology

It is useful to distinguish between elements of difficult situations that are relatively acute and perhaps treatable and those that are better regarded as chronic and thus in need of management. Most axis I psychopathology falls under the treatable component of the difficult clinical situation, while somatoform disorders and personality pathology usually require management. Despite its amenability to treatment, axis I psychopathology is just as likely to be unrecognized in difficult clinical situations as it is in primary care practice in general, in which only 40% to 60% of mental disorders are detected and an even smaller proportion is adequately evaluated and treated. Diagnostic aids are discussed broadly in Chapter 3 and specifically in the chapters pertaining to particular disorders.

Patients who have situational adjustment disorders may present with difficult or unpleasant symptoms and behaviors that also can be found in more endogenous axis I disorders. These patients are likely to improve in time or with some judicious support. In the face of certain stresses (acute illness or other major life events), some patients regress in more unpleasant ways, but their history may suggest that they will reconstitute to their usual, less problematic interpersonal style.

Similarly, axis I disorders can transiently generate behavior more often thought of as resulting from personality pathology. Table 16-1 shows some axis I conditions and their corresponding interpersonal presentations often mistaken for personality disorders. These may respond well to pharmacologic or other therapies, generally with lysis of the interpersonal difficulties. Personality disorders, by contrast, are enduring, and their interpersonal problems will be seen longitudinally over time rather than only in cross-section.

Somatoform Disorders or Patterns of Somatization

Some axis I disorders, such as somatization disorder and hypochondriasis, do not lend themselves to a treatment-oriented approach. Instead, they require a longer-term management approach. It is useful to explicitly diagnose the presence of a somatoform disorder or pattern of somatization so models for assessing and managing somatization (discussed in Chapter 15) can be used appropriately.

Abrasive Personal Style

Patients with marked personality traits or frank personality disorders require long-term management. As is the case with chronic illnesses, the physician must accept that the interpersonal problems won't simply go away and that the patient and physician must find a best way to accommodate one another. In addition to examining one's own emotional reaction and behavioral response to the patient (discussed later in this chapter), the physician may find three general principles to be useful.

TABLE 16-1 Axis I Disorders and Their Corresponding Interpersonal Presentations

Disorder	Interpersonal Problems
Depression	Dependency, irritability, poor compliance (decreased concentration, motivation)
Mania	Irritability, seductiveness, antisocial behaviors, poor compliance, grandiosity, depreciation
Panic disorder	Dependency, reassurance-seeking
Obsessive-compulsive disorder	Demanding (requests for many facts, details, time)
Posttraumatic stress disorder	Irritability, hostility, impulsivity
Attention deficit hyperactivity disorder	Poor compliance (impaired concentration), impulsivity
Schizophrenia	Poor compliance (lack of understanding, impaired motivation)
Paranoia	Hostile, demanding
Substance abuse disorders	Poor compliance, demanding, hostile

TABLE 16-2 Well-Described Personality Types in Medical Management

- Dependent, overdemanding clingers (oral personality)
- Orderly, controlled (compulsive personality)
- Dramatizing, captivating (histrionic personality)
- Long-suffering, self-sacrificing (self-defeating, masochistic personality)
- Guarded, querulous (paranoid) person
- Uninvolved, aloof (schizoid) patient
- Superior, entitled demanders (narcissistic)
- Manipulative help-rejecters
- Self-destructive deniers

Recognize common patterns. Certain personality types are well described in the medical literature (see Groves; Kahana and Bibring). Being able to recognize that a patient is exhibiting a previously described, known pattern may be helpful in itself. In addition, the physician can read up on the dynamics and suggestions for dealing with certain personality styles. Table 16-2 lists some of the types that are particularly well described in the literature. Note that some descriptions conform to more standard diagnostic nomenclature (eg, DSM-IV), whereas others derive from other descriptive models or even from psychodynamic models. Note also that these are not discrete, non-overlapping categories.

Talk to the patient about the process and limits. Patients frequently find themselves distressed by, and uncomprehending of, a difficult situation. They may have only a vague sense of something going wrong between themselves and the physician. They might have little awareness of their impact on the physician, and they seldom see how the interaction may echo other interpersonal problems they have. The situation often can be improved considerably by the physician's tactful acknowledgment that the problem exists. The patient thus can be invited to join a collaboration in understanding what has gone wrong and how the relationship might be repaired.

The model proposed here is the one used in the field of conflict resolution. It consists of four elements:

1. Identify the problem(s) in a nonjudgmental way.
2. Understand the patient's perspective.
3. Establish mutually beneficial goals.
4. Negotiate a settlement or plan.

This procedure provides the patient and physician an opportunity to air what often has been *sub rosa* resentment or ill will, and it allows the physician a chance to model how to discuss these resentments constructively. The discussion involves reclarifying the roles, boundaries, and limits of the relationship. Physicians have the opportunity to more clearly define the rules under which they wish to work with the patient and how they should handle any rule violations. The discussions should follow these guidelines:

1. Present to the patient that he or she is sad, not bad; focus on the defensive nature of his or her behavior rather than imply any malice or deliberate intent to harm.

2. Acknowledge the patient's impact on you, the physician, without necessarily revealing the full intensity or adding any personal information that might burden the patient (eg, how his or her behavior reminds you of your stepfather or how it has given you chest pain).

3. When invoking limits, try to avoid portraying the limits as punishment, and offer something in place of anything you take away (eg, "I'm stopping the codeine because it was making you nauseated and constipated, but I've arranged for some physical therapy to help those tender spots.").

Many physicians are reluctant to impose limits or deny patients what they are requesting unless the request is wildly inappropriate. This is often a reaction to persistence or guilt-induction on the patient's part. Nonetheless patients with difficult personalities, like children and adolescents, often benefit from the structure of clear, nonpunitive rules and limit-setting.

Recognize and use your own emotional reaction and behavioral response. Physicians are admonished repeatedly, during training and beyond, to be sensitive to patients' feelings. Unfortunately, physicians seldom are encouraged to pay much attention to their own feelings, in particular the feelings that certain patients engender. Monitoring feelings provoked by patients may play a role in accurately assessing difficult patient situations. Recognizing the existence and nature of one's own distress may contribute important clues to the type of interpersonal traits the patient brings to the relationship. Looking forward especially to seeing a certain patient or finding oneself sprucing up for a certain patient, for example, should prompt the physician to consider that he or she may be dealing with a histrionic or seductive patient.

The physician's emotional response plays a role in management as well. Many times a patient-physician situation proves to be difficult because of a pattern of behavioral responses and counter-responses by both parties. Many patient behaviors that seem provocative to the physician are actually covert requests for having additional needs met. Many physicians respond with emotional withdrawal, criticism of the patient, or angry use of setting limits. The patient then perceives this response as further rejection, which mobilizes additional neediness and an increase in the original provocative style. The physician, increasingly angry that the patient is not "getting it," may in turn escalate his or her use of counter-provocations.

The cycle may repeat itself until one or both participants decide to change tactics or abandon the relationship. Physicians who recognize their emotional reactions and their behavioral responses to those reactions are in a far better position to offer an alternative response to the patient.

The last reason for physicians to attend to their own feelings is their own mental health. Difficult patient situations add to any other stresses the physician is facing, so reducing the number and intensity of these situations constitutes good preventive medicine. Also, most physicians derive considerable satisfaction from solving clinical problems, helping patients, and experiencing themselves as being seen in a positive light. Thus, overcoming difficult patient situations may be satisfying in multiple ways.

The Context and Process of Care

As discussed earlier, difficult patient care situations exist within a context in which the patient's family system and the dynamics of the patient-physician relationship are dominant features. Physicians should systematically assess the quality of communication in the patient-physician relationship by examining hidden conflicts with the patient's explanatory model of the disease; reflect on the adequacy of the attention they have paid to the patient's subjective experience of the illness (see Kleinman); evaluate the power relationship within the patient-physician relationship; and empower the patient (or set limits) as necessary.

Finally, to examine potential subversion of the health care process by conflict or dysfunction in the patient's family system, the physician may employ methods of family systems assessment and intervention that have been developed and modified for use in the primary care setting (see Doherty and Baird; Hahn, Chapter 1). The use of a genogram-based interview (see McGoldrick and Gerson), meetings with families, and determination of whether a dysfunctional compensatory alliance has been established in the patient-family-physician relationship are particularly useful. Those who are interested in taking these approaches and who have not had training in this area are encouraged to read the cited references. Many primary care physicians, however, feel more comfortable obtaining consultation with clinicians who are experienced in family evaluations and therapy.

Consultation, Referral, and Support

As with any difficult clinical problem, sometimes an interpersonal situation becomes so complicated that an outside party is needed to review it or to intervene. A curbside consultation with a primary care colleague or a psychiatrist with whom the physician is comfortable may yield useful advice at times. The colleague may recognize a pattern from his or her own patients, suggest a missed axis I or other diagnosis, or help the physician better see his or her own reaction and contribution to the impasse. In addition, the physician may be helped by being able to ventilate that a patient is distressing and to receive some peer support and encouragement.

At other times a more formal psychiatric consultation or referral is warranted. Many patients with difficult personalities are loath to seek psychiatric care. They tend to feel that others, rather than they themselves, are marching to the wrong drumbeat, so why do they need to see someone? Several approaches may facilitate the patient's acceptance and the physician's getting useful feedback:

- Promoting the consultation as needed to address anxiety, depression, weight loss, pain, or some other process the patient would like to improve
- Emphasizing that you are asking the consultant for feedback about the patient that will enable understanding, leading to better patient care
- Being careful not to present the referral as punishment for misbehavior
- Stressing that you will remain the patient's physician (ie, you are not transferring the patient's care to the psychiatrist)
- Referring the patient to a psychiatrist with knowledge about, and interest in, these types of problems [a consultation–liaison psychiatrist, a family (systems) psychiatrist, or a psychoanalyst probably will be more helpful than a psychopharmacologist]
- Supporting the patient's expression of the pain and unhappiness caused by underlying family and psychological conflict so a suggestion of referral feels like an emotionally logical consequence of the patient's expressed distress

Case Vignette (continued)

Dr Carlson arranges to have coffee with his friend and colleague Dr Reston, a general psychiatrist, to discuss Mr Henry. They both quickly see Mr Henry as most fitting the pattern of a superior, entitled demander. Dr Reston tells Dr Carlson something about his experience with similar patients and gives Dr Carlson some things to read. The heart of the matter seems to be that Mr Henry makes Dr Carlson feel belittled. Dr Reston suggests a firm but empathic confrontation, playing to Mr Henry's narcissism. Dr Carlson realizes that he can live with Mr Henry's noncompliance and boasting if he and his staff are not under constant attack, so the focus will be on the deprecation first.

SPECIFIC DIFFICULT SITUATIONS

The following discussion covers patients who are nonadherent, hostile or angry, demanding or entitled, dependent or clinging, and seductive. Somatizing patients, who certainly may be among the most difficult patients, are discussed in Chapter 15.

The Nonadherent Patient

The term *nonadherent* is preferred to *noncompliant*. The latter suggests a patient's failure to follow a physician's mandated prescription, while the former implies a patient's deviation from a more mutually agreed-on course. Again, the emphasis here must be on the reciprocal interaction between patient and physician rather than on patient shortcomings, psychopathology, or obstreperousness. About 7% of patients in primary care settings have been shown to sabotage their own care, which includes nonadherence along with other behaviors, including failing to seek needed care.

There are many reasons that patients do not follow a physician's recommendations. Some of the most common are shown in Table 16-3. Understanding the reasons will clarify the interventions required. The physician has to identify carefully his or her own contributions and to assess the contributions the patient brings that might be remediable. Cognitive and practical barriers usually can be identified fairly readily by asking appropriate questions (eg, having the patient restate the instructions or spell out in detail how the treatment plan might be carried out). It also is important to ask the patient how he or she understands the illness, its cause, and how he or she believes it is best treated. These inquiries probe for patient misunderstandings, idiosyncratic etiologic explanations, and interest in alternative or complementary therapies.

The reasons given above generally involve factors that are known to the patient (although he or she may be reluctant to acknowledge them). Other reasons may be thought of as more psychological—involving feelings about the illness, the treatment, or the physician—that may be less accessible to the patient. In many cases, tactful probing will identify one or more fears that are affecting the patient's cooperation. The fears revolve around the course of the illness, proposed treatment, treatment failure, or the physician himself or herself. Oppositional patients, for example, may fear being dominated or controlled by the physician, while paranoid patients may be concerned that the physician is withholding information or has ulterior motives for his or her suggestions.

The last aspect of nonadherence pertains to its ability to affect physicians. Of the reasons for this, which are shown in the following list, certain ones strike closest to home

TABLE 16-3 Common Reasons for Patient Nonadherence to Medical Advice

Information Deficit or Cognitive Problem
- Patient is inadequately informed by physician
- Patient has intellectual deficits, cannot comprehend
- Proposed regimen is too complex
- Distortion by depression, psychosis, etc

Practical Barriers to Implementation
- Financial limitations or restrictions
- Recommended services are not available (eg, substance-abuse services)
- Transportation or other logistical impediments
- Another person is needed to implement

Denial of Illness or Seriousness of Illness
- Patient is afraid of treatments (eg, surgery, certain medications)
- Patient has had adverse effects from the treatment
- Secondary gain (disability, family support, etc)
- Patient wants alternative treatment (vitamins, folk treatment, etc)
- Patient doesn't believe treatment will work
- Patient doesn't trust or believe physician
- Someone else (family member, other doctor) is telling patient to do something else
- Patient has oppositional personality style
- Patient's life too chaotic to follow through

for each physician (another reason that physicians need to be aware of their own emotional responses):

- The physician fears that the patient will suffer unnecessarily or have a bad outcome.
- The physician fears that he or she will be blamed for a bad outcome.
- The physician feels that the patient is being disrespectful.
- The physician feels that the patient is being hostile.
- The physician feels that his or her competence or knowledge is being called into question.

The Hostile, Angry Patient

Hostile, angry patients fall into several categories:

- *Realistic disappointments.* Many of these patients are angry because the physician or the health care system has not done well by them. Patients who do not receive enough time, information, answers to questions, or concern about their emotional well-being will feel cheated. Physicians, like most people, often respond to anger by avoidance or additional withholding behavior, and this may lead to the patient's further resentment.
- *Displacement.* Some patients displace onto the physician their anger over their illness, their other life problems, or other people in their lives. If their life is not going well,

this can easily become an enduring pattern. Anger about mistreatment by other providers in the health care system often is displaced onto the primary provider.

- *Paranoid traits*. Patients with paranoid personality styles may chronically feel that the physician does not have their best interests at heart. They may express concern about being cheated, wonder whether the physician knows what he or she is doing, believe that they are being experimented on or receiving second-rate care, or worrying that information will not be kept confidential.
- *Narcissistic or borderline problems*. Patients with narcissistic or borderline features may be more reactive to the vicissitudes of the interaction with the physician. These patients may react with cold rage if they feel they are being demeaned or slighted, whereas borderline patients often express intense hostility around issues related to separation or abandonment. Narcissistic patients are discussed in the section on entitled and demanding patients.

The most critical approach to dealing with angry patients is for the physician to acknowledge the patient's anger and ask what it is all about. At times, adding some version of "If I've done anything that angers you, please tell me what it is" may be helpful as well. This maneuver draws attention to the anger as an issue, allows the patient to complain, offers the physician as willing to discuss the anger nondefensively in the context of the patient-physician relationship, and invites collaboration to change things for the better. The patient's response generally will help clarify which of the situations above is at work and suggest a therapeutic approach.

Patients who identify bona fide shortcomings are entitled to an apology and a promise to work together to change things. If the patient has unrealistic expectations, this can be clarified and appropriate limits noted or substitutes offered. The physician should encourage the patient to express directly any dissatisfaction that arises in the future rather than letting resentment simmer.

Patients using displacement typically either rationalize about their anger or are unable to explain it. Rationalizations consist of finding things about which to criticize the physician in which the severity is out of proportion to the anger (eg, "Your receptionist was too brusque when I called last month"; "You seemed rushed the last few times we met"). An empathic comment about a known stress ("You must be disappointed that all of the feeling hasn't returned to your hand after the surgery") can be used to suggest the true target of the anger without confronting the patient about the false target.

Dealing with paranoid patients can be demanding. Underlying most paranoia is the fear of being hurt or abandoned, and there is a projection of the patient's hostile feelings onto others. Paranoid patients generally resist proposals for psychiatric evaluation. They interpret the recommendation as abandonment and criticism. Suggestions for working with paranoid patients include:

- scrupulous honesty on the part of the physician (openness and full disclosure about finances, diagnosis, plans, prognosis, etc);
- acknowledging that the patient is struggling to trust the physician;
- encouraging the patient to review his or her interactions with the physician over time to decide if the physician is trustworthy;
- offers of second opinions, additional sources of information, and so forth to confirm the physician's recommendations;

- taking extra care in issues of confidentiality;
- involving the patient in any third-party interactions (utilization reviewers, insurers, family members, employers, etc).

Managing borderline patients is complex. Because many borderline patients have mood instability, suicidal or other self-destructive urges, identity disturbances, and a generally chaotic life, psychiatric referral is appropriate, and it is often acceptable to the patient. The primary care physician must stress his or her ongoing involvement to avoid mobilizing the patient's fears of abandonment. Effective pharmacotherapy and newer psychotherapies may modulate the episodes of rage or dysphoria. The primary care physician has to stress continually his or her interest and concern with these patients, yet set firm limits on the patients' behavior. Coordination of care with the psychiatrist is essential to avoid problems of splitting care between the psychiatrist and the primary care physician.

The Demanding or Entitled Patient

Demanding or entitled patients generally fall into the spectrum of what are often called narcissistic disorders. These include, in addition to narcissistic personality disorder itself, some patients with borderline and antisocial personality disorders. These patients are characterized by a strong sense of self-importance, typically treating others (including physicians) as inferiors or servants to their own needs. They may be quite charming and even flattering so long as the physician is doing what they ask, but the physician's expressions of autonomy or disagreement frequently are met with intense, haughty disdain or expressions of rage.

Demanding or entitled patients seem to be inordinately concerned about how others perceive them. They frequently decide on actions based on how others will view the action rather than by any true, internalized sense of good or bad. They often are preoccupied with features that make them appear special, whether in intellect, looks, powerful contacts, or income.

These patients are difficult for a physician because they expect the patient-physician relationship to be managed by their rules—mainly that they are in charge and the physician is a subordinate. They may use a deft combination of charm, compliments, threats, and insults to maintain their superior position. They may expect physicians to treat them as if the physicians had no other patients, unlimited time, and no nonprofessional life they wish to call their own. Demanding or entitled patients are deflated when they are asked to limit their stay, pay their bills, follow directions, or otherwise be reminded that they are patients (ie, of their ordinariness). Mr Henry, the patient in the vignette, illustrates many of these features.

Case Vignette (continued)

The confrontation discussed by Drs Carlson and Reston will emphasize that Dr Carlson wants the best for Mr Henry, that Mr Henry is entitled to the best care, and that things such as regularly scheduled appointments, which are planned with some extra time allotment, would give Mr Henry the special treatment he deserves. In exchange, the insinuations about Dr Carlson's competence and the threats to fire him have to stop, for how can Dr Carlson give Mr Henry his full attention and support if he is continually being put down and threatened?

Dr Carlson and Dr Reston decide to see how this initial approach works before trying other steps. In particular, they decide not to propose a consultation to Mr Henry, who likely will see it as an insult and as threatened abandonment. When Dr Carlson and Mr Henry are working more cooperatively, Dr Carlson might propose a referral for help in dealing with tension and perhaps weight loss and drinking control as well.

Underlying the grandiosity and vanity of these patients is a fragile sense of self-esteem. The manifestations of this personality are all thought to be defensive maneuvers designed to shore up this vulnerability. Thus, physician demands and criticisms threaten the patient's self-esteem and lead to compensatory increases in narcissistic behaviors. The physician therefore must address these patients' fears of failing to measure up and their need to feel special, or even better than others. This was the reason for the approach taken with Mr Henry. By reaffirming his need for specialness and offering him modest concessions, Dr Carlson may be able to reduce Mr Henry's need for defensive grandiosity and thereby obtain a reduction in his attacks.

The Dependent or Clinging Patient

The dependent or clinging patient has three main variants:

- Patients with a dependent personality style have a strong need to attach themselves almost slavishly to those whom they see as powerful parental or authority figures. They seek frequent contact with the physician, need a great deal of reassurance, worry excessively about whether they are liked, and often wish for the physician to make decisions for them. They may be extremely grateful for whatever they receive, but their sycophancy, passivity, and clinginess is often off-putting.
- Those with obsessive-compulsive personalities, by contrast, are less needy and passive but, rather, crave time and attention because of their doubting and indecisiveness. They, too, may seek frequent reassurances about their health, but they are less likely to cede decision-making to the physician. If the physician tries to impose something on the patient, the patient may become quite oppositional.
- Some patients with schizoid personalities become attached to physicians because they lack other interpersonal relationships in their lives. They may seek additional time and attention, but the physician often feels puzzled by their lack of emotional expression or willingness to share personal information. Their social skills are often deficient, and they appear awkward, eccentric, or even bizarre.

The underlying reasons for the attachment behavior in these three types is quite different. The truly dependent patient is terrified of rejection and abandonment. The compulsive patient seeks an intellectualized form of assistance to deal with life's uncertainties and hazards by an increased sense of control. The schizoid patient primarily seeks the superficial façade of a close relationship without the emotional sharing or vulnerability.

Despite the differing dynamics, each type of patient needs firm but supportive limit-setting by the physician. The physician has to be explicit about length of visit time available, availability for phone calls, and willingness to make decisions for the patient. These have to be presented in a way that expresses:

- ongoing involvement and concern (ie, not abandonment),
- lack of punitive intent (ie, not criticism),

- understanding that the patient wants something more or different,
- the advantages to the patient of adhering to the limit (eg, "When our office visits run over time, I begin to think about running late, and then I'm not giving you the full attention you deserve"),
- the physician's willingness to stick to an agreed-on or imposed limit ("I'm hanging up now—our 5 minutes to discuss this have elapsed").

Also, it often is helpful to involve family members or surrogates in offering the patient support, reassurance, or decision-making rather than having the physician fill this role alone. Dependent patients frequently are willing to accept psychotherapy referrals (where they may do best in group settings). Compulsive and schizoid patients tend to be more reluctant, often unable to identify a good reason why this might be helpful.

The Seductive Patient

We use the term *seductive* here broadly, referring not only to patients who explicitly seek a sexual relationship with the physician but to any patient who tries to induce the physician to breach his or her professional role. This may cause a "boundary crossing," which is a minor lapse in the patient-physician role boundaries. Although these overtures are not inherently improper, the physician should be attentive to boundary crossings because they might represent precursors to more serious boundary violations (see Gabbard and Nadelson, 1995). These boundary violations may include things such as:

- physical contact between the physician and the patient (other than the physical exam or a handshake),
- providing care to the patient out of office hours or in nonclinical settings,
- giving or accepting gifts,
- disclosing personal information about the physician to the patient,
- giving the patient advice about nonclinical matters (legal, financial, etc),
- deliberately recording inaccurate medical data in a chart or report.

The seductive patient typically begins by making small, apparently innocuous requests of or offers to the physician. Examples include the patient asking about the physician's home life, requesting a hug or a kiss, prolonging office visits for no clear reason, or offering or soliciting stock tips. These matters typically are presented in such a way that it seems churlish or prudish to refuse. In addition, the patient often is grateful, expresses his or her appreciation, and may compare the physician favorably to others (such as other physicians or an intimate partner).

Over time the requests tend to escalate in small, incremental ways that seem to draw patient and physician into a closer emotional relationship. Some physicians do not find the early stages of this continuum difficult at all, and they may even enjoy working with their "special" patients or feeling special themselves. Other physicians become upset because of what they perceive as increasing demands, threats or guilt-induction, and phony flattery. Whether the physician enjoys these patients or finds them difficult at this stage is a function of the physician's personality and the patient's charm.

Eventually, most physicians reach a point of feeling progressively more uneasy as they become aware of being drawn into one or more boundary crossings. Then they may feel embarrassed, angry, and/or fearful for their professional and personal reputations. At that point the patient certainly will be labeled as difficult, and the physician will attempt to withdraw emotionally. The physician usually does this abruptly and without any explanation to the patient. In return, the patient tends to feels hurt and abandoned, reacting with increased, cruder forms of seductiveness or rage, and possibly threatening public disclosure, retaliation, or even lawsuits.

We are emphasizing the course of this relationship because early recognition and prevention are far better than after-the-fact repair or damage control. Physicians need to be keenly aware of even the smallest boundary crossings and use them as guideposts to watch for potentially troubling patterns. A friendly hug or a kiss on the cheek may be appropriate with certain patients under certain circumstances but always should be flagged for the physician's early-warning system.

Boundary crossings are a breach of the physician's fiduciary duty to the patient and thus always represent a potential or actual ethical violation. Physicians who find themselves rationalizing atypical behavior with a patient usually are heading for trouble and should seek consultation with a colleague. Physician behaviors that fail the colleague disclosure test (Would I be willing to tell what I have done to a colleague?) are almost certainly unethical.

Why are patients seductive? Some patients have a strong need to feel special, different, or chosen by parental figures (or others, more broadly), and they have found that exchanging confidences, gifts, and affection will often yield such a relationship. Others have had sexualized experiences (either explicitly or implicitly) in childhood and continue to associate parental figures with sexual expression. Many of these patients have marked disturbances in self-esteem and may feel that sex (or some version of it) is all they have to offer others. They also may have a persistent neediness, sometimes in the open and sometimes latent, that leads them to be driven in their seductive behavior.

When physicians come to realize that they are dealing with a seductive patient, whether boundaries have or have not been violated, the following steps are called for:

- Physicians should gently but firmly reaffirm the professional and fiduciary nature of the relationship and their wish that it remain that way.
- If boundary crossings have occurred already, physicians should indicate that having thought back on the violations, they felt they were not wise in the context of a patient-physician relationship and that similar events must not occur.
- Physicians should stress that they want to care as best they can for the patient within the boundaries of the professional relationship and that maintaining that relationship is the best way to care for the patient.
- Physicians must emphasize that their rejecting certain types of interactions between themselves and the patient does not mean the physician does not care for or wish to work with the patient.
- Physicians must take pains not to blame the patient for any boundary crossings that may have occurred.
- If the patient becomes angry and threatens to expose the physician, he or she should express the hope that the patient won't do so, as this would truly make it difficult for the physician and the patient to work together in a more appropriate way.
- Physicians should not use a psychiatric consultation or referral as a way of punishing or banishing the patient.

SUMMARY

Patients whom the physician experiences as interpersonally difficult are best conceptualized using a systems framework. This approach looks at the contribution of the patient, the physician, their respective role expectations, the nature of their relationship, and the involvement of other parties who may be affecting the interaction. Physicians who are attentive to their own emotional reactions to patients may use these reactions diagnostically, therapeutically, and even prophylactically to anticipate difficult situations.

Assessment of difficult situations includes adequate consideration of treatable situational or axis I disorders. Management involves taking a long-term approach with modest goals, recognition of certain well-described personality types and issues, imposition of reasonable limits on the patient, and attention to the underlying mechanisms that drive patient behavior. Well-described patient types include nonadherent, hostile, dependent, demanding, and seductive patients, and there are often effective approaches to working with such patients when they are recognized.

ADDITIONAL READINGS

Barsky AJ. Patients who amplify bodily sensations. *Ann Intern Med*. 1979;91:63-70.

Doherty WJ, Baird MA. *Family Therapy and Family Medicine*. Guilford, Conn: Guilford Press; 1983.

Gabbard GO, Nadelson C. Professional boundaries in the physician-patient relationship. *JAMA*. 1995;273:1445-1449.

Gillum RF, Barsky AJ. Diagnosis and management of patient noncompliance. *JAMA*. 1974;228:1563-1567.

Groves JE. Taking care of the hateful patient. *N Engl J Med*. 1978;298:883-887.

Groves JE. Management of the borderline patient on a medical or surgical ward: the psychiatric consultant's role. *Intl J Psychiatry Med*. 1976;6:337-348.

Hahn SR. Physical symptoms and physician-experienced difficulty in the doctor-patient relationship. *Ann Intern Med*. 2001;134:897-904.

Hahn SR. Family assessment. In: Feldman M, Christensen J, eds. *Behavioral Medicine: A Primary Care Handbook*. Norwalk, Conn: Appelton & Lange; 1998.

Hahn SR, Kroenke K, Spitzer RL, et al. The difficult patient: prevalence, psychopathology, and functional impairment. *J Gen Intern Med*. 1996;11:1-8.

Hahn SR, Feiner JS, Bellin EH. The doctor-patient-family relationship: a compensatory alliance. *Ann Intern Med*. 1988;109:884-889.

Kahana RJ, Bibring GL. Personality types in medical practice. In: Zinberg N, ed. *Psychiatry in Medical Practice*. New York, NY: International University Press; 1964:108-123.

Kleinman A. *The Illness Narratives: Suffering, Healing, and the Human Condition*. New York, NY: Basic Books; 1988.

Kleinman A, Eisenberg L, Good B. Culture, illness, and care: clinical lessons from anthropological and cross-cultural research. *Ann Intern Med*. 1978;88:251-258.

Lieberman JA. Compliance issues in primary care. *J Clin Psychiatry*. 1996;57(supp 7):76-82.

McGoldrick M, Gerson R. *Genograms in Family Assessment*. New York, NY: WW Norton & Co, Inc; 1985.

Nisselle P. Difficult doctor-patient relationships. *Aust Fam Physician*. 2000;29:47-49.

Parson T, Fox R. Illness, therapy, and the modern American family. *J Soc Issues*. 1952;8:31.

Perry JC, Vaillant GE. Personality disorders. In: Kaplan HI, Sadock BJ, eds. *Comprehensive Textbook of Psychiatry*. 5th ed. Baltimore, Md: Williams & Wilkins; 1989:1352-1386.

Rolland JS. *Families Illness, & Disability: An Integrative Treatment Model*. New York, NY: Basic Books; 1994.

Chapter **17**

Women's *Mental Health*

Marjorie Greenfield, MD
Miriam B. Rosenthal, MD

Throughout the world, men and women have mental disorders at equal rates, but their patterns often differ. These differences deserve the attention of primary care physicians, as well as that of mental health professionals. Much of our current knowledge is not yet sufficient to understand why these differences are present or to fully comprehend the variations in incidence, prevalence, etiology, diagnoses, clinical presentations, treatment responses, and effective prevention strategies.

From adolescence through menopause, women have twice the rate of depressive disorders (major depression, dysthymia, rapid-cycling bipolar disease, and seasonal affective disorder). Women have a higher incidence of anxiety disorders (simple phobias, agoraphobia, panic disorder, generalized anxiety disorder, and posttraumatic stress disorder) and somatization disorders. Men have higher rates of substance abuse (alcohol and other drug abuse or dependence) and antisocial personality disorders.

Schizophrenia, obsessive-compulsive disorder, and bipolar disorder occur at similar rates in men and women, though times of onset, clinical course, and treatment responses may differ. Little is known about people with subthreshold diagnostic conditions, which may also cause considerable emotional distress and social disruption.

EXPLANATIONS FOR GENDER DIFFERENCES IN MENTAL DISORDERS

Although the causes of gender differences in mental illnesses, especially depression, remain elusive, some theories have been offered. Women may be more likely than men to recall past episodes of mental illness, go to physicians more often, or present with subthreshold forms of disorders. Another theory suggests that the observed discrepancies have a biological basis, such as genetic differences or hormonal influences including menstrual cycle fluctuations and menopausal effects. A third theory emphasizes psychological and cultural circumstances. All of these factors are likely to play a role.

Evidence for Hormonal Effects

Gender differences in the prevalence of mood disorders begin at puberty and decline at menopause, giving support to the concept that hormones contribute to these differences. Mood and behavior are known to fluctuate during the menstrual cycle, with 5% of women experiencing symptoms severe enough to interfere with interpersonal relationships and occupational functioning. Women are more likely to undergo mood and behavioral changes during and after a pregnancy than at any other time. Of new mothers, 10% to 15% experience postpartum major depression, and 1% develop postpartum psychosis, usually an exacerbation or new onset of bipolar illness, major depression, or schizophrenia. Many women have mood disturbances during the perimenopause, possibly related to sleep disturbances from hot flashes.

Psychological and Cultural Factors

Psychological and cultural factors may contribute substantively to gender differences in mental illnesses. Some evidence shows that women have different cognitive styles and ruminate more than men do. These differences may influence their response to psychotherapy and also contribute to the prevalence of certain diagnoses.

Culturally, women face more social and economic difficulties than men, more physical and sexual abuse, and differing role expectations and responsibilities for balancing child-care and careers. In cross-cultural research, women's social status at all ages contributes to their psychological well-being.

Work-related status is an important predictor of mental health for a woman, whether she is a homemaker or is employed outside her home. Discrimination in the workplace, sexual harassment, and having a spouse who does not support a working wife all increase the risk for mental disorders. Women who have young children at home are at increased risk for mental disorders, especially depression and anxiety.

In general, women may attain greater satisfaction than men from relationships with partners, children, and friends. Disruption of these ties may make women more vulnerable to psychological problems. For men, marriage seems to provide a protective factor against depression, whereas married women are more likely to be depressed than are those who are single or separated. Women who feel helpless or victimized, have lost a parent at an early age, have less than a high school education, have no close friends, and/or have unstable marriages are all at higher risk for psychological problems.

PRESENTATIONS OF MENTAL ILLNESSES

For most mental illnesses, the clinical presentations are similar for men and women, although age of onset seems to differ. Symptom patterns of depressive illnesses differ by gender, with women having more atypical depressions including sleepiness, overeating, weight gain, seasonal variations, and somatization. Milder depressive illnesses are more common in women, along with presentation at younger ages. Although women are at higher risk for becoming depressed, they are not at greater risk for staying depressed.

In schizophrenic illnesses, men have an earlier onset of disease and poorer premorbid personalities, with more schizoid features. The data comparing male and female clinical symptomatology remain unclear and require more research, although literature on this subject is increasing. Because, historically, most research on mental illness used men as the standard, it is useful to focus here on facets of mental health and illness specific to women, including issues throughout the reproductive life cycle.

ASSESSMENT OF WOMEN FOR PSYCHOLOGICAL PROBLEMS

When assessing women for psychological problems, it is important to inquire about emotional, behavioral, and cognitive changes related to menses, use of contraceptives, pregnancy and postpartum, pregnancy loss, abortion, infertility, and menopause. Excessive preoccupation with physical symptoms (including pain) may indicate a psychological overlay obscuring real biological disorders. Patients often fear that if they admit to their medical caretakers that they are anxious or depressed, the physicians will not believe their symptoms and may abandon them. The physician must try to tease apart, without any bias, what is physical and what is psychological. Understanding the patient's personality and coping style can help the physician identify problems and plan treatment strategies.

TABLE 17-1   Positive Responses to Domestic Violence Screening: What to Do

Screening for domestic violence can be intimidating to the practitioner who hasn't been trained to deal with positive responses. If the patient is a minor, the law requires health care workers, teachers, and others in positions of responsibility for children to make a report to the Department of Human Services, usually through the child abuse hotline in your community. The same requirements do not apply to health care practitioners and other professionals with a competent adult who shares this sort of information with you. Consider taking these steps:

1. Ask the patient for details of what has happened to her, and try to get a sense of how acute her risk is. Ask about psychological, physical, and sexual abuse.

2. Tell her that she does not deserve to be treated this way. Everyone deserves to feel safe in her home and with those who claim to care about her.

3. Give her information about resources for battered women and safe houses. Many communities have a hotline for victims of domestic violence that can hook them up with services. Posters or flyers in the office containing this information also can be helpful.

4. Ask her if she has thought about leaving her situation. Hiding some money and planning ahead about what she might do can help a woman to escape when she feels ready to leave.

5. Many women who eventually get away from severely abusive partners take a long time to take action or even go back numerous times after leaving. These relationships are complex, with psychological, financial, and child-custody implications. Even though it is frustrating for the practitioner, continued support is empowering and ultimately may save a life.

The best predictor of psychological disturbance is a past history of such conditions, especially at times of transitions and following sexual, physical, or emotional traumas. Family history of mental disorders also predicts risk. It is important to assess the quality of relationships, especially social supports, and the home and occupational environment. Questions such as, How are things at home? Have you ever felt unsafe in your home? and Have you ever been injured or threatened by another person? can help identify victimization, whether physical, sexual, or verbal (Table 17-1). It is helpful to know about a person's schooling, whether the patient was in "special classes," whether she went to college, and so forth. Financial strain may contribute to overall distress. In addition, women tend to have more than one psychiatric condition, so evaluation for coexisting morbidities, such as depression and self-medication with drugs or alcohol, is prudent. One must specifically ask about herbal supplements, as these often are not considered medications.

SPECIFIC PSYCHOLOGICAL DISORDERS IN WOMEN

While the preceding sections discussed manifestations of common psychiatric conditions in women compared with men, several psychiatric diagnoses are unique to women. These include premenstrual dysphoric disorder, issues related to infertility and its treatment, psychological changes of the menopause, and postpartum depression. Since some psychological stress is normal during these life stages, the primary care physician must be aware of the normal range of responses to these transitions and how to diagnose, treat, and appropriately refer disorders when they occur.

Menstruation-Related Psychological Disorders

Case Vignette

Mrs Arnold, a 32-year-old married woman in good health, presents to her primary care physician because "I need anger management or something." She notes that each month before her period she gets very irritable. She says that she "flies off the handle over nothing," screaming and harshly criticizing her subordinates at work, her husband, and her two school-age children over things "that normally don't bother me—and shouldn't." This moodiness lasts for over a week and is usually gone by the second or third day of her period. The rest of the month she says that her life is pretty good and that she enjoys her work and her family. Her behavior at work has earned her some negative reviews from her supervisors, and she is worried about her future in this job if she can't control her behavior. She is also worried that her behavior is damaging to her children.

Mrs Arnold's menstrual periods are regular and are characterized by 3 or 4 days of bloating and breast tenderness before the onset of bleeding. She and her husband use condoms as their method of contraception. The physical examination is unrevealing, and the mental status exam shows a frustrated woman with a great deal of self-blame but no hopelessness or suicidal ideation.

The patient is asked to complete a daily PMS symptom chart for 2 months and to return for another appointment. The chart supports the physician's clinical impression that Mrs Arnold is suffering from premenstrual dysphoric disorder with the absence of symptoms for the week following her menstrual period each month.

Premenstrual syndrome (PMS) occurs in about 75% of normal women. It is experienced as a variety of physical and psychological changes that start in the days prior to the onset of menses and remit with the beginning of bleeding. Physical symptoms, such as breast tenderness, water retention, and bloating, are caused by circulating progesterone. The psychological manifestations usually include depression, irritability, emotional lability, and occasionally elation. Most women can function despite these symptoms.

Premenstrual dysphoric disorder (PMDD) is a more serious form of PMS, occurring in about 5% of women, with severe, distressing symptoms that interfere with activities and relationships. The disorder currently is included in *Diagnostic and Statistical Manual of Mental Disorders,* fourth edition (DSM-IV), as Appendix B. Although the symptoms may be distressing, PMS and PMDD are indicative of normal ovulatory cycles and are not thought to represent abnormal hormone levels.

For about half of the women who present to a physician or mental health professional with premenstrual symptoms, the symptoms represent an exacerbation of another problem such as depression, anxiety, eating disorder, substance abuse, or psychosis. The menstrual cycle may make a psychiatric disorder worse, can initiate the expression of a disorder, or may exacerbate a condition premenstrually. Accurate diagnosis of PMS and PMDD requires keeping careful prospective diaries and noting at least 1 week free of symptoms in each cycle (Figure 17-1).

The etiologies of PMS and PMDD are not clearly known except for their relationship to sex hormones. Premenstrual disorders may have other causes as well. Research is under way to further elucidate the relationship of PMS to neurotransmitters, adrenocorticoid hormones, thyroid function, and psychosocial variables. The symptoms of premenstrual

FIGURE 17-1 Eli Lilly's Premenstrual Daily Symptom Chart

Name _____   Month _____

1. Circle the days of your menstraul period in the row labeled Day of Month
2. Begin your ratings today. If today is the 12th of the month, mark your symptoms in the column labeled 12. At the same time each day, use a marker or pen to fill in the correct numbered box to show how severe each symptom was over the past 24 hours. Leave the symptom blank if you had no problem with that symptom. See example bar on the right. If you forgot to fill in a day, place an X in the Day of the Month bar to signify that you did not fill in the chart for that day.
3. Continue on new page on the first day of the next month.

Example:

	None	Mild	Moderate	Severe
	3	3	3	3
	2	2	2	2
	1	1	1	1

Day of Month	1	2	3	4	5	6	7	8	9	10	11	12	13	14	15	16	17	18	19	20	21	22	23	24	25	26	27	28	29	30	31
Irritability																															
Sudden mood changes																															
Tension																															
Sadness																															
Decreased interest in usual activities																															
Feeling overwhelmed																															

Day of Month		1	2	3	4	5	6	7	8	9	10	11	12	13	14	15	16	17	18	19	20	21	22	23	24	25	26	27	28	29	30	31
Difficulty concentrating	3																															
	2																															
	1																															
Bloating	3																															
	2																															
	1																															
Breast tenderness	3																															
	2																															
	1																															
Food cravings	3																															
	2																															
	1																															
Lack of energy	3																															
	2																															
	1																															
Change in sleep	3																															
	2																															
	1																															
Relationship problems	3																															
	2																															
	1																															
Other:	3																															
	2																															
	1																															

syndrome or premenstrual dysphoric disorder may increase with age, after having a baby, after starting or stopping oral contraceptives, or following pelvic surgery.

Mild PMS usually does not require treatment. Treatments for PMDD have included diet, vitamins, exercise, relaxation training, group support, cognitive-behavioral or interpersonal psychotherapy, and use of antidepressant or antianxiety agents (Table 17-2). PMS and PMDD are not indications of hormonal abnormalities and generally do not benefit from hormonal manipulations. Studies have shown some benefit from supplemental calcium carbonate (500 mg bid) taken during the 2 weeks prior to menstruation. Selective serotonin reuptake inhibitors (SSRIs) have been helpful to some patients when taken at usual dosages all month or for the week or two prior to menses. For underlying disorders exacerbated by the menstrual cycle, treating the primary problem is usually the best approach.

Psychiatric Disorders in Pregnancy and the Puerperium

Pregnancy is a major developmental transition that involves biological, psychological, and social changes. Many women appear more emotionally distressed without meeting the

TABLE 17-2 Treatments Used for Physical and/or Emotional Symptoms of PMS and PMDD

Lifestyle Alteration
- Diet

    Regular meals

    Reduced salt, alcohol, caffeine, sugar, fat

    Carbohydrate-rich foods

- Dietary supplements:

    Calcium (1200 mg/day)

    Magnesium

    Vitamin E (mastalgia)

    Vitamin B$_6$

- Aerobic exercise
- Relaxation techniques
- Adequate sleep

Psychotherapy
- Supportive therapy
- **Cognitive-behavioral**

Anxiolytics
- **Alprazolam**
- Buspirone hydrochloride

Antidepressants
- Bupropion hydrochloride
- **Venlafaxine hydrochloride**
- **SSRIs**

    Continuous use

    Luteal phase only

- Tricyclic antidepressants

Hormonal Treatment
- Oral contraceptives
- Progesterone
- **Danazol**
- **GnRH agonists**
- Oophorectomy

Other
- NSAIDs
- **Spironolactone**
- Herbal treatments

    Evening primrose oil

    Agnus cactus fruit extract

Note: Boldfaced entries have been shown to be effective in randomized controlled trials.

criteria for any mental illness during this period. Normal psychological changes include anxiety, mood lability, and extreme concerns about bodily changes and the well-being of the fetus. Although mood disorders associated with pregnancy and the puerperium have been described for centuries, they have become a focus of research in recent years because of women's apparent vulnerability to depressive and anxiety disorders, especially around pregnancy.

Case Vignette

Ms Thomas is a 21-year-old single woman with a 2-year-old child and a newborn. At her 6-week postpartum checkup, her obstetrician, noting that she appeared quite sad, obtained the history that she has been feeling quite down since the death of her mother 2 years ago. She became more depressed after the birth of her first baby and feels that this new baby has made things even worse.

Ms Thomas has had no prior psychiatric diagnosis or treatment. Currently the symptoms include anhedonia, increased fatigue, sleeplessness with frequent wakenings even when the baby is asleep, decreased appetite with 15 pounds weight loss since she was discharged from the hospital, lack of concentration and memory, lessened sexual interest to the dismay of her boyfriend, and suicidal thoughts and ideas about harming her children. Ms Thomas said she did not use alcohol or drugs. She confided to the social worker in the clinic that she had been hearing voices in the past month telling her to hurt her 2-year-old in addition to herself. She and her two children live alone, although she has relatives in town. The father of both of these children was living with her but moved back with his mother during Ms Thomas's pregnancy and has not been very helpful. There is a family history of depression and alcoholism.

This woman has several high-risk factors for mental illness. She has a past history of depression, a positive family history for mental illness and alcoholism, a significant loss with the death of her mother (exacerbated by the loss of the boyfriend and father of her pregnancies), and a lack of social supports. She needs immediate hospitalization, mobilization of family and social supports, psychotropic medications in addition to psychotherapy (supportive, cognitive-behavioral or interpersonal), and help from community resources such as visiting nurses and others.

Postpartum blues are the least severe of the pregnancy-related affective reactions. Up to 70% of puerperal women have this condition. Postpartum blues occur cross-culturally, start within 48 hours of delivery, and last 2 days to 3 weeks. The condition is characterized by emotional lability, elation or tearfulness, sadness, anxiety, irritability, insomnia, and fatigue. In most women, these feelings resolve spontaneously. The etiology is thought to be a reaction to the marked fall in gonadal steroids that follows delivery. No treatment is indicated.

Postpartum depression is a major depression that may begin during pregnancy but often starts afterward, with an onset during the first 3 months following childbirth. Postpartum depression affects 10% to 15% of new mothers and as many as 30% of women who have had a prior depression. The symptoms are those of a major depression, although there are more features of guilt related to the baby and, at times, obsessional thoughts about harming the baby. The role of sleep deprivation in postpartum depression has not been well studied. The likelihood of postpartum depression is increased by a personal history of depression, family history, depressive symptoms during the pregnancy, and psychosocial stressors such as conflicts with partner, concerns about child care, death in the family, and inadequate social supports.

Adolescents are often more vulnerable. Perinatal loss, birth of twins or more, and babies with congenital anomalies or severe illness also increase the risk for postpartum depression. Perinatal loss is accompanied by symptoms of bereavement and may coexist with a depressive illness. Another period of vulnerability for onset of depression is at the time of weaning from breastfeeding. Milder forms of depressive illnesses in the postpartum period sometimes have been referred to as adjustment reactions with depressed mood.

Evaluation for postpartum depression should always include a physical exam with thyroid studies. It is important to inquire about suicidal feelings, as well as issues related to the safety of the baby and any other children. Alcohol and drug use also are prevalent with this condition. The Edinburgh Postnatal Depression Scale, which also can be used during pregnancy, is a helpful screening tool.

Psychotherapy, support groups, and self-help organizations such as Depression after Delivery (1-800-944-4PPD or www.depressionafterdelivery.com) and Postpartum Support International (1-805-967-7636 or www.chss.iup.edu/postpartum) have been used successfully with and without medications. Cognitive-behavioral and interpersonal psychotherapies have been found to be helpful. Light therapy also is being used with some success. Obsessive ruminations respond well to treatment with cognitive-behavioral therapy and antidepressant medications, especially the SSRIs and clomipramine, a tricyclic antidepressant. At this time no conclusive data are available pertaining to the use of ovarian hormones such as estrogen and progesterone in treating postpartum depressions, although estrogen is being studied. There has been interest in the use of sex hormones to address the possible role of steroid deprivation as an etiology for postpartum mood disorders, and in some cases of depressive illness in women estrogen has been effective.

The benefits of psychotropic medications (Table 17-3) must be weighed against the potential risks of their use during pregnancy and breastfeeding. All psychotropic drugs do cross the placenta, and none has been approved by the US Food and Drug Administration for use in pregnancy. These drugs should be tapered when ready to discontinue and not be withdrawn suddenly when pregnancy is diagnosed. Even though gradual

---

TABLE 17-3 Guidelines for Use of Psychotropic Medications in Pregnancy and Postpartum

- Be certain to obtain informed consent, including risks, benefits, and alternatives.
- Use medications that have some documented safety data.
- If patient has been on a medication that helped, try using it again.
- Use the lowest effective dosage of a single medication.
- Encourage good health habits such as avoiding cigarettes, alcohol, illicit drugs, and herbs that have not been proved safe.
- Include psychotherapies as the first line in milder cases, then include with medications to minimize dose of drugs needed.
- Always include close family members in treatment decisions if woman agrees.

tapering is usually the safest approach, consideration should be given to continuing needed medications or to switching to drugs with better fetal safety profiles during pregnancy. Safety concerns relate to anatomic or behavioral teratogenicity, toxicity to the fetus or mother, and long-term neurobehavioral effects.

Further study and follow-up of babies exposed in utero to psychotropic medications is currently under way. Decision-making about treating mental illness during pregnancy and breastfeeding must weigh the effects of the medications against the suffering from untreated illness. Breastfeeding infants of mothers on psychotropic medications should be followed by their care providers for behavior changes and any other possible adverse drug effects.

Untreated depressive illnesses may last as long as 9 months, with profound effects on the infant and family. Even relatively short-term treatment of postpartum depression can provide long-lasting benefits for the entire family.

Of women with postpartum depression, 50% will experience a recurrence within 4 years. Studies have demonstrated the effectiveness of preventive treatment with antidepressant medications that are begun immediately after delivery for women at high risk for recurrence of postpartum depressions. Risk factors for postpartum depression should be assessed during prenatal care.

Postpartum psychosis, the most severe mental illness related to pregnancy and the puerperium, occurs in 1 or 2 women per 1000 deliveries. More than half of these women have depressive disorders, and others are schizophrenic or have other psychotic conditions, including organic conditions. Schizophrenia may have its onset, exacerbate, or remit during or after pregnancy. Those at most risk for postpartum psychosis have personal or family histories of mental illness. Women at high risk for postpartum psychosis should be observed closely during their pregnancies and afterward. They should not be left alone postpartum.

In addition to hallucinations, delusions, and loss of reality, there may be confusion, distractibility, sensory clouding, and problems with attention. Suicide or neonaticide are concerns with postpartum psychosis. If you suspect that a patient has a postpartum psychosis, keep in mind that these women require immediate consideration for hospitalization in a psychiatric unit.

Treatment for postpartum psychosis consists of appropriate antipsychotic medications and occasionally electroconvulsive therapy, which can be safe and effective when appropriately administered.

Anxiety disorders, especially obsessive-compulsive disorder, may start with or without depression in the postpartum period. Panic attacks also may begin postpartum. Treatment with SSRIs and psychotherapy, especially cognitive-behavioral therapy, is often helpful.

Disorders of mother–infant attachments are included in some classifications of postpartum disorders and should be considered by primary care providers. Some of the maternal attitudes that indicate the possibility of disordered attachment are lack of interest in the newborn, refusal to look at or hold the infant, hostile verbal expressions about the newborn, extreme disappointment in the sex or appearance of the baby, lack of social support (especially from the partner or mother), inadequate living arrangements, the mother's own rejection by her parents, young maternal age, and denial of the pregnancy with no prenatal care.

Infertility-Related Psychological Disorders

The primary care physician frequently is the first to learn about a fertility problem. There is no evidence that women who are infertile are any more likely to have psychiatric conditions than is the population at large. Nevertheless, some psychological disturbances can interfere with reproduction. For example, with appropriately sensitive questioning, the physician may learn that the couple has an unconsummated sexual relationship. Depressive syndromes and eating disorders may interfere with the functioning of the hypothalamic–pituitary–gonadal axis and affect ovulation. Some antipsychotic medications, such as risperidone, increase prolactin, leading to disturbances in ovulatory cycling. Behaviors such as smoking and alcohol or drug use can affect fertility by interfering with sexual functioning and also by disturbing neuroendocrine activity.

Fertility treatment commonly taxes the relationship and the emotions of the individuals involved. In addition, fertility drugs can cause mood disturbances. Assisted reproductive technologies, such as in vitro fertilization and its variations (both with and without collaborative reproduction with donor gametes or surrogate carriers), can be emotionally, physically, and financially draining. Psychological reactions to infertility depend on a number of factors, including the age at which reproductive problems are first recognized; the individual's stage of development, personality structure, coping styles, and preexisting psychopathology; support of family and friends; the medical problems causing the infertility; cultural and religious influences; and the skills and empathy of the medical staff caring for the individual and couple. The patient's reactions may include anger, grief, sadness, guilt, blame, feelings of lack of control and helplessness, and possibly sexual problems or problems with the partner.

The urban legend that fertility improves in couples who decide to adopt has been shown to be a reporting bias and is not true. Although some studies suggest that treatment of depressive illnesses does improve female fertility, more research has to be done. Mind–body programs that teach relaxation techniques have been helpful in controlling pain during fertility treatments. These techniques are being studied to see if pregnancy rates improve for patients receiving this training, but the data are not yet in. Psychiatric syndromes, including eating disorders and depression, must be recognized by the fertility team and suitably treated or referred because treatment is important for the patient's overall health, regardless of any causal relationship to the infertility. For depressive illnesses that require psychotropic medications, the SSRIs have been found to be the safest for women trying to conceive or who have just become pregnant.

Menopause and Psychiatric Disorders

Although no data have suggested that menopause, the time after the last menstrual period, is associated with any increase in psychiatric disorders for women who have not had problems before, some of the newer epidemiological information suggests that there is a small increase in depressive disorders during the perimenopause.

The perimenopause—the years that surround the transition to menopause—often presents with a change in the menstrual cycle. Cycles may be shorter or longer and menstruation lighter or heavier. Hot flashes and sleep disturbances may be noted, particularly around the menses. Although a number of excellent long-term studies have been done on the biological and psychosocial aspects of the menopausal transition, these have focused mainly on white middle-class women in Western cultures, where it is hard to separate the effects of the strong mythology about menopause from its biology. Other difficulties in the research on depressive illnesses include misdefining the symptom of depressed mood as an actual diagnosis of depression, not correlating hormonal status with symptoms, and confusing association with causation.

Hot flashes and vaginal dryness are the most frequently reported physiological symptoms of menopause, but they are influenced by diet, body weight, cultural expectations, and other variables. The most common psychological symptoms include irritability, labile mood, anxiety, depression, and decrease in short-term memory. The most common psychiatric diagnoses noted at this time are major depression, dysthymia, anxiety disorders, and alcohol and other substance abuse.

Risk factors for these syndromes, especially the affective conditions, are similar to those at other times of life, including a personal and/or family history of psychiatric disorders, life stressors, physical or sexual abuse, alcohol or drug use, anxiety, physical illness, and sleep problems. Women may be more vulnerable to mood disorders during the menopausal transition because of estrogen withdrawal (with its presumed effects on brain neurotransmitters); the effects of unpleasant symptoms such as hot flashes, vaginal dryness, or psychological changes; sleep disturbance from nighttime hot flashes; and/or midlife stressors such as partner problems, adolescent children, aging parents, and physical illnesses.

Assessment and management of the midlife and menopausal woman includes physical and psychological assessment, education about this transition, counseling, and psychotherapy when indicated. The decision about hormone replacement is based on individualized assessment of the risks and benefits. Estrogens often are useful because they resolve hot flashes, enhance mood, improve sleep, expand short-term memory, enhance sexual functioning, and lead to an overall sense of well-being. If systemic estrogen is given, a progestin must be added either continuously or cyclically to protect the uterus from the carcinogenic risk of unopposed estrogen. Progestins themselves may have PMS-like mood-altering effects.

Research from the Women's Health Initiative of the National Institutes of Health has questioned the safety of long-term use of estrogen–progestin combinations. Possible risks include breast cancer and heart disease. Short-term risks include deep venous thrombosis and vaginal bleeding. Hormone replacement therapy was shown to protect women from osteoporosis and hip fracture and from colon cancer. Questions as to whether estrogen delays the onset of Alzheimer disease (AD) remain to be answered. New information does not support the delay in AD, but more research and data are needed. Ultimately, the decision as to whether long-term estrogen treatment is in the best interest of an individual will depend on her underlying risk factors and how the estrogen-deprivation symptoms affect her quality of life. Many of the benefits of systemic estrogen can be obtained with alternative treatments, such as bisphosphamates, SSRIs, transvaginal estrogen, and others.

Although estrogen may improve well-being and may augment antidepressants, it is not an effective treatment for severe depressive illness. If depression is identified, mood symptoms may be modified by diet, exercise, social supports, and education about what changes to expect. Coexisting medical problems, such as hypothyroidism, can have psychiatric manifestations. Psychiatric syndromes should be treated the same as at other times in the life cycle. Referral to a mental health professional, as always, is indicated if the woman or her family requests it; a second opinion is needed; the patient responds poorly to adequate trials of medication; the woman is suicidal; one suspects psychosis, bipolar disease, or dual diagnoses; or the primary care physician is not comfortable with the amount of psychological discomfort the patient is experiencing. The goal of menopausal management is to enhance coping, to help the woman feel better physically and mentally, and, when possible, to improve overall health.

TREATMENT ISSUES FOR WOMEN WHO HAVE PSYCHIATRIC DISORDERS

Treatment has to be directed at problem-solving and helping patients to develop a sense of mastery and competency. There are gender differences in the pharmacokinetics of antidepressants and other psychotropic medications, although these have not yet been well studied. Women are thought to secrete less gastric acid, have a slower gastric emptying rate, have more body fat, and have greater liver enzyme activity than men. Therefore, women may show a higher plasma level of a given medication than men would, given similar dosages. Women may have more side effects from drugs than men. Drug dosages may have to be adjusted during the premenstrual phase of the menstrual cycle or during pregnancy and the puerperium. Oral contraceptives may alter dosage requirements of some psychotropic medications.

SUMMARY

Women with mental health conditions are likely to present differently than men. Depression and anxiety disorders are particularly prevalent in women, whereas substance abuse problems and some types of personality disorders are more common in men.

The many psychological, biological, and cultural influences on a person's mental health require a biopsychosocial approach to evaluation and treatment. Understanding the differences between men and women is one step in this approach. Assessing the patient in the context of individual psychological make-up, response to hormonal fluctuations, and the impact of social relationships provides a more holistic picture of the patient's mental state.

Several mental health conditions are unique to women. The primary care physician must be able to differentiate the normal premenstrual emotional changes from the disruption of premenstrual dysphoric disorder. A new mother may need assessment for postpartum depression or psychosis, and her primary care physician must be able to differentiate those diagnoses from the normal baby blues and exhaustion that commonly follow childbirth. Menopause also presents challenges for the physician, with the need to balance quality of life, which may be improved with hormone replacement therapy, with possible long-term health risks of hormone use. Thus, comprehensive primary care of women requires knowledge about gender issues in health and disease, skills at assessing the patient's concerns in the context of this knowledge, and sensitivity to the ways in which a female patient with emotional or behavioral problems may present herself.

Our understanding of gender differences in mental health is just beginning. As more research becomes available, it is hoped that many of the unanswered questions about differences in diagnoses, presentations, severity of illness, somatization, treatment response, and, most important, prevention, will be answered.

ADDITIONAL READINGS

ACOG Practice Bulletin: Clinical Management Guidelines for Obstetrician-Gynecologists. *Premenstrual Syndrome*. 2000(April);15:1029-1037.

Burns LH, Covington SN, eds. *Infertility Counseling: A Comprehensive Handbook for Clinicians*. New York, NY: Parthenon Publishing Group; 1999.

Burt VK, Altschuler LL, Ragon N. Depressive symptoms in the perimenopause: prevalence, assessment, and guidelines for treatment. *Harv Rev Psychiatry*. 1998;6(3):121-132.

Burt VK, Suri R, Altshuler LL, Stowe Z, Hendrick VC, Muntean E. The use of psychotropic medications during breast-feeding. *Am J Psychiatry*. 2001;58:1001-1009.

Chambers CD, Johnson KA, Dick LM, et al. Birth outcomes in pregnant women taking fluoxetine. *N Eng J Med*. 1996;335:1010-1015.

Cox J, Holden J, Sagovsky R. Detection of postnatal depression: development of the Edinburgh Postnatal Depression Scale. *Brit J Psychiatry*. 1987;150:782-786.

Ernst CL, Goldberg JF. The reproductive safety profile of mood stabilizers, atypical antipsychotics, and broad-spectrum psychotropics. *J Clin Psychiatry*. 2002;63(Suppl 4):42-55.

Frank E, ed. *Gender and its Effects on Psychopathology*. Washington, DC: American Psychiatric Press, Inc; 2000.

Glaze R, Cox JL. Validation of a computerized version of the 10 item (self rating) Edinburgh Postnatal Depression Scale. *J Affective Disorders*. 1991;22:73-77.

Leibenluft E, ed. *Gender Differences in Mood and Anxiety Disorders: From Bench to Bedside*. Washington, DC: American Psychiatric Press, Inc; 1999.

Leon IG. *When a Baby Dies: Psychotherapy for Pregnancy and Newborn Loss*. New Haven, Conn: Yale University Press; 1990.

Lewis–Hall F, Williams TS, Panetta JA, Herrera JM, eds. *Psychiatric Illness in Women: Emerging Treatments and Research*. Washington, DC: American Psychiatric Press, Inc; 2002.

McGrath E, Keita GP, Strickland BR, Russo NF, eds. *Women and Depression: Risk Factors and Treatment Issues*. Washington, DC: American Psychological Association; 1990.

McKinlay SM. The normal menopause transition: an overview. *Maturitas*. 1996;23:137-145.

Miller LJ, ed. *Postpartum Mood Disorders*. Washington, DC: American Psychiatric Press, Inc; 1999.

Rosenthal MB, Goldfarb J. Infertility and assisted reproductive technology: an update for mental health professionals. *Harvard Rev Psychiatry*. 1997;5:169-172.

Schmidt PJ, Roca CA, Rubinow DR. Clinical evaluation in studies of perimenopausal women: position paper. *Psychopharmacol Bull*. 1998;34(3):309-311.

Stowe ZN, Nemeroff CB. Psychopharmacology during pregnancy and lactation. In: Schatzberg A, Nemeroff CB, eds. *American Psychiatric Press Textbook of Psychopharmacology*. Washington, DC: American Psychiatric Press, Inc; 1998.

Wisner KL, Gelenberg AJ, Leonard H, Zarin D, Frank E. Pharmacologic treatment of depression during pregnancy. *JAMA*. 1999;282:1264-1269.

Chapter **18**

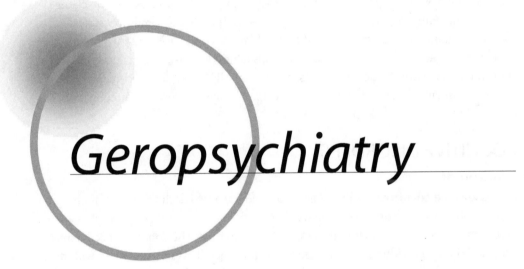

Geropsychiatry

Sanford Finkel, MD

In 1900, 4% of Americans were over the age of 65. This number increased to 13% by 2000 and will increase to approximately 17% by the year 2020. For the average person, longevity has increased from 47 years to 76 years in only one century. Further, subjective and objective data confirm that the elderly are healthier than their parents were at the same age. On a given day, 95% of those over the age of 65 are living in noninstitutional settings, and almost 90% function independently.

Opportunities for older people continue to increase. Many return to school, taking courses or even obtaining academic degrees. Others participate in volunteer activities; some choose new career paths. However, the aging process brings less positive changes for some, including physical health problems; loss of friends and family, possibly a spouse; economic problems; retirement from a familiar workplace; and involuntary relocation to a new home. Psychiatric illnesses, such as depression, dementia, and anxiety, can interfere with the quality of these individuals' lives. Yet, for most mentally ill elderly, treatments are available to manage symptoms and improve functioning and quality of life.

COGNITIVE DISORDERS

Syndromes

Age-associated cognitive decline. Age-associated cognitive decline (AACD) is characterized by subjective memory problems, which include increased difficulty recalling words, problems remembering names and faces, and forgetfulness. The condition occurs in as many as 80% of individuals over the age of 65 and generally is not associated with dementia. Individuals with AACD generally score 28 to 30 on the 30-point Mini-Mental State Examination (MMSE) but score one standard deviation below the mean of young adults on a standardized memory test. Individuals with AACD need to be reassured that they do not have Alzheimer disease (AD). For those who are open to new experiences and willing to work on improving their memory on an ongoing basis, nonpharmacologic cognitive enhancement techniques have been shown to be useful. Examples include relaxation techniques to diminish anxiety, use of mnemonics (memory tricks), and visual imagery.

A significant decrease in the use of memory strategies as one ages is one of the primary reasons for AACD. Although cognitive tests are performed more slowly with advanced age, some aspects of memory function such as forgetting rates, immediate memory, search processes, and susceptibility to interference do not change. The presence of anxiety or unrealistically low expectations also interferes with memory performance.

Mild cognitive impairment. Mild cognitive impairment (MCI), which is characterized by additional memory deficits, is sometimes described as pre-AD. During this phase, clear evidence of memory impairment is present, although the person may function adequately in work and social situations. However, although each year approximately 15% of people with MCI will develop AD, approximately 20% will never develop AD.

Dementias. Dementia is a syndrome, not a specific diagnosis. It is characterized by symptoms that are found in a variety of dementing illnesses. Symptoms include memory impairment, aphasias, apraxias, agnosias, and impairment of executive functioning in decision-making. The most common type of dementia is AD. However, the following constitute at least 10% of all dementing illnesses: vascular dementia, frontotemporal dementia, and Lewy body dementia. AD and other dementias are commonly overdiagnosed in certain populations, eg, those with sensory deficits, depression, and schizoid personalities; those over age 90; those in nursing homes; and those with severe preexisting developmental disorders (eg, Down syndrome).

Cognitive decline, impaired functioning, and behavioral and psychological symptoms are manifest in all the dementing illnesses. Pharmacologic treatments with cholinesterase inhibitors slow progression of the illness, increase time to nursing home placement, and increase time of functioning ability in activities of daily living. Issues such as driving and financial and legal matters ideally are best dealt with early in the course of the illness. Also, special attention must be given to the caregiver. Caregivers often suffer significant psychological and emotional distress as the disease progresses. A quarter of the spouses of people with AD develop major depression over the course of the illness. One study indicated that caregivers who receive counseling experience improved well-being and are able to delay placing the AD patient in a nursing home. See Chapter 10 for more information about dementias.

Evaluation of Cognitive Impairment

The primary care physician's role is critical in the evaluation of cognitively impaired patients for four reasons:

- The cognitively impaired patient is likely to show up in the primary care physician's office.
- The longitudinal relationship between the patient and the physician provides a unique opportunity to observe changes over time.
- The longitudinal relationship generates confidence that may encourage the patient and family to report any concerns to the physician.
- All interventions in this field are best if done toward the earliest possible stage of the illness.

By the time patients are brought to the attention of specialists (eg, geriatricians, psychiatrists, neurologists), they may be significantly affected and beyond the scope of any strategies currently under investigation. Primary care physicians who are fully aware of the diagnostic strategies can help increase the number of elderly patients who can benefit from early treatment.

Patient history. Questions on the patient history should reflect the definition of dementia, ie, progressive deterioration in cognition to a level lower than the patient baseline involving memory, language, and other cognitive functions, which impairs activities of daily living (ADLs) but is associated with a normal level of consciousness. To assess whether cognitive deficits exist, the primary care physician should use standard mental status cognitive screens such as the MMSE (see Chapter 3) or the 7 Minute Screen (7MS) (see Solomon) to look for deficits and to establish a baseline for future evaluation. It is critically important to obtain collateral history from a family member or other reliable source inasmuch as the patient's information may be inaccurate.

Physical examination. In the physical examination, the primary care physician seeks evidence of neurologic or systemic illness. Important clues include the presence of hypertension and evidence of end-organ damage, such as bruits, which would suggest cardiovascular illness, stigmata of thyroid disease, neurological focal findings, peripheral neuropathy, apraxia of gait or ADLs, signs of infection, or other illnesses in which cognition can be adversely affected (eg, Parkinson disease or multiple sclerosis).

Diagnostic studies. Standardized laboratory studies consist of complete blood count, chemistry screen, folate and vitamin B_{12}, thyroid function, and urinalysis. Computed tomography (CT) scan may be helpful if diagnosis is in doubt. In addition to an MSE, a functional assessment is needed. Can the homemaker bake to her previous standard? Can the patient write checks accurately? Is the patient taking his or her medications appropriately? Medication compliance can be determined in collaboration with pharmacies as to frequency of prescription refill, via co-count, or via even more sophisticated electronic or computer-driven devices placed in the home.

Neuropsychological testing can offer objective evidence of cognitive impairment, distinguish depression from dementia, and correlate functional deficits to a location of probable impaired portions of the brain. This testing can be valuable when the diagnosis is in question, when documentation is required for legal proceeding, and as an assessment of a patient's functional strengths and weakness as a guide to the safest, least restrictive living environment. A depression screen is often valuable in determining coexisting depression.

Treatment is focused on slowing progression of illness by use of cognitive-enhancing medication, eliminating excess disability caused by comorbid and medical and/or psychiatric illness, maximizing functioning, providing support, and educating family members and other caregivers.

Behavioral and Psychological Symptoms of Dementia

The behavioral and psychological symptoms of dementia (BPSD) (Table 18-1), previously referred to as behavioral disturbances of dementia, result in patient and caregiver suffering, premature institutionalization, excess disability, and socioeconomic loss. In many instances, caregivers can tolerate the functional and cognitive declines that occur with dementia, but they are distressed and even overwhelmed by the behavioral and psychological symptoms. The primary care physician can offer the caregiver counseling to help him or her manage these symptoms when they appear as the disease progresses. Among these symptoms are delusions, eg, patients may believe that people are stealing, that the family is planning for institutionalization, that family and friends are impostors, that their

TABLE 18-1 Common Behavioral and Psychological Symptoms of Dementia

- Delusions
- Hallucinations
- Aggression, verbal and/or physical
- Agitation
- Apathy, poor motivation
- Insomnia, disrupted sleep-wake cycle
- Wandering

home is not their own, or that their spouse is guilty of sexual infidelity. The accompanying agitation and the "real" qualities of delusions sometimes result in verbally and even physically abusive behavior toward family members and the caregiver. The primary care physician can counsel the caregiver to refrain from contradicting the patient and to instead reassure the patient ("I won't let anything happen to you") or distract the person ("Let's go watch some television").

Delusions occur in the majority of Alzheimer patients over the course of the illness. However, hallucinations are less frequent and may be less severe than those experienced with other psychiatric illnesses. For example, patients may relate that they see individuals, such as children, in their home when none exist. Visual hallucinations are more common in people with visual impairment or who have Lewy body dementia. Arguing about these hallucinations results in little benefit. If these types of hallucinations generally are not disturbing, no direct treatment may be necessary. Instead, the physician should suggest that the caregiver empathize with the patient and offer comfort and reassurance, if necessary. This is in contrast to hallucinations with other psychoses in late life where medication is generally mandatory.

AD causes disturbances in the circadian rhythms, and sleep problems may result with both the Alzheimer patient and spouse being up for the better part of the night. The patient's wandering can also add to caregiver anxiety and suffering. Sleep medication for the AD patient may be warranted. A depressive affect, including tearfulness and statements of wanting to be dead, occurs early in the illness and may be accompanied by agitated symptoms of depression (eg, insomnia, anorexia, and weight loss). Patients may benefit from antidepressant treatment. Verbally abusive behavior, which includes screaming and cursing, as well as physically abusive behavior, such as hitting, pushing, and kicking, are more common occurrences as the illness progresses. Other behaviors include sexual disinhibition; hoarding food, valuables, or newspapers; and culturally inappropriate behavior.

Nonpharmacologic approaches should be tried as the first interventions whenever possible. Redirection of attention, reassurances, and rechanneling energy are among the best initial approaches for the caregiver to use in these circumstances. However, these approaches do not work uniformly well with all demented patients, or they may work variably with a patient depending on the environment or the patient's internal psychological state. Other techniques that have been shown to be effective in some individuals include background music and recreational therapy. The danger of wandering may be diminished by applying electronic bracelets or by using internal door locks. All AD patients should be enrolled in the Safe Return Program sponsored by local Alzheimer associations.

For those who require medication to manage their psychotic and aggressive symptoms (Table 18-2), the atypical antipsychotic medications are especially important. Risperidone (Risperdal), which has been studied extensively, has been shown to be effective in patients with psychotic and aggressive symptoms. Daily doses range from 0.25 to 2 mg, with the mean dose of 1 mg. Risperidone must be used with caution in people with a history of cerebral vascular illness. Smaller studies have suggested that olanzapine (Zyprexa) may be helpful in doses of 5 mg. Although data are currently lacking, quetiapine fumarate (Seroquel) may also be helpful in doses ranging from 25 to 250 mg. As

TABLE 18-2 Pharmacologic Treatment of Behavioral and Psychological Symptoms of Dementia

Drug	Typical Daily Dosing (mg)	Precautions
Risperidone	0.25 to 2.0	Extrapyramidal effects, sedation, and possible cerebral vascular events
Olanzapine	2.5 to 10	Sedation, glycemic control
Quetiapine fumarate	25 to 250	Sedation
Sertraline	50 to 200	SIADH
Citalopram hydrobromide	10 to 40	SIADH
Benzodiazepines*	Varies with drug	Sedation, worsened cognition, falls
Buspirone hydrochloride	10 to 40	
Carbamazepine	400 to 1600	Sedation, falls, SIADH, hematologic, skin problems
Divalproex	125 to 1000	Sedation, nausea, dehydration

*Shorter-acting drugs such as lorazepam, oxazepam, and chlordiazepoxide hydrochloride are preferred to avoid accumulation.

with all older patients, start with a low dose and increase gradually, if possible. Benzodiazepines, particularly short-acting ones like lorazepam, may be of benefit for short-term use or when other medications are not effective. These drugs must be used judiciously because of the possibilities of falls or worsened cognition. The selective serotonin reuptake inhibitors (SSRIs) have also been shown to be helpful in decreasing anxiety and agitation, as well as depression associated with dementing illnesses. Controlled studies with sertraline (Zoloft, 25 to 100 mg/day) and citalopram (Celexa, 10 to 40 mg/day) have demonstrated effectiveness for symptoms of anxiety, depression, and agitation. In general, patients with BPSD whose symptoms have failed to respond quickly or whose symptoms are severe should be referred to a geriatric psychiatrist.

DEPRESSION

Case Vignette

Mrs Jones, a 76-year-old woman with hypertension, osteoarthritis, and coronary artery disease, comes to see her primary care physician 3 months after she underwent emergency coronary-artery bypass grafting. The surgery was without complications. She complains that "my brain just isn't working since that operation." When asked if she feels sad, she says, "Who wouldn't with their mind starting to go like this?" Previously a very active, outgoing woman,

Mrs Jones reports becoming virtually housebound "because I don't want my friends to see how dumb I am now." When family comes to visit, she finds she has little energy or enthusiasm to play with her grandchildren, formerly a great joy for her. She falls asleep easily but wakes up regularly at 4:00 AM and cannot go back to sleep. She eats "as little as my husband will let me get away with" and has maintained her weight. Her physical examination is uninformative. On mental status exam, Mrs Jones sits slumped over and avoids eye contact with the physician, both in contrast to her preoperative pattern of behavior. When asked cognitive questions, she initially answers, "I don't know" or "What difference does it make," but if pressed, generally answers appropriately. When she makes small errors (eg, initially incorrectly reciting serial 7s when she gets to the 50s), she not only catches the error and corrects it but also adds, "See, doctor, I told you I am a dope these days."

Depressive symptoms are more common in the elderly than younger patients, but rates of major depression appear to be somewhat lower. The symptom picture in the elderly is generally similar to that of younger patients and may include insomnia, anorexia, low energy, poor concentration, psychomotor retardation, inability to derive pleasure from usually pleasurable activities, depressed mood, and suicidal ideation or intent. There may be atypical presentations in late life, which include apathy and pseudo-dementia, a condition in which cognitive deficits play a prominent part in the clinical presentation; the deficits may even simulate a dementia syndrome. Although these cognitive deficits may be "reversible" when the depression is treated, the pseudodementia is highly correlated with developing a dementing illness years later. Pseudodementia (and depression) may be distinguished from dementia by several features:

- Presence of a full, major depressive syndrome that has gone on for more than 2 weeks.
- Poor effort when answering cognitive questions. The person with pseudodementia will say, "Who cares," "Why bother," or "I don't know." However, their performance increases with effort. The person with AD may try to answer the question but may not give an answer to the question that is being asked.
- Inconsistent pattern of performance (eg, knowing all recent presidents but unable to give the season).
- Drawing attention to poor performance on the cognitive exam, often with a self-deprecatory attitude.

Biological factors and neurotransmitter abnormalities may be precipitants for late-life depression. Losses, particularly interpersonal and physical ones, may also contribute. Major depression must be distinguished from normal grieving. Marked functional impairment, suicidal ideation, and notable self-criticism or guilt are less common in bereavement. Suicide is an important potential complication, particularly in men, those who have current depression, those who have a history of depression, or those who have a current excessive use of alcohol. Twenty percent of elderly males who commit suicide have seen a primary care physician within 24 hours, 40% within a week, and 70% within a couple of months of their death.

Treatment follows the same outlines as for younger patients. Psychotherapy plays an important role in management, particularly in offering hope and modifying negative thinking. All antidepressive drugs used for younger patients may be used in the elderly.

Controlled studies suggest that the SSRIs—particularly sertraline (Zoloft) and fluoxetine hydrochloride (Prozac)—are as effective as the more traditional tricyclic medications (eg, amitriptyline hydrochloride [Elavil], imipramine hydrochloride [Tofranil]). However, SSRIs have a much better and safer side-effect profile, particularly for the elderly, although certain infrequent side effects such as syndrome of inappropriate secretion of antidiuretic hormone (SIADH) are more commonly seen in the elderly. Tricyclics also can be sedating, causing orthostatic hypotension and anticholinergic effects, as well as His-ventricular conduction delay effects. Other commonly used antidepressants include bupropion hydrochloride (Wellbutrin), venlafaxine hydrochloride (Effexor), and mirtazapine (Remeron).

For individuals with psychotic symptoms, those who are suicidal, and those who are severely withdrawn, electroconvulsive therapy (ECT) may be useful.

PSYCHOSIS

Late-onset schizophrenia (sometimes called paraphrenia) is a psychotic disorder characterized by bizarre delusions without the personality deterioration that is commonly seen in earlier onset schizophrenia. It occurs predominantly in women and is associated with auditory and visual sensory deficits, a history of personality disorder, social isolation, lower social class, and bearing no children. The illness is often characterized by bizarre delusions with sexual content ("The landlord is coming into my apartment at night to have sex with me.") or paranoid ideas ("The FBI is sending electronic beams through the wall to affect my brain.").

Case Vignette

Mrs Batson is an 80-year-old widow in good health who has lived alone for several years since the death of her husband. She presents to her primary care physician's office demanding a referral to an otorhinolaryngologist because of irritation and burning in her nose and the back of her throat. She attributes these sensations to "some kind of nasty gas" that her upstairs neighbor, "a handsome guy, but a lady-killer type, if you know what I mean," has been piping in through her plumbing whenever she gets undressed to take a bath. She has confronted the neighbor several times, but "he looks me over like a cat looks at a mouse and says he has no idea what I'm talking about." She has asked her landlord to send a plumber on several occasions, and she has even called the police to file a complaint against the neighbor. "Those men—the landlord, the plumber, and the policeman—don't believe me; they're all in cahoots." Examination of her eyes, ears, nose, and throat is normal. Mrs Batson is calm but angry at being so mistreated, and her cognitive examination demonstrates am MMSE score of 30/30.

These patients can be helped with antipsychotic medication and supportive therapy; however, they often mistrust physicians and other health care professionals and may not seek assistance. Because they generally are not a danger to themselves or others, they are not certifiable for psychiatric hospitalization and therefore may not receive treatment, much to the consternation of their neighbors, family, landlord, and police.

In contrast, patients with early-onset schizophrenia may have a long history of institutionalization that requires special supports (eg, specialized residential care or adult daycare). Nevertheless, approximately 20% demonstrate significant improvement in late life. Further, the positive signs of schizophrenia, such as delusions and hallucinations, diminish; however, the negative symptoms, such as apathy and withdrawal, often increase.

ANXIETY DISORDERS

Generalized anxiety disorder and panic disorder occur in late life. Some anxiety disorders are part of a lifetime pattern from earlier in life, whereas others arise for the first time later in life. Medications including pseudoephedrine, calcium channel blockers, and bronchodilators may precipitate feelings of anxiety. Caffeine, which can have a markedly longer half-life in the elderly, is another potential offender. A range of medical illnesses— endocrinologic, neurologic, pulmonary, cardiovascular, and hematologic—can all produce anxiety symptoms as well. Conversely, anxiety disorders may contribute to a range of medical illnesses, including hypertension, asthma, and regional ileitis. High levels of anxiety are also associated with increased risk for myocardial infarction in older men.

Although benzodiazepines continue to be used, they are being replaced with the SSRIs, such as sertraline (Zoloft) and paroxetine hydrochloride (Paxil), which have been shown to be effective in treating panic disorders and obsessive-compulsive disorders. Nonpharmacologic interventions include cognitive-behavioral psychotherapy, biofeedback, relaxation techniques such as progressive muscle relaxation or visual relaxation, transcendental meditation, yoga, background music, and recreational therapy (see Chapter 8 for more information on anxiety disorders).

SLEEP DISORDERS

Sleep disorders are very common in the aged. Approximately half of those over the age of 65 complain of problems falling asleep, maintaining sleep, and experiencing early-morning awakening; 25% regularly use sleep medications. Sleep apnea occurs in more than 25% of older patients and is associated with snoring, obesity, and cognitive impairment. Slow-wave sleep (stages 3 and 4 of nonrapid eye movement sleep) diminishes markedly with age, thereby increasing the percentages of stage 1 and stage 2 sleep. Total rapid eye movement (REM) sleep remains stable. With age-related alterations and circadian rhythm patterns, older people demonstrate decreased alertness and sleepiness in the late afternoon and early evening. Bright lights and/or structured recreational activities have been shown to normalize circadian rhythms and improve late afternoon alertness. Other factors that contribute to sleep problems include psychiatric disorders (especially depression), pain, side effects to medication, infections, and respiratory illness.

Sleep apnea, which is generally associated with upper airway occlusion, results in interruption and cessation of airflow. It is also a risk factor for both sudden death due to nocturnal cardiac arrhythmias and for dementia. Eighty percent of patients who can tolerate continuous positive airway pressure benefit from treatment, and up to 75% of surgically treated patients benefit. Other sleep problems in late life include nocturnal myoclonus, which is characterized by intense leg movements during sleep, and restless leg syndrome, which may continue for 45 minutes at a stretch, awakening both the individual and the spouse.

Whenever possible, treatment for insomnia should be geared toward environmental modification—attention to lighting, temperature, noise, exercise, and special light used for reading or watching television—treating underlying psychiatric or medical disorders with short-term hypnotics. Temazepam (Restoril) 7.5 to 15 mg or zolpidem tartrate (Ambien) 5 to 10 mg are commonly used for insomnia. See Chapter 11 for more information about sleep disorders.

ALCOHOL AND CHEMICAL ABUSE AND DEPENDENCY

Approximately 10% of Americans over the age of 65 have a drinking problem, and 50% of those are alcohol dependent. These patients may present medically with lacerations and abrasions as a result of falls and with malnutrition and cognitive deficits. In the emergency department, they may be diagnosed as having AD. Hygiene is often poor with self-neglect evident. The Brief Michigan Alcohol Screening Test (MAST) or the CAGE questionnaire are useful screening tests that take only a couple of minutes to administer.

Treatment focuses on both detoxification and subsequent rehabilitation. Detoxification supports physiologic homeostasis through adequate hydration, vitamin B supplements (especially thiamin), treatment of agitation (eg, with an antipsychotic), and environmental support (eg, quiet, adequate lighting) to maintain the patient's safety. Coexisting medical and psychiatric illnesses should be treated. Illnesses commonly associated with alcohol disorders include depression, dementia, sleep disorders, congestive heart failure, osteoporosis, pneumonia, anemia, and diabetes mellitus. Insomnia, low energy, and impotence also occur. Rehabilitative treatment is generally not available in specialized programs for the elderly, and existing treatment programs usually focus on younger adults or adolescents. Disulfiram (Antabuse) is potentially dangerous in the elderly because it may produce severe cardiovascular and autonomic side effects in combination with alcohol. Individual and/or group therapy may be helpful, and referral to an addiction specialist is indicated. One third of all members of Alcoholics Anonymous (AA) are over the age of 50. AA provides useful support for many elderly alcoholics. Treatment and family involvement, as well as social service intervention, are generally advisable. See Chapter 8 for more information on treating alcoholism and other addictions.

Illicit drugs generally are not a problem for the aged, who rarely begin such use after the age of 65. However, benzodiazepines are commonly used, especially for anxiety and sleep problems. Although they have demonstrated marked efficacy and are generally less toxic and addictive than their predecessors, abuse and habituation to these drugs are common, as is the potential for falls or cognitive impairment. Many elderly experience significantly decreased anxiety and are reluctant to discontinue the medications. For many, the problems of insomnia or anxiety begin again as the medication is withdrawn. Nevertheless, after the initial symptoms subside, gradual reduction and discontinuation is generally advisable and possible.

SPECIAL PROBLEMS WITH MEDICATION

The elderly are high users of medications. Over two thirds of those over age 65 take an over-the-counter drug each day. Many elderly see more than one physician and do not always communicate what medications they may be taking for various medical conditions, allowing the potential for negative drug interactions. Similarly, they may fail to communicate that they are taking over-the-counter medications, vitamins, herbal preparations, or other "health" preparations with substantial potential for adverse effects or drug interactions. They may also have difficulty understanding or remembering directions for taking their medications. Medication-related mistakes are not uncommon and are often preventable.

In general, because of impairments in both renal and hepatic clearance of drugs compared to younger populations, elderly patients should have more cautious initiation and adjustment of medications. Starting doses of psychotropic medications in the elderly should generally be one third to one half of the usual recommended initial doses, and dose increases should be carried out in smaller increments and with more time between adjustments than is typically done for younger patients. The primary care physician can thus be especially helpful in addressing the increasing complexity of managing the elderly patient's medicines, especially when both general medical and psychiatric problems are being treated.

SUMMARY

Although people are living longer and are healthier later in life, mental illness is still common in the elderly. Treatment of dementing illness is in the early stages of development, but even better treatments can be expected in the years ahead. Psychotropic medications can reduce, alleviate, and/or effectively treat the behavioral and psychological symptoms of dementia, depression, psychosis, and anxiety. Major depression and other depressive disorders continue to occur in late life and remain treatable through a variety of therapies, as they do for younger people. Some of the more flagrant symptoms of schizophrenia often ameliorate, and late-life schizophrenia is treatable with antipsychotic medication, supportive psychotherapy, and psychosocial programming. Sleep complaints and sleep disorders are generally common but can be treated with environmental adjustment, bright lights, altered schedules, or medication. Alcoholism and chemical dependency occur and may present in subtle forms, which requires careful history-taking, screening via brief scales, physical exam, and laboratory and toxicology testing. Referrals may be made to geriatric psychiatrists who specialize in diagnosing, treating, and preventing late-life mental disorders.

ADDITIONAL READINGS

American Medical Association. *Alcoholism in the Elderly: Diagnosis, Treatment, Prevention, Guidelines for Primary Care Physicians.* Chicago, Ill: American Medical Association; 1995.

Finkel SI, Burns A. Behavioral and psychological symptoms of dementia (BPSD): a clinical and research update. *Int Psychogeriatrics.* 2000;12(Suppl 1).

Finkel SI, Woodson C. History and physical examination of elderly patients with dementia. *Int Psychogeriatrics.* 1997;9(Suppl 1):71-75.

Mace N, Rabins P. *The 36-Hour Day: A Family Guide to Caring for Persons with Alzheimer Disease, Related Dementing Illnesses, and Memory Loss in Later Life.* New York NY: Warner Books, Inc; 2001.

Mittelman M, Epstein C, Pierzchala A. *Counseling the Alzheimer's Caregiver.* Chicago, Ill: AMA Press; 2003.

Quality Standards Subcommittee of the American Academy of Neurology. Practice parameter for diagnosis and evaluation of dementia. *Neurol.* 1995;44:2203-2209.

Reisberg B, Burns A. Diagnosis of Alzheimer's disease. *Int Psychogeriatrics.* 1997;9(Suppl 1).

Scharf MB, Jennings SW. Sleep disorders. In Bienenfield D, ed. *Verwoerdt's Clinical Geropsychiatry.* 3rd ed. Baltimore, Md: Williams & Wilkins; 1990:178-194.

Solomon P, Hirschoff A, Kelly B, et al. A 7 minute neurocognitive screening battery highly sensitive to Alzheimer's disease. *Arch Neurol.* 1998;55:349-355.

Chapter 19

Somatic Treatments

Prakash S. Masand, MD
Greg Clary, MD
K.N. Roy Chengappa, MD
K. Ranga Krishnan, MD

Somatic treatments have become an increasingly important component in the treatment of many psychiatric illnesses, including mood disorders, anxiety disorders, psychotic disorders, and, most recently, personality disorders. Recent advances in the understanding of neurobiology and pharmacology have led to development of many exciting compounds. Most notable are the selective serotonin reuptake inhibitors, which have revolutionized the treatment of mood and anxiety disorders, and the newer generation of antipsychotics, which represent an important advance in the treatment of many disorders. This chapter presents a discussion of somatic treatments for psychiatric illnesses, including antidepressants, anxiolytics and hypnotics, mood stabilizers, antipsychotics, psychostimulants, electroconvulsive therapy, hypnotherapy, biofeedback, and light treatment, among others.

ANTIDEPRESSANTS

Most effective antidepressants increase synaptic levels of norepinephrine and/or serotonin and, in some cases, dopamine. They accomplish this by inhibiting reuptake of these compounds or by preventing their metabolism. In many cases the drug itself is metabolized to pharmacologically active compounds that act differently from the parent compound. As a result, the *in vivo* effects of the drug include the effects of both the parent compound and its metabolites. Antidepressant drugs are classified by pharmacologists into five main categories: selective serotonin reuptake inhibitors (SSRIs), tricyclic antidepressants (TCAs), monoamine oxidase inhibitors (MAOIs), serotonin/norepinephrine reuptake inhibitors (SNRIs), and other antidepressant drugs (Table 19-1).

The beneficial effects of imipramine hydrochloride (a TCA) on depressed patients were noticed in 1958, and from the 1960s until the late 1980s, TCAs were the drugs of choice for depression in the United States. MAOIs were first identified as effective antidepressants in the late 1950s. They are still used in a limited fashion because of side effects and food and drug interactions. In the last few years there has been a renewed interest in the development of MAOIs less likely to cause these problems. Dissatisfaction with TCA side effects led to development of the SSRIs, which in turn has driven much basic and clinical research on serotonin. Fluoxetine hydrochloride, the first SSRI, was approved for clinical use in the United States in 1987. Other agents with different biochemical profiles have subsequently been developed in attempts to further reduce adverse drug effects. A comparison of side-effect profiles for different antidepressants is shown in Table 19-2.

General principles for managing the side effects from all antidepressants include:

- educating patients about the illness, medications, and side effects, including medication discontinuation issues, before initiating treatment;
- starting initially with a low dose of better-tolerated antidepressants like SSRIs;
- regular follow-up and asking patients about side effects, including sexual ones;
- taking side effects seriously; and
- dose reduction or waiting for tolerance to develop.

The indications for antidepressant drugs in major depression (Table 19-3) include moderate to severe, chronic, psychotic, and melancholic forms. Patients with recurrent

TABLE 19-1 Antidepressants Available in the United States

Drug	Brand Name*	Usual Number of Doses/Day	Common Dose Range (mg/day)	Therapeutic Plasma Levels (ng/mL)
SSRIs				
Citalopram hydrobromide	Celexa	1	20–60	—
Escitalopram oxalate	Lexapro	1	10–40	—
Fluoxetine hydrochloride	Prozac	1	5–80	—
Fluvoxamine maleate	Luvox	≥2	50–300	—
Paroxetine hydrochloride	Paxil	1	10–50	—
	Paxil CR	1	12.5–62.5	—
Sertraline hydrochloride	Zoloft	1	50–200	—
TCAs				
Amitriptyline hydrochloride	Elavil	1	50–300	> 200[†]
Amoxapine	Asendin	1	50–300	—
Clomipramine hydrochloride	Anafranil	1	50–250	—
Desipramine hydrochloride	Norpramin	1	50–300	> 125
Doxepin	Sinequan	1	50–300	—
Imipramine hydrochloride	Tofranil	1	50–300	> 200[‡]
Maprotiline hydrochloride	Ludiomil	1	50–200	—
Nortriptyline hydrochloride	Pamelor	1	25–150	50–150
Protriptyline hydrochloride	Vivactil	1	10–60	—
Trimipramine	Surmontil	1	50–300	—
MAOIs				
Phenelzine	Nardil	≥ 2	15–90	> 80%[§]
Tranylcypromine sulfate	Parnate	≥ 2	10–90	—
SNRIs				
Venlafaxine hydrochloride	Effexor	≥ 2	75–450	—
	Effexor XR	≥ 1	37.5–300	—
Others				
Bupropion hydrochloride	Wellbutrin	≥ 2	75–450	> 50[‖]
	Wellbutrin SR	≥ 1	75–450	> 50[‖]
Mirtazapine	Remeron	≥ 1	15–60	—
Nefazodone hydrochloride	Serzone	≥ 2	100–600	—
Trazodone hydrochloride	Desyrel	1	100–600	—

* Some antidepressants are available under more than one proprietary name.

[†] Amitriptyline hydrochloride + nortriptyline hydrochloride levels.

[‡] Imipramine hydrochloride + desipramine hydrochloride levels.

[§] More that 80% of platelet MAO inhibition is generally necessary for therapeutic response.

[‖] In one study, 10 to 29 ng/mL was the therapeutic window.

TABLE 19-2 Comparison of Side-Effect Profiles of Antidepressants

Drug	Orthostatic Hypotension	Anti-cholinergic	Sedation	Gastro-intestinal*	Sexual
SSRIs					
Citalopram hydrobromide	0	0	0	++	+++
Escitalopram oxalate	0	0	0	++	+++
Fluoxetine hydrochloride	0	0	0	++	+++
Fluvoxamine maleate	0	0	+	++	+++
Paroxetine hydrochloride	0	0	+	++	+++
Paroxetine hydrochloride CR	0	0	+/0	+	+++
Sertraline hydrochloride	0	0	0	++	+++
TCAs					
Amitriptyline hydrochloride	+++	+++	+++	+	+++
Amoxapine	++	+	+	+	+++
Clomipramine hydrochloride	+++	+++	+++	+	+++
Desipramine hydrochloride	++	++	+	+	++
Doxepin	++	+++	+++	+	+++
Imipramine hydrochloride	+++	++	++	+	+++
Maprotiline hydrochloride	++	+	++	+	+++
Nortriptyline hydrochloride	+	++	+	+	++
Protriptyline hydrochloride	+	+++	+	+	+++
Trimipramine	++	+++	+++	+	+++
MAOIs					
Phenelzine sulfate	+++	0	+	0	+++
Tranylcypromine sulfate	+++	0	0	0	+++
SNRIs					
Venlafaxine hydrochloride	0†	0	+	++	+++
Venlafaxine hydrochloride XR	0†	0	+	++	+++
Others					
Bupropion hydrochloride	0	0	0	+	+/0
Bupropion hydrochloride SR	0	0	0	+	+/0
Mirtazapine	++	0	+++	+	++
Nefazodone hydrochloride	+	0	++	+	+
Trazodone hydrochloride	++	0	+++	+	++

Note: 0 = minimal to none; + = low; ++ = moderate; +++ = high.

* Excluding constipation due to anticholinergic effects.

† Venlafaxine hydrochloride can cause a dose-dependent increase in blood pressure.

TABLE 19-3 Indications for Antidepressants in Major Depression

- Moderate to severe depression

- Chronic depression

- Psychotic depression (in conjunction with antipsychotics)

- Failure to respond to psychotherapy (<50% improvement after 8 weeks)

- Strong family history of affective illness

- Previous response to antidepressants

depression, two or more episodes, or those with a strong family history should be considered candidates for long-term maintenance antidepressant drug therapy. Patients who have failed to respond to psychotherapy (ie, those with less than 50% improvement after 8 weeks) should also be considered as candidates for antidepressants.

It is important to bear in mind that all antidepressants have roughly the same efficacy in major depression and they all have the same 2- to 6-week delay in onset of action. There are some differences in efficacy among the drugs for other conditions, particularly anxiety disorders and chronic pain syndromes. The varying classes and individual agents do, however, differ in their side-effect profiles, half-lives, and frequency of dosing.

Table 19-4 lists other disorders for which antidepressants have been shown to be helpful. These include bipolar depression, dysthymia, panic disorder, obsessive-

TABLE 19-4 Psychiatric and Nonpsychiatric Indications for Antidepressants

Psychiatric Indications

• major depression	• social anxiety disorder
• minor depression	• posttraumatic stress disorder
• bipolar depression	• body dysmorphic disorder
• dysthymia	• attention-deficit hyperactivity disorder
• panic disorder	• paraphilias
• obsessive-compulsive disorder	• compulsive gambling
• bulimia nervosa	• hypochondriasis
• some personality disorders	• impulsive aggression

Nonpsychiatric Indications

• neuropathic pain	• enuresis
• cataplexy due to narcolepsy	• pathologic weeping and laughing
• organic personality disorders	• insomnia
• fibromyalgia	• irritable bowel syndrome

Note: Not all antidepressants are equally effective for these conditions; only some specific drugs or classes have been studied or found to be effective.

compulsive disorder (OCD), bulimia nervosa, social anxiety disorder, and posttraumatic stress disorder (PTSD). Note that these drugs have clinical value in a number of nonpsychiatric conditions.

The contraindications (absolute and relative) to the use of antidepressants are listed in Table 19-5. These include certain medical conditions as well as concurrent use of particular medications.

Drug Interactions

Physicians should be aware of potential drug interactions because most medically and surgically ill patients take several drugs. The potential risks of drug interactions include poor outcome, increased adverse effects, toxicity, increased medical and psychiatric costs, and destabilization of other medical illnesses. The physician may need to titrate dosages

TABLE 19-5 Contraindications to Antidepressants	
Drug/Class	**Contraindications**
SSRIs	Concurrent use of MAOIs
TCAs	Concurrent use of MAOIs*
	Benign prostatic hypertrophy*
	History of urinary retention*
	Closed angle glaucoma*
	Second-degree atrioventricular block*
	Bundle-branch block*
MAOIs	Concurrent use of TCAs*
	Concurrent use of SSRIs
	Concurrent use of certain other drugs and foods
Venlafaxine hydrochloride	Concurrent use of MAOIs
	Uncontrolled hypertension
Nefazodone hydrochloride	Concurrent use of MAOIs
	History of hepatic disease*
	Concurrent use of terfenadine, astemizole, cisapride
Bupropion hydrochloride	History of seizures
	History of eating disorder
	CNS tumors or lesions
	Active alcohol abuse
	Concurrent use of drugs that lower seizure threshold

* Relative contraindications.

or monitor blood levels in some patients who are at risk for drug–drug interactions. These include the elderly and debilitated, patients on multiple drug regimens (particularly involving drugs that may inhibit or induce the metabolism of concomitant medications), and patients who might be deficient in certain cytochrome isoenzymes.

Both pharmacodynamic (what the drug does to the body) and pharmacokinetic (what the body does to the drug) interactions are important to the physician. There is great variation in the absorption, distribution, and excretion of the individual drugs, causing clinically meaningful differences in plasma levels following administration. Most of the TCAs, SSRIs, and SNRIs are metabolized through hepatic microsomal systems. It may be important to know which cytochrome P450 enzyme is responsible for the metabolism of a drug in order to assess the potential influence of drugs that inhibit these enzymes. Table 19-6 lists the substrates, inducers, and inhibitors of these isoenzymes that are relevant to drug interactions with antidepressants.

Selective serotonin reuptake inhibitors. All SSRIs are not equally likely to produce drug–drug interactions. The physician must carefully monitor the use of other drugs that are metabolized by the P450 enzymes, such as the TCAs or venlafaxine hydrochloride. The SSRIs inhibit several P450 isoenzymes, which are important (particularly, 3A3/4, 2C9, 2C19 but also 2D6) for drug interactions (fluvoxamine maleate > fluoxetine hydrochloride > paroxetine hydrochloride > sertraline hydrochloride > citalopram hydrobromide, escitalopram oxalate). Paroxetine hydrochloride primarily inhibits the 2D6 isoenzyme.

Even though all the SSRIs are tightly bound to plasma proteins, they do so to the α_1 acid glycoproteins rather than serum albumin, making SSRIs less likely to interact with other tightly plasma-protein-bound drugs like digoxin, which binds to serum albumin. Cimetidine may impair first-pass SSRI metabolism, increasing the plasma concentration of the parent SSRI. The SSRIs should not be used in combination with MAOIs.

Tricyclic antidepressants. TCAs are metabolized by the cytochrome P450-2D6 isoenzyme. When a TCA is used in combination with SSRIs, particularly fluoxetine hydrochloride, paroxetine hydrochloride, or sertraline hydrochloride, plasma concentrations of the TCA can increase up to two- to fourfold.

Administration of adrenergic drugs to patients taking TCAs can lead to unexpectedly large increases in blood pressure and a higher incidence of arrhythmias. TCAs decrease the effectiveness of clonidine and guanethidine sulfate. TCAs (including clomipramine hydrochloride) should be used with the MAOIs in the treatment of refractory depression only by clinicians experienced in the use of this combination to avoid development of the "serotonin syndrome," which is characterized by tachycardia, hypertension, hyperpyrexia, myoclonus, ocular oscillations, confusion, convulsions, and even death.

The anticholinergic effects of the TCAs (eg, dry mouth, blurred vision, constipation, delirium, and urinary hesitation or retention) may be increased in patients also taking phenothiazines or other anticholinergic drugs (eg, gastrointestinal [GI] antispasmodics). This is particularly likely to be a problem in the elderly. Barbiturates can increase the metabolism of TCAs, requiring higher than usual doses of the antidepressant. TCAs may elevate plasma concentrations of phenytoin and increase the activity of warfarin sodium. Cimetidine, haloperidol, methylphenidate, and phenothiazines can block the metabolism of TCAs, possibly raising plasma concentrations to nontherapeutic or toxic levels.

TABLE 19-6 Cytochrome P450 Drug Interactions

Isoenzyme	Substrates	Inhibitors	Inducers
1A2	caffeine	fluvoxamine maleate	cigarette smoking
	phenacetin		charcoal-broiled foods
	theophylline		omeprazole
	aminophylline		cabbage
	TCAs (demethylation)		brussels sprouts
	propranolol hydrochloride		
	tacrine hydrochloride		
	verapamil hydrochloride		
2C9/19	diazepam	fluvoxamine maleate	—
	TCAs (demethylation)	fluoxetine hydrochloride	
	warfarin sodium	sertraline hydrochloride	
	tolbutamide		
	phenytoin		
	NSAIDs (ibuprofen)		
	omeprazole		
2D6	antipsychotics	quinidine	—
	TCAs, venlafaxine hydrochloride	paroxetine hydrochloride	
	paroxetine hydrochloride	fluoxetine hydrochloride	
	codeine	sertraline hydrochloride	
	propranolol hydrochloride, timolol	citalopram hydrobromide	
	metoprolol	phenothiazines, escitalopram	
	encainide hydrochloride	levopromazine	
	flecainide acetate	vincristine sulfate	
3A4	alprazolam, midazolam hydrochloride	ketoconazole	glucocorticoids
	triazolam	fluvoxamine maleate	rifampin
	carbamazepine	nefazodone hydrochloride	phenytoin

TABLE 19-6 (continued)			
Isoenzyme	Substrates	Inhibitors	Inducers
3A4	dapsone	fluoxetine hydrochloride	carbamazepine
	clarithromycin	sertraline hydrochloride	phenylbutazone
	lidocaine	erythromycin	sulfinpyrazone
	lovastatin	grapefruit juice (naringenin)	
	oral contraceptives		
	calcium channel blockers		
	erythromycin		
	quinidine		
	steroids		
	loratadine		
	TCAs		

Monoamine oxidase inhibitors. MAOIs should not be administered to patients who are taking TCAs, SSRIs, buspirone hydrochloride, or opioids such as meperidine hydrochloride and dextromethorphan hydrobromide. This combination of drugs may lead to the serotonin syndrome. Several foods and over-the-counter pain medications, cold medications, nasal decongestants, cough medications, and stimulants are also contraindicated in patients taking MAOIs.

Serotonin/norepinephrine reuptake inhibitors and other antidepressants. Venlafaxine hydrochloride is metabolized by cytochrome P450-2D6 and is also a weak inhibitor of this isoenzyme. Drugs such as SSRIs that inhibit this enzyme may increase serum concentrations of venlafaxine hydrochloride. Venlafaxine hydrochloride should not be given in combination with MAOIs. Nefazodone hydrochloride inhibits the cytochrome P450-3A4 isoenzyme (see Table 19-6). Clinical experience with drug–drug interactions involving mirtazapine is limited, although the drug is known to be a substrate (but not inhibitor) of P450-2D6, 1A2, and 3A4.

The metabolism of bupropion hydrochloride may be affected by drugs that induce or inhibit the cytochrome P450 isoenzymes. The combination of bupropion hydrochloride and an MAOI should be avoided. Bupropion hydrochloride may augment the activity of antiparkinsonian medications, allowing the dose of the antiparkinsonian medication to be decreased, but this combination should be used with care.

Patients taking trazodone hydrochloride in combination with SSRIs or MAOIs (eg, to treat insomnia) may experience mental clouding. Patients taking the combination of trazodone hydrochloride and an MAOI should be followed carefully. Trazodone hydrochloride can potentiate the effects of other central nervous system (CNS) depressants, such as hexobarbital, phenytoin, and alcohol. Trazodone hydrochloride inhibits the effects of clonidine; these two drugs should not be used in combination.

Selective Serotonin Reuptake Inhibitors

Despite their significant structural differences, the six drugs in this class (fluoxetine hydrochloride, citalopram hydrobromide, escitalopram oxalate, fluvoxamine maleate, paroxetine hydrochloride, and sertraline hydrochloride) have similar side effects and a similar spectrum of action. Some SSRIs, particularly paroxetine hydrochloride and sertraline hydrochloride, are also approved for treating generalized anxiety disorder, panic disorder, OCD, PTSD, and social anxiety disorder. It is premature to conclude that all SSRIs are equally effective in the treatment of anxiety disorders. The SSRIs are the treatment of choice for most indications calling for antidepressants because of their superior side-effect profile, tolerability, patient compliance, and safety in overdose. Several recent studies have shown that patients on SSRIs are more likely to receive an adequate dosage and less likely to discontinue the drug than are patients treated with TCAs. Even though the SSRIs cost more than TCAs, studies have shown that the total cost of treating an episode of major depression (outpatient and inpatient care for management of adverse effects, blood work, electrocardiogram [ECG], and other tests) is less overall with the SSRIs than with the TCAs.

Pharmacology. All six SSRIs are metabolized in the liver and eliminated in the urine. Fluoxetine hydrochloride and sertraline hydrochloride have active metabolites, both of which are also SSRIs. The range of half-lives is very broad, ranging from 15 hours for fluvoxamine maleate to 48 hours for fluoxetine hydrochloride (Table 19-7). The active metabolite of fluoxetine hydrochloride, norfluoxetine, has a half-life of 146 hours. The advantage of a longer half-life is a lower likelihood of withdrawal symptoms when the patient occasionally forgets a dose. The disadvantage is the persistence of any untoward drug effects.

Mechanism of action. SSRIs selectively inhibit neuronal uptake of serotonin in the brain, which allows serotonin released into the synapse to act for a longer time. In one sense, SSRIs have an effect similar to that of direct-acting agonists, except that the action of SSRIs depends on neuronal release of serotonin. Paroxetine hydrochloride has modest NE (norepinephrine) reuptake inhibition. Sertraline hydrochloride also has some dopamine reuptake properties.

Indications. All six SSRIs are equally effective in the treatment of major depression, whether unipolar or bipolar, although there is some evidence that paroxetine hydrochloride may be less likely to induce hypomania or mania in bipolar patients. Several trials have shown that SSRIs are effective in treating TCA- or MAOI-resistant depression. SSRIs are also effective in treating depression with anxious features. There is no evidence to support any SSRI being better for agitated or retarded depression.

All the SSRIs are as effective in treating OCD as is the TCA clomipramine hydrochloride but with fewer side effects. SSRI therapy generally requires higher doses than are used for treating depression, and it may be necessary to treat anxiety for 10 to 12 weeks to observe a response. SSRIs are also effective in treating dysthymia, panic disorder, bulimia nervosa, social anxiety disorder, PTSD, generalized anxiety disorder, and certain personality disorders (especially those characterized by impulsivity, aggressivity, and irritability). SSRIs may be more efficacious than TCAs for the treatment of atypical depression, body dysmorphic disorder, and paraphilias. Paroxetine hydrochloride CR (controlled release) and venlafaxine hydrochloride XR (extended release) may be

TABLE 19-7 Half-lives and Active Metabolites of Antidepressants °

Drug	Half-life*	Active Metabolites
SSRIs		
Citalopram hydrobromide	35 hours	No
Escitalopram oxalate	27–32 hours	No
Fluoxetine hydrochloride	1–3 days	Yes
Fluvoxamine maleate	13.6–15.6 hours	No
Paroxetine hydrochloride CR	21 hours	No
Sertraline hydrochloride	26 hours	Yes
TCAs		
Amitriptyline hydrochloride	24 hours	Yes
Amoxapine	8 hours	Yes
Clomipramine hydrochloride	32 hours	Yes
Desipramine hydrochloride	36 hours	No
Doxepin	28–52 hours	Yes
Imipramine hydrochloride	10 hours	Yes
Maprotiline hydrochloride	51 hours	Yes
Nortriptyline hydrochloride	28 hours	No
Protriptyline hydrochloride	8–12 hours	No
Trimipramine	9 hours	No
MAOIs		
Phenelzine	16 hours	No
Tranylcypromine sulfate	24 hours	No
SNRIs		
Venlafaxine hydrochloride XR	5 hours	Yes
Others		
Bupropion hydrochloride SR	14 hours	Yes
Mirtazapine	14 hours	Yes
Nefazodone hydrochloride	2–4 hours	Yes
Trazodone hydrochloride	3–6 hours	No

* Parent compound including slow-release preparations.

effective in treating neuropathic pain. There is some evidence that paroxetine hydrochloride and citalopram hydrobromide may also be effective for irritable bowel syndrome.

Dosing and interactions. Typical dose ranges and frequency of dosing for the SSRIs are shown in Table 19-1. All SSRIs inhibit the hepatic P450 isoenzymes and can cause clinically significant increases in drugs metabolized by this system (Table 19-6).

All six SSRIs are potentially lethal when combined with MAOIs, and these drugs should not be taken together. Fluoxetine hydrochloride should be discontinued at least 6 weeks before an MAOI is initiated, and other SSRIs should be discontinued at least 2 weeks prior to MAOI administration. MAOI therapy should be discontinued for at least 2 weeks prior to the initiation of an SSRI. The combination of SSRIs and MAOIs has been associated with the serotonin syndrome.

Side effects and toxicity. Treatment with SSRIs may be associated with CNS symptoms such as agitation, anxiety, sleep disturbance, tremor, sexual dysfunction, or headache. All SSRIs are equally likely to cause sexual side effects. SSRIs may also cause dry mouth, sweating, weight change, or GI disturbances, including nausea and diarrhea. SSRIs, unlike the TCAs, do not typically cause anticholinergic side effects, orthostatic hypotension, or cardiac symptoms. The SSRIs appear to be safe in overdose if they are the only drug ingested.

Although the six SSRIs are similar in action and in side effects, there are some differences in their side-effect profiles that are unexplained by current knowledge. Fluvoxamine maleate is more sedating while fluoxetine hydrochloride is more activating. Paroxetine hydrochloride and fluvoxamine maleate are more likely to lead to a withdrawal syndrome when discontinued abruptly. This syndrome is characterized by dizziness, paresthesias, lethargy, nausea, insomnia, and anxiety. Patients will need instructions on how to taper off these drugs to avoid the syndrome successfully. If withdrawal is abrupt, the syndrome can last up to 3 weeks and can be relieved by restarting of the medication. Tips for managing side effects are shown in Tables 19-8 and 19-9.

TABLE 19-8 Management of Common Antidepressant Side Effects I

Insomnia*
- Lower dose; wait for tolerance to develop
- Give entire dose in AM
- Zolpidem tartrate (10 mg at bedtime)
- Trazodone hydrochloride (25 to 300 mg at bedtime), doxepin (25 to 100 mg at bedtime), clonazepam (0.5 to 2.0 mg at bedtime)

Activation or Jitteriness†
- Start with low doses, especially in patients with panic disorder
- Lower dose; wait for tolerance to develop
- Lorazepam (0.5 to 3 mg/day), clonazepam (0.5 to 2 mg/day), alprazolam (0.75 to 3 mg/day)

Gastrointestinal
- Lower dose; wait for tolerance to develop
- Cisapride (5 to 15 mg), famotidine (20 to 40 mg), nizatidine (150 to 300 mg) for nausea
- *Lactobacillus acidophilus* capsules for diarrhea

Headache
- Rule out substance use or abuse
- Lower dose; wait for tolerance to develop

TABLE 19-8 (continued)

Headache—(continued)
- Relaxation exercises

- Ibuprofen (400 to 800 mg), amitriptyline hydrochloride (25 to 100 mg), divalproex sodium (1000 to 1500 mg)

- Sumatriptan succinate

Paresthesias
- Lower dose

- Pyridoxine (50 to 150 mg)

Sexual Dysfunction
- Wait for tolerance to develop (unlikely)

- Sildenafil citrate (50 to 100 mg/day), 1 hour before sexual intercourse (effective in males)

- Bupropion hydrochloride SR (150 to 300 mg/day), stimulants (5 to 20 mg/day)

- Amantidine hydrochloride (100 to 400 mg/day), yohimbine hydrochloride (2.7 to 10.8 mg/day), buspirone hydrochloride (20 to 40 mg/day)

- Bethanechol chloride (10 to 20 mg before sex), cyproheptadine hydrochloride (4 to 12 mg 1 to 4 hours before sex)

- Switch to bupropion hydrochloride or nefazodone hydrochloride (not usually recommended)

Discontinuation Syndrome
- Restart discontinued drug at full dose; taper dose down over 1 to 2 weeks

- Alternatively, switch to equivalent dose of different drug with longer half-life (eg, fluoxetine hydrochloride)

---

* Rule out nocturnal myoclonus, akathisia, hypomania, worsening of depression, or anxiety.

† Rule out nocturnal myoclonus, akathisia, sleep panic attacks, hypomania, worsening of depression/anxiety.

Tricyclic Antidepressants

TCAs provide a reliable antidepressant response for moderate to severe nondelusionally depressed patients, especially those with major depression of the endogenous or melancholic type who may be candidates for hospitalization. With the availability of SSRIs and SNRIs, TCAs are considered second-line therapy for mood and anxiety disorders.

Pharmacology. TCAs are readily absorbed after oral administration, but there is considerable variation in resulting plasma levels. Most TCAs have a half-life of approximately 24 hours (except protriptyline hydrochloride), which allows once-a-day dosing. The TCAs with secondary-amine side chains, desipramine hydrochloride, nortriptyline hydrochloride, protriptyline hydrochloride, and maprotiline hydrochloride, are metabolized in the liver by hydroxylation and glucuronidation and then excreted by the kidneys. The tertiary-amine TCAs, imipramine hydrochloride, amitriptyline hydrochloride, trimipramine maleate, and doxepin, are demethylated in the liver and converted to secondary-amine active metabolites.

TABLE 19-9 Management of Common Antidepressant Side Effects II

Anticholinergic
- Dry mouth: hard candy, sugar-free gum, PO pilocarpine hydrochloride (5 to 10 mg/day)

- Blurred vision: artificial tears, PO pilocarpine hydrochloride (5 to 10 mg/day)

- Constipation: exercise, increase fluid/fiber intake, stool softener, PO pilocarpine hydrochloride (5 to 10 mg/day)

- Urinary hesitancy: PO bethanechol chloride (10 to 50 mg/day)

- Dry eyes: artificial tears, PO pilocarpine hydrochloride (5 to 10 mg/day)

- Impaired memory: lower dose, switch drugs

- Tachycardia: lower dose

- Delirium: discontinue (D/C) drug; physostigmine (ie, 2 mg IV) under careful monitoring

Cardiovascular
- Orthostatic hypotension: rise slowly, increase fluids, use stockings or abdominal binders:

    Fludrocortisone acetate (0.025 to 0.1 mg/day)

    Methylphenidate (10 to 15 mg/day)

    Dextroamphetamine (5 to 10 mg/day)

- Hypertension: D/C antidepressant

- Arrhythmias: D/C antidepressant

- Prolonged cardiac conduction:* D/C antidepressant

Sedation†
- Lower dose; wait for tolerance to develop

- Give entire dose at bedtime

- Caffeine

- Methylphenidate (10 to 15 mg/day), dextroamphetamine (5 to 10 mg/day)

Weight Gain‡
- Exercise, nutritional counseling

- Lower dose

- Switch to drug less likely to cause weight gain (bupropion hydrochloride)

- Add bupropion hydrochloride (300 to 400 mg)

Impaired Memory and Apathy
- Lower dose; wait for tolerance to develop

- Methylphenidate (5 to 20 mg), dextroamphetamine (5 to 20 mg), bupropion hydrochloride (75 to 300 mg)

Excessive Perspiration
- Lower dose; wait for tolerance to develop

- Terazosin hydrochloride (2 mg at bedtime), clonidine (0.1 to 0.3 mg)

---

* Monitor if QT_c > 440 m/sec; D/C TCA if QT_c > 500 m/sec or > 25% increased over baseline.

† Rule out pharmacokinetic interactions, worsening of atypical depression, and medical disorders.

‡ Rule out hypothyroidism, residual atypical depression, and comorbid eating disorder.

The rate of metabolism of TCAs varies 30- to 40-fold within the population. Seven to 9% of Caucasians are "low hydroxylators" because they have a mutated form of the P450-2D6 enzyme that is responsible for the metabolism of imipramine hydrochloride, desipramine hydrochloride, and probably the other TCAs. Other medications also affect the P450 enzymes and will affect plasma TCA levels (Table 19-6). It may be useful to monitor plasma concentrations of imipramine hydrochloride, nortriptyline hydrochloride, and desipramine hydrochloride in some patients. Indications for monitoring blood levels of TCAs include these:

- The patient is not responding to adequate doses.
- The patient has disabling side effects at low doses.
- Compliance is an issue.
- The patient is elderly or at high risk for side effects or toxic levels because of underlying cardiac or liver disease.
- The patient is at risk for pharmacokinetic interactions.

Mechanism of action. The precise mechanism of action of TCAs is unknown. It is known, however, that these drugs block reuptake of various neurotransmitters, especially NE and 5HT, at receptor sites in the brain and other tissues. Different TCAs affect the reuptake of these biogenic amines to varying degrees, which may account for their differential efficacy in individual patients. TCAs have a broader array of effects on neurotransmitter systems than do SSRIs and may also have a different spectrum of clinical effects. TCAs also increase stage 4 sleep and inhibit rapid eye movement (REM) sleep, which may contribute to their antidepressant actions.

Desipramine hydrochloride, nortriptyline hydrochloride, protriptyline hydrochloride, and maprotiline hydrochloride act primarily as norepinephrine reuptake inhibitors, while imipramine hydrochloride, amitriptyline hydrochloride, trimipramine, and doxepin hydrochloride act on both norepinephrine and serotonin reuptake. Amoxapine is a norepinephrine reuptake inhibitor and a potent blocker of dopamine D_2 and serotonin $5\text{-}HT_2$ receptors. Clomipramine hydrochloride has several pharmacologic properties that raise questions about its mechanism of action. It is a tertiary-amine TCA and a potent serotonin reuptake inhibitor with significant D_2 antagonist properties, and it is metabolized to a potent secondary-amine norepinephrine reuptake inhibitor, norclomipramine.

Indications. The TCAs are all effective in the acute treatment of major depression in both inpatient and outpatient populations. They are effective in 80% of nonpsychotic patients with unipolar depression and melancholia who have an illness duration of less than 1 year if the plasma levels of the drug are maintained for 4 to 6 weeks. TCAs are less effective than MAOIs or SSRIs at treating major depression with atypical features (mood reactivity, increased appetite or weight gain, hypersomnia, heaviness of arms and legs, interpersonal rejection sensitivity). TCAs are more effective than SSRIs in hospitalized depressed patients, arguing that drugs that affect both 5HT and NE may be better in this subpopulation.

TCAs are less effective (with the exception of clomipramine hydrochloride) in the treatment of OCD than are SSRIs or MAOIs. Clomipramine hydrochloride is unique among the TCAs in that it is an effective treatment for OCD. It has also been successfully used in depression refractory to other TCAs. TCAs are generally less effective (with the exception of imipramine hydrochloride and clomipramine hydrochloride) in the treatment of panic disorder than are SSRIs or MAOIs. Imipramine hydrochloride and clomipramine hydrochloride are effective in the treatment of panic disorder, and amitriptyline hydrochloride and doxepin are particularly effective in the treatment of chronic pain syndromes. Imipramine hydrochloride can be helpful for generalized anxiety disorder. Desipramine hydrochloride has been found to be useful by itself or in combination with stimulants for attention deficit hyperactivity disorder (ADHD).

Amoxapine is effective in the treatment of major depression with psychotic features. It may be as effective as the combination of other TCAs with an antipsychotic drug, although its use does not allow for individual titration of the antipsychotic and antidepressant dose. Hence, its use for this condition should be discouraged.

Dosing and drug selection. See Table 19-1 for dosing guidelines. Secondary amine TCAs (desipramine hydrochloride, nortriptyline hydrochloride) are generally preferable over tertiary (imipramine hydrochloride, amitriptyline hydrochloride) because of their more favorable side-effect profile. An exception might be made when a side effect can be turned to particular therapeutic advantage, eg, exploiting the potent antihistaminic properties of doxepin for managing pruritus, gastric reflux, or decreased appetite in cancer or AIDS.

Side effects and toxicity. All of the TCAs have prominent side effects related to their anticholinergic, antihistaminic, and alpha-adrenergic blocking properties. The side effects include sedation, dry mouth, constipation, orthostatic hypotension, blurred vision, urinary retention, and excessive perspiration. Doxepin and amitriptyline hydrochloride are the most difficult of the TCAs to tolerate. Tips for managing common TCA side effects are shown in Table 19-9.

Nortriptyline hydrochloride is generally better tolerated in elderly patients than the other norepinephrine reuptake inhibitors. At equivalent doses, nortriptyline hydrochloride is slightly more anticholinergic than desipramine hydrochloride. However, it is used at about one half the dose of desipramine hydrochloride; consequently, at the doses used in clinical practice, nortriptyline hydrochloride is less anticholinergic. Nortriptyline hydrochloride is also less likely to cause orthostatic hypotension than other TCAs, which also makes it more tolerable in elderly patients and those with preexisting cardiac illness.

TCAs may be significantly toxic when blood concentrations are two to six times higher than therapeutic concentrations. Concentrations of 500 to 1000 ng/mL are associated with prolongation of the QT interval, although specific pharmacodynamic properties that might contribute to fatal arrhythmia in humans are not clearly established. TCA blood concentrations may remain elevated for several days after overdose, presenting a cardiac risk even after apparent clinical improvement, particularly if the ECG has not normalized. CNS toxicity, including coma, shock, respiratory depression, delirium, seizures, and hyperpyrexia, may occur with overdose. A 1-week supply of a TCA may be fatal if taken all at once, and patients with suicide potential should be given special consideration when TCAs are being prescribed.

Amoxapine may cause extrapyramidal reactions and tardive dyskinesia. It also causes seizures and is lethal in overdose. Clomipramine hydrochloride has prominent side effects that often limit dosing. It causes sedation and anticholinergic side effects, making gradual dose escalation necessary. It frequently causes sexual dysfunction.

Monoamine Oxidase Inhibitors

MAOIs are effective in treating a wide variety of psychiatric disorders, but their use has been somewhat limited because they have potentially severe side effects. Patients taking MAOIs are subject to dietary and over-the-counter drug restrictions. MAOIs are seldom used as a first-line therapy in treatment-naive patients. Hypertensive crisis may occur in some patients from the potentiation of the pressor effects of amines in food. These drugs are infrequently used currently, even by most psychiatrists, and their use in primary care practice is extraordinary.

Serotonin/Norepinephrine Reuptake Inhibitors

Venlafaxine hydrochloride is a novel bicyclic compound that is chemically unrelated to the TCAs. It has demonstrated antidepressant activity and a relatively mild side-effect profile. It is the only SNRI currently available in the United States. Venlafaxine hydrochloride is rapidly absorbed after oral administration, with peak plasma levels being achieved in less than 2 hours. Its half-life is short, from 3 to 5 hours, although an active metabolite, *O*-desmethylvenlafaxine, has a half-life ranging from 9 to 11 hours. It can be dosed once daily, although some patients may need twice-daily dosing. The extended release formulation, venlafaxine hydrochloride XR, is better tolerated than the immediate release (IR) formulation.

Venlafaxine hydrochloride acts on both serotonin and norepinephrine reuptake mechanisms. It is more selective for serotonin than for norepinephrine at doses less than 150 mg/day. It is as potent as imipramine hydrochloride at blocking serotonin reuptake but is weaker at blocking norepinephrine reuptake. Venlafaxine hydrochloride does not inhibit MAO and does not significantly bind to serotonin, norepinephrine, dopamine, muscarinic cholinergic, alpha$_1$-adrenergic, or histamine H$_1$ receptors.

Venlafaxine hydrochloride is effective in inpatients and outpatients with major depression. There is some evidence to indicate that it may lead to higher rates of remission compared to some SSRIs like fluoxetine hydrochloride. Venlafaxine hydrochloride is particularly effective in patients with treatment-refractory depression (those that have failed treatment with SSRIs or TCAs). It is also effective in chronic pain patients and preferred to the TCAs like amitriptyline hydrochloride in this population because of its better side-effect profile. Venlafaxine hydrochloride has fewer side effects than the TCAs, probably because it has no receptor antagonistic properties. The most common side effects are nausea, somnolence, dizziness, headaches, and increased perspiration (see Tables 19-8 and 19-9). Sexual dysfunction has also been reported. Venlafaxine hydrochloride may cause dose-related hypertension in some patients, so blood pressure monitoring is important during treatment, particularly at doses greater than 300 mg/day. Venlafaxine hydrochloride appears to be as safe as SSRIs in overdose, inducing drowsiness and lethargy in patients who intentionally overdosed.

Other Antidepressants

Bupropion hydrochloride is structurally related to phenylethylamines and is unrelated to TCAs, SSRIs, or MAOIs. It is rapidly absorbed following oral administration, with peak blood levels occurring within 2 hours. Bupropion hydrochloride has no significant potency at blocking reuptake or binding to any known neurotransmitter receptors. It is, however, a weak blocker of dopamine reuptake, and its primary metabolite has significant norepinephrine reuptake blocking properties. The mechanism of action for bupropion hydrochloride remains unclear. Bupropion hydrochloride acts in animals and humans as a CNS stimulant and an indirect dopamine agonist.

Bupropion hydrochloride is effective in the treatment of major depression. It is as effective as SSRIs or TCAs in treating depression in inpatients and outpatients and may be useful in treating patients refractory to TCAs. It may also be useful in treating bipolar depression and attention-deficit disorder. It is one of the few antidepressants that is not effective in treating panic disorder or PTSD. It is thought to be somewhat less likely than other antidepressants to precipitate mania in bipolar patients.

Bupropion hydrochloride can cause restlessness, insomnia, and anorexia. It lacks anticholinergic effects, is not sedating, has minimal sexual side effects, and has a favorable cardiovascular profile. Physicians should be aware that bupropion hydrochloride may induce seizures, especially at higher doses (greater than 450 mg/day); otherwise it is relatively safe in overdose. The risk of seizures in patients taking bupropion hydrochloride at doses of less than 450 mg/day is 0.48%, compared to 0.1% in patients taking TCAs or SSRIs. The incidence of seizures with bupropion hydrochloride may increase 10-fold at doses between 450 and 600 mg/day. The risk increases substantially in patients with prior history of seizures, head trauma, brain tumor, bulimia nervosa, or anorexia nervosa. Bupropion hydrochloride should not be taken by patients receiving medications that lower seizure threshold (such as clozapine), in patients who are abusing alcohol or benzodiazepines (BZPs), and those with a history of eating disorders. Precautions to avoid seizures include using divided doses, with the maximum single dose not exceeding 150 mg. The slow-release formulation of bupropion hydrochloride SR is better tolerated than the immediate release formulation. The risk of seizures with bupropion hydrochloride SR is similar to the SSRIs.

Trazodone hydrochloride is structurally unrelated to TCAs or other classes of antidepressants. It is well absorbed after oral administration, with peak blood levels occurring about 1 to 2 hours after administration. Trazodone hydrochloride is a serotonin receptor antagonist with weak serotonin reuptake inhibitor properties. Its metabolite, m-chlorophenylpiperazine (m-CPP), acts as an agonist at some serotonin receptor subtypes and as an antagonist at others.

The primary indication for trazodone hydrochloride is in the treatment of major depression. It is as effective as TCAs in the treatment of major depression in inpatients and outpatients. Trazodone hydrochloride also exhibits anti-anxiety properties, and some clinicians use low-dose trazodone hydrochloride as a sleep-promoting agent, particularly with the SSRIs.

Side effects associated with trazodone hydrochloride include sedation, orthostatic hypotension, dissociative feelings, increased myocardial irritability, and, rarely, priapism. Priapism caused by trazodone hydrochloride is a medical emergency: it may require surgical intervention and may lead to permanent impotence. Trazodone hydrochloride has a wider therapeutic margin than TCAs, MAOIs, and some other second-generation antidepressants. It is relatively safe in overdose situations, especially when it is the only therapeutic agent, although there have been some reports of ventricular irritability.

Nefazodone hydrochloride is chemically related to trazodone hydrochloride and has similar pharmacologic properties. It lacks the significant alpha$_1$-adrenergic antagonist properties of trazodone hydrochloride, which may account for its better side-effect profile (ie, less sedation and orthostasis). Nefazodone hydrochloride, like trazodone hydrochloride, is metabolized to *m*-CPP. Nefazodone hydrochloride is a serotonin receptor antagonist ($5HT_2$) with weak serotonin reuptake inhibitor properties.

Nefazodone hydrochloride has a therapeutic profile similar to that of trazodone hydrochloride. It inhibits the hepatic enzyme 3A4 and may cause clinically significant increases in the concentrations of drugs metabolized by this enzyme (see Table 19-6). Nefazodone hydrochloride has efficacy similar to trazodone hydrochloride but with fewer side effects, particularly less sexual dysfunction. It is also less likely to cause priapism.

Unlike most antidepressants (except bupropion hydrochloride), nefazodone hydrochloride either increases or has no effect on REM sleep in humans. It has been reported to improve memory function and does not potentiate the depressant effects of alcohol. Nefazodone hydrochloride–associated side effects include sedation, headache, asthenia, dry mouth, nausea, and constipation. In rare instances it can cause hepatic dysfunction and should be avoided in patients with preexisting hepatic disease. It does not alter cardiac conduction or electrocardiographic indices. It is less sedating than the tertiary amine TCAs and may not cause as much sexual dysfunction as the SSRIs. It appears to have no effect on seizure threshold. Nefazodone hydrochloride is relatively safe in overdose.

Mirtazapine is an antidepressant with a unique pharmacologic profile. It acts as an antagonist on the presynaptic α_2-adrenergic and serotonergic autoreceptors, increasing the availability of norepinephrine and serotonin in the synapse. It also antagonizes the postsynaptic $5HT_2$ and $5HT_3$ receptors. Mirtazapine is indicated for the treatment of major depression, particularly that associated with insomnia and weight loss. The most common side effects of mirtazapine therapy are somnolence, appetite increase, and weight gain.

ANXIOLYTICS AND HYPNOTICS

The use of sedative/hypnotic/anxiolytic agents remains a major controversy within the primary care community. Since their introduction in the late 1950s, benzodiazepines (BZPs) have been considered a safe alternative to the barbiturates for sleep disturbances and anxiety disorders (Table 19-10). BZPs quickly became the most frequently prescribed psychotropic agent worldwide. For many years, anxiety and sleep disorders were treated carte blanche with BZPs. With this high use came a great deal of previously unrecognized knowledge about these compounds not available from preclinical trials. Dependency, withdrawal, and abuse potential were commonly encountered, and many physicians became frightened by these aspects and generally refused to prescribe agents of this class. Advocates against the use of BZPs pointed to research that demonstrated the efficacy of cognitive-behavioral therapy in the treatment of insomnia as well as anxiety; and the use of alternative agents such as buspirone hydrochloride and the SSRIs, as well as information that demonstrated a decline in cognitive function and increased motor vehicle collisions in patients using these agents. Proponents of BZPs pointed to research that demonstrated the efficacy of BZPs in patients with clearly diagnosed anxiety and sleep disorders and the fact that those who became dependent or abused these medications comprised a small minority of patients compared to those who benefited from treatment

TABLE 19-10 Anxiolytics

Drug (trade name)	Duration of Action	Rate of Absorption	Dose (mg/day)	Need to Taper	Clearance	Indications
Benzodiazepines						
Alprazolam (Xanax)	Short	Medium	0.75–1.5	Yes	H	GAD, PD, phobias
Chlordiazepoxide hydrochloride (Librium)	Long	Medium	15–40	No	H	GAD, alcohol withdrawal
Clonazepam (Klonopin)	Long	Rapid	1.5–10	No	H	GAD, PD, seizures, phobias
Clorazepate dipotassium (Tranxene)	Long	Rapid	15–60	No	H	GAD, seizures
Diazepam (Valium)	Long	Rapid	2–40	No	H	GAD, alcohol withdrawal
Halazepam (Paxipam)	Long	Medium	60–160	No	H	GAD
Lorazepam (Ativan)	Short	Medium	2–6	Yes	R	GAD, alcohol withdrawal, adjunct in medical illness*
Oxazepam (Serax)	Short	Slow	30–60	Yes	R	GAD, alcohol withdrawal
Prazepam (Centrax)	Long	Slow	20–40	No	H	GAD
Nonbenzodiazepines						
Buspirone hydrochloride (BusPar)	Short	Rapid	15–30	No	H	GAD

Note: H = hepatic, R = renal, GAD = generalized anxiety disorder, PD = panic disorder.
* See text.

with these compounds. No matter which side you take in this argument, BZPs and agents similar to BZPs remain a highly prescribed class of medication within the psychiatric and primary care sector, and the need for a clear understanding of BZPs is necessary for all practicing physicians.

The major complicating factor in the use of BZPs is the addiction and dependence potential which, despite being lower than that of barbiturates, clearly has ramifications in treatment choices and duration of treatment for many patients.

Benzodiazepines

Even though most patients on BZPs may develop physiological dependence (withdrawal symptoms on discontinuation), a very small minority develop psychological dependence (craving, escalation of dose, etc) and hence addiction.

BZPs are generally classified into two basic categories (Table 19-10). The first relates to biological half-life; the second relates to their degree of potency or the rate at which the patient notices a response to the medication. BZPs have high, intermediate, or low potency. Except for clorazepate dipotassium, the rate-limiting factor of the onset of action of the BZPs is their absorption by the GI tract. Once absorbed by the GI system, the BZPs as a class are highly lipophilic and rapidly absorbed into brain tissue.

Mechanism of action. BZPs are considered to exert their primary action in the treatment of anxiety by binding to the gamma aminobutryic acid (A [GABA-A]) receptor. GABA-A receptors are found in many regions of the brain including the cortex, limbic system, locus coeruleus, and cerebellum. BZPs have widespread effects on the brain including sedation, muscle relaxation, anxiety reduction, and an increase in seizure threshold. BZPs also lower sympathetic tone through both central and peripheral mechanisms. Although not clearly understood, BZPs are thought to exert their biochemical action by stimulating an increased affinity of the receptor for GABA, which in turn leads to an increase in the opening of chloride channels, allowing chloride ions to flow into the neuron, making it more resistant to excitation. These receptors are not felt to be exclusively sensitive to the BZPs and also react to barbiturates and alcohol. In an indirect way, this may explain the site at which withdrawal and dependency take place.

Therapeutic indications. The major indication for BZPs in psychiatry and general medical practice are for adjustment disorder with anxious mood, the anxiety disorders (including generalized anxiety disorder, social anxiety disorder, panic disorder), and insomnia. Use of these agents requires a clear diagnosis and consideration of alternative treatments such as behavioral therapy and SSRIs, in many cases prior to treatment with these agents. BZPs are often the first line of treatment, in a time-limited fashion, when an adjustment disorder with anxiety is present or the symptoms of anxiety or sleep disturbance require quick resolution.

The anxiolytic efficacy of BZPs is similar across this class of medications. The long-term treatment of anxiety disorders with BZPs may be complicated by a degree of tolerance that may develop if the action is not as robust as initially experienced. The initial effect of these medications leads to changes of arousal and somatic anxiety. Much of the symptomatic relief experienced by patients involves relief from the somatic complaints, such as increased muscle tension, palpitations, increased perspiration, or hyperactivity of the GI tract, usually with the constant worry or depressive symptoms from which they also suffer.

Contraindications and drug interactions. Relative contraindications to the use of BZPs include situations where sedation, hypoventilation, or decreased sensorium or cognition could be problematic. This would include such conditions as the concomitant use of other sedating or depressant medications (particularly alcohol), marked respiratory disease, obstructive sleep apnea, dementia, or delirium. Use of BZPs in the elderly is associated with an increased risk of falls and fractures. Drug interactions, though theoretically described, are surprisingly rare except in the case of additive effects from other CNS depressants, especially alcohol. The risk of fatality or suicide is extremely low when BZPs are used alone; however, the risk increases dramatically when other sedating drugs are also taken.

Abuse and withdrawal. Concern regarding the addictive potential and difficulty in discontinuing use of BZPs frequently leads to failure to use an appropriate medication for a given diagnosis and undertreatment when the BZPs are prescribed. As with any medical condition, the ratio of risk to benefit must be considered, and there must be an understanding of the consequences of nontreatment.

Insomnia and benzodiazepines. BZPs may offer symptomatic relief for transient and short-term insomnia (Table 19-11). They are generally not recommended as long-term treatment for chronic insomnia or in patients with sleep apnea. Long-acting BZPs are not usually recommended for the treatment of insomnia because they may lead to oversedation during the day and some residual cognitive symptoms (Table 19-10). In some instances, long-acting BZPs may be somewhat effective in patients who suffer nocturnal awakenings or late-onset insomnia. In general, the shorter half-life agents such as estazo-

TABLE 19-11 Hypnotics					
Drug (trade name)	Duration of Action	Half-life (hours)	Absorption	Dose (mg)	Accumulation Potential
Benzodiazepines					
Estazolam (Prosom)	Short	10–24	Rapid	1–2	Low
Flurazepam hydrochloride (Dalmane)	Long	24–72	Rapid	15–30	High
Quazepam (Doral)	Long	39	Rapid	7.5–15	High
Temazepam (Restoril)	Short	6–11	Less rapid	7.5–30	Low
Triazolam (Halcion)	Short	1–3	Rapid	0.125–0.25	Low
Nonbenzodiazepines					
Zolpidem tartrate (Ambien)	Long	2	Rapid	5–10	Low
Zaleplon (Sonata)	Short	1	Rapid	5	Low

lam and temazepam are preferred in the treatment of insomnia because of their short
duration of action and lack of accumulation of drug.

Buspirone Hydrochloride

Long-term treatment of anxiety disorders generally requires use of alternative psychopharmacologic treatments. Recently, the treatment of choice is the SSRIs, particularly
paroxetine hydrochloride and sertraline hydrochloride, which have been approved by
the US Food and Drug Administration (FDA) for most anxiety disorders. Buspirone
hydrochloride, a non-BZP and non-SSRI, has been demonstrated to have efficacy in the
treatment of generalized anxiety disorder (Table 19-3). Buspirone hydrochloride is an
azapirone anxiolytic that acts as a partial 5-HT1A agonist, which appears to be as effective
in treating generalized anxiety as BZPs. However, in contrast to the BZPs, buspirone hydrochloride has a slower onset of action and lack of effect in the acute anxiety period.
These effects may lead to treatment failures because the patient previously treated with
BZPs may not believe the drug is effective in the early course of treatment. Unfortunately,
buspirone hydrochloride is ineffective for depressive symptoms or anxiety disorders other
than generalized anxiety disorder, limiting its use in most patients. Buspirone hydrochloride has demonstrated a good side-effect profile: it has no sedation, no memory or
psychomotor impairment, no interaction with alcohol, no abuse potential, and no disinhibition phenomenon. Buspirone hydrochloride does require tid dosing and it does tend
to be more expensive when compared to the BZPs.

Zolpidem Tartrate

Zolpidem tartrate is an imidazopyridine with a chemical structure unrelated to the
BZPs. Released as a nonbenzodiazepine, it was felt to be a medication for insomnia that
had essentially no muscle relaxant, anxiolytic, or anticonvulsant properties (Table
19-11). Zolpidem tartrate may be the medication of choice in patients with pulmonary
comorbidity because it has essentially no effect on nocturnal respiration. In addition,
zolpidem tartrate neither interferes with sleep stages 3 and 4 nor decreases REM sleep.
Reportedly there is no evidence of tolerance or withdrawal from this compound,
although case reports do exist stating that some withdrawal symptoms do occur with
discontinuation.

Zaleplon

Another relative newcomer in the treatment of insomnia, zaleplon is a pyrazolopyrimi-
dine class and interacts with the GABA receptor complex (Table 19-11). Its half-life is
only 1 hour, making it particularly helpful in the treatment of sleep initiation problems
and for patients who wake up at night and have trouble returning to sleep. Zaleplon also
may be of benefit in the elderly, in whom long half-life medications may lead to drug interactions or side effects. Like zolpidem tartrate, it has not been shown in the research
literature to demonstrate any tolerance or withdrawal symptoms. Also like zolpidem tartrate, zaleplon decreases sleep latency and has essentially no effect on the sleep architecture. Zaleplon has also been demonstrated to cause essentially no impairment of cognitive
or psychomotor skills.

MOOD STABILIZERS (THYMOLEPTICS)

Far fewer treatments are available for stabilizing mood in bipolar and related disorders than there are for treatment of depressive, anxiety, or psychotic disorders. The FDA has approved lithium for acute mania, acute depression, and the maintenance phase of bipolar illness. The FDA has also approved sodium divalproex (Depakote) and olanzapine (Zyprexa) for acute mania. Carbamazepine (Tegretol), another anticonvulsant mood stabilizer, has no FDA-approved indication for bipolar illness, even though it has been used as a standard treatment for certain forms of this illness for more than two decades. Lithium, divalproex, and carbamazepine are used in a narrow therapeutic range and have a number of critical drug–drug interactions; hence, particular attention should be paid to patient and family education. These medicines must be used with special precautions in certain populations such as pregnant and lactating women and the elderly. Certain other agents that are used as off-label in refractory cases are discussed below.

Table 19-12 summarizes key facts about lithium, valproic acid, carbamazepine, oxcarbazepine, lamotrigine, topiramate, and gabapentin. In general, primary care physicians are unlikely to be providing primary management of bipolar disorders that call for these agents, but they should be familiar with common adverse effects and drug interactions. See the American Psychiatric Association's practice guidelines on bipolar disorder (1995) for additional information, including monitoring of plasma levels and checking of laboratory parameters.

Lithium

Since description of lithium's antimanic properties in 1949 by the Australian Cade, its use has spread across the world. In acute mania, blood levels often need to be in the 0.8 to 1.5 mEq/L range; similar levels are required for acute bipolar depression. Maintenance treatment blood levels are often in a somewhat lower range, from 0.6 to 1.0 mEq/L.

In the older literature, overall response rates with monotherapy in acute mania and bipolar depression ranged from 60% to 80%, although newer studies suggest a range of 40% to 60%. It has been suggested that lithium might be much more effective in the so-called classic, euphoric, or elated mania with moderate agitation as opposed to more atypical (dysphoric, mixed-state) or rapid-cycling (four or more episodes in a year) presentations. The response in acute mania is generally seen in 7 to 10 days with lithium, although in bipolar depression it may take longer.

Although there is generally no tolerance or psychological dependence seen with lithium, there is increasing evidence that abrupt withdrawal (over less than 2 weeks) may be associated with a fairly rapid and severe recurrence of an episode. Sometimes these recurrences do not readily respond to lithium at the previous dose levels and often are more protracted in their course. On the other hand, gradual withdrawal (over 2 to 4 weeks or longer) is associated with a less severe reemergence of symptoms, though of course symptoms eventually recur. Absent an emergency (eg, acute lithium toxicity), it is best to consult with the patient's psychiatrist before stopping lithium. Lithium has antisuicidal benefits even in patients who do not respond well for continued bipolar symptoms.

Lithium is best suited to those patients who can be educated about the narrow therapeutic index of lithium, the careful need to monitor levels, thyroid and kidney functions,

TABLE 19-12 Mood Stabilizers

Factor	Lithium (Eskalith, Lithobid, etc)	Valproic Acid (Depakene, Depakote)	Carbamazepine (CBZ) (Tegretol)	Oxcarbazepine (OXC) (Trileptal)	Lamotrigine (LTG) (Lamictal)	Topiramate (TPM) (Topamax)	Gabapentin (GBP) (Neurontin)
Serum plasma levels	0.8–1.5 mEq/L acute, 0.6–1.0 mEq/L maintenance	50–125 ng/mL	4–12 ng/mL	NA	NA	NA	NA
Usual daily dosage	600–1800 mg/day	750–2500 mg/day	400–1600 mg/day	900–2400 mg/day	100–600 mg/day	100–600 mg/day	900–2400 mg/day
Onset of action	5–14 days	3–15 days	3–15 days	2–4 weeks	4–8 weeks	2–4 weeks	2–4 weeks
Protein binding	Not bound to plasma proteins	90%, ↓ with higher concentration	76%	40%	55%	13%–17%	3%
Half-life (hour)	24 (average); increase with age and/or decreased renal function	6-16 (average); increase with age and/or decreased hepatic function	Initially 25–65; with repeated dosing, 12–17	8–10	25–30	19–23	6
Metabolic pathway(s)	Not metabolized; primarily excreted; unchanged in urine	Hepatic (glucuronidation, mitochondrial B oxidation, microsomal oxidation)	Hepatic, CYP P450- 3A4, possibly 2D6	Hepatic, mainly glucoronidation, minor via CYP3A4	Hepatic, mainly glucoronidation	Minimal hepatic, primarily excreted unchanged in urine	Minimal metabolism, primarily excreted unchanged in urine

(continued)

TABLE 19-12 (continued)

Factor	Lithium (Eskalith, Lithobid, etc)	Valproic Acid (Depakene, Depakote)	Carbamazepine (CBZ) (Tegretol)	Oxcarbazepine (OXC) (Trileptal)	Lamotrigine (LTG) (Lamictal)	Topiramate (TPM) (Topamax)	Gabapentin (GBP) (Neurontin)
Elimination route(s)	Renal	Renal	Renal (70%), fecal (30%)	Renal	Renal	Renal	Renal
Common drug interactions	↑ Lithium serum concentrations (fluoxetine hydrochloride, ACE inhibitors, diuretics, NSAIDs) ↓ lithium serum concentrations (acetazolamide, diuretics, theophylline) antipsychotics may increase lithium neurotoxicity	Interacts with many drugs that are hepatically metabolized (cimetidine hydrochloride, erythromycin, etc)	↓ Half-life of phenytoin, warfarin sodium, doxycycline, theophylline CBZ levels ↓ by phenobarbital, phenytoin, or primidone CBZ ↓ levels of haloperidol and valproic acid, ↓ oral contraceptive efficacy	↓ Calcium channel blockers by 30% ↓ oral contraceptive efficacy	↑ LTG levels by valproate sodium ↓ LTG levels by CBZ, phenytoin	↓ Digoxin levels by TPM ↓ oral contraceptive efficacy by TPM ↓ TPM levels by CBZ, phenytoin, phenobarbital	Minimal
Common adverse effects	Nausea, vomiting, diarrhea, polyuria, polydipsia, tremor, hypothyroidism, acne, dry skin, weight gain	GI distress, diplopia, sedation, tremor, alopecia, weight gain and thrombocytopenia	Dizziness, drowsiness, unsteadiness, SIADH, rashes, hyponatremia, hematological (rare)	Hyponatremia, sedation and ataxia in combination treatment	Skin rashes, GI distress	Cognitive side effects, paresthesias, weight loss, rare: renal stones, very rare: angle closure, glaucoma	Weight gain sedation

pregnancy status, and drug interactions. These patients must also be willing and able to adhere to the treatment recommendations. Lithium can be quite problematic during pregnancy and lactation: it has been associated with cardiac anomalies in the developing fetus and fluid shifts that make maintenance later in pregnancy difficult; it can also cause acute neurotoxicity in the newborn.

Valproate Sodium (divalproex sodium, valproic acid)

The anticonvulsant (antikindling) and GABAergic activities and the blocking of voltage-dependent sodium channels and repetitive action potentials on neurons are postulated to explain the actions of valproate sodium in both seizure disorders and bipolar disorders.

Valproate sodium is used for acute mania, and it has increasingly been applied to atypical presentations of mania including dysphoric mania, rapid-cycling forms of the disorder, and where there is a seizure history. It has been less well studied for acute bipolar depression and maintenance treatment, although it has been used for these indications as well. The one controlled maintenance study in bipolar disorder vs lithium and placebo failed to separate both lithium and valproate sodium from placebo, arguing for the need for rational polypharmacy in the maintenance treatment of bipolar disorder.

Some early effects include benign hepatic transaminase elevations, hyperammonemia, and sedation, as well as GI side effects. There is a potential risk for serious hepatatoxity in a few vulnerable individuals. Leukopenia and thrombocytopenia, which are often reversible on drug discontinuation, are rare events. Due to its highly protein-bound nature and extensive metabolism by the liver, several drug–drug interactions are possible with valproate sodium, though surprisingly not that many have been reported. There is some concern about polycystic ovarian syndrome in women with long-term use of valproate sodium. Unlike lithium, data on valproate sodium withdrawal are sparse. The use of valproate sodium in the first trimester of pregnancy has been associated with neural tube defects in the fetus.

Carbamazepine

Carbamazepine (CBZ) is an anticonvulsant drug like valproate sodium that is believed to act through the BZP receptor and by inhibiting kindled seizures in the limbic brain. Like valproate sodium, CBZ blocks voltage-dependent sodium channels and high-frequency repetitive action potentials in neurons. In spite of its lack of FDA approval for a bipolar indication, it has been used for acute mania, acute bipolar depression, and maintenance bipolar treatment. As with valproate sodium, it is preferred for certain atypical presentations of bipolar disorder.

Side effects include blurred vision, ataxia, nausea, and rashes. Less frequent are mild leukopenia, mild thrombocytopenia, hyponatremia, and transient liver enzyme elevations. Due to several hepatic enzyme interactions, particular attention needs to be paid when other drugs are added or removed in a patient receiving carbamazepine, especially decreased oral contraceptive efficacy in women. The use of carbamazepine in the first trimester of pregnancy has been associated with neural tube defects in the fetus.

Oxcarbazepine

Oxcarbazepine (OXC) is an anticonvulsant related to CBZ that has been used in Europe for more than two decades and has been introduced into the United States recently.

Two double-blind studies of small numbers of bipolar and schizoaffective bipolar subjects done in Europe several years ago concluded equal efficacy for OXC vs lithium or haloperidol. The off-label use of this agent in bipolar disorder has increased in view of a much cleaner drug interaction profile relative to its predecessor carbamazepine. Nonetheless, some induction at CYP3A4 occurs, and caution should be exercised for loss of oral contraceptive efficacy. Cross-sensitivity to carbamazepine should be borne in mind while prescribing OXC. Hyponatremia as a side effect should also be kept in mind. It is weight neutral.

Lamotrigine

Lamotrigine (LTG) is an anticonvulsant drug that has shown efficacy in bipolar depression and in rapid cycling bipolar II disorder but not in mania. The slow titration (starting at 25 mg per day and increasing it by 25 mg every week to reach a target of 50 to 200 mg a day) required to reduce the risk of serious dermatologic reactions may preclude antimanic efficacy. Bipolar depression and rapid cycling disorder are particularly difficult to treat. It is less likely than the usual unimodal antidepressants (tricyclic, MAOI, SSRI, SNRI, etc) to switch the subject into the manic pole and also induce a rapid cycling course and may offer an attractive alternative, either as monotherapy or as an add-on. Slow titration of LTG is necessary in the presence of valproate sodium (where the dose of LTG is cut by 50%), and pediatric use of LTG is associated with rashes, which rarely can be life threatening in the form of Steven-Johnson syndrome. In adults with bipolar disorder, the incidence of rash is less than 5% with gradual dose titration.

Topiramate

Topiramate (TPM) is an anticonvulsant with a broad spectrum of activity (inhibition of the sodium and calcium channels, increase in cerebral GABA, antagonization of AMPA/kainate glutamate receptors, and carbonic anhydrase inhibition). It is being used off label in psychiatry as an adjunctive mood stabilizer and weight loss or weight-stabilizing agent in bipolar disorder, schizoaffective disorder, binge eating disorder, etc. Monotherapy with topiramate is not efficacious in acute mania. Preliminary data suggest efficacy of TPM in binge-eating disorder and in alcoholism. Weight loss is a feature of TPM that has driven its recent use in psychiatry. Cognitive side effects and paresthesias may be limiting in some subjects. A 1% to 2% incidence of renal stones with very rare reports of bilateral angle closure glaucoma are worth mentioning to patients prior to initiation. Preliminary data also suggest low doses of TPM (25 to 50 mg per day) may help PTSD.

Gabapentin

Gabapentin (GBP) is an anticonvulsant that is used primarily as add-on treatment in bipolar illness or in agitation in dementia patients. Randomized controlled trials in bipolar disorder have been negative; nonetheless, open data and fairly extensive off-label use in psychiatry has led to its use in bipolar patients with comorbid panic and anxiety syndromes. GBP may also be effective for socially phobic subjects. Due to the minimal drug interactions and good tolerability, practitioners have added GBP to other mood stabilizers or psychotropic agents.

Other Anticonvulsants

Zonisamide has been evaluated in one open study in psychiatric patients in Japan; manic patients in general showed improvement. However, it has not been evaluated adequately in psychiatry, although a recent study found weight loss superior to placebo in primary obesity. Levetiracetam has been used anecdotally in bipolar illness but has not been adequately evaluated in psychiatry. Similarly, the case reports regarding tiagabine hydrochloride in bipolar disorder have been too mixed at best to recommend use.

ANTIPSYCHOTICS AND ANTIPARKINSONIAN AGENTS

The modern era in the treatment of psychosis began with the success of chlorpromazine in treating schizophrenia in the mid-1950s, which led to the development of a number of other phenothiazines. Approximately 70% of patients with schizophrenia taking phenothiazines and drugs of other classes (eg, butyrophenones, thioxanthenes, dibenzoxazepines, and dihydroindolones) experience clinically significant relief of their positive symptoms (delusions and hallucinations) and decreases in disorganization and bizarre behavior, but few patients are restored to complete functional abilities. Dissatisfaction with the side effects produced by these "typical" antipsychotics encouraged the development of "atypical" antipsychotics such as clozapine, risperidone, olanzapine, quetiapine fumarate, ziprasidone hydrochloride, and aripiprazole.

Side Effects

All of the typical antipsychotic drugs are similar in efficacy, differing only in potency and side-effect profile. Each patient may respond differently to a given drug, both in terms of therapeutic efficacy and side effects experienced (Table 19-13). Physicians should therefore be familiar with several different drugs. The choice of a drug for the treatment of psychosis should mainly be based on the physician's familiarity with the drug, the side-effect profile, the required route of administration, and patient preference. Many aspects of antipsychotic treatment are covered in Chapter 9.

Typical Antipsychotics

These drugs are absorbed adequately when administered orally, but food or antacids may decrease absorption. All are metabolized in the liver, so there is a significant first-pass effect with oral administration. Peak effect of an oral dose occurs at 2 to 4 hours after administration, 30 to 60 minutes after intramuscular administration. Drugs administered parenterally are not subject to a first pass through the portal circulation; this route of administration results in significantly higher serum levels than does oral administration of an equivalent dose.

The typical antipsychotics block neurotransmitter dopamine (D_2 receptors). Blockade of postsynaptic dopaminergic receptors located in the mesolimbic and mesocortical tracts appears to be the main mechanism by which these drugs have their therapeutic effects. They also block D_2 receptors in the striatum, which causes the extrapyramidal symptoms (EPS) that are the major side effects of these drugs. The tubero-infundibular dopaminergic tract is also blocked by several typical antipsychotics, leading to hyperprolactinemia, galactorrhea, and menstrual irregularities.

TABEL 19-13 Comparison of Side Effects of Antipsychotics

Drug	Extrapyramidal Symptoms	Anticholinergic	Sedation	Orthostatic Hypotension	Weight Gain/Diabetes Mellitus*
Conventional					
Chlorpromazine	++	++	+++	+++	+++
Fluphenazine hydrochloride	+++	+	++	++	+
Haloperidol	+++	0	+	++	+
Loxapine hydrochloride	++	+	++	+	+
Mesoridazine besylate	+	+++	+++	++	++
Molindone hydrochloride	+	+	++	+	+
Perphenazine	++	++	++	++	+
Thioridazine	++	+++	+++	+++	+++
Thiothixene hydrochloride	+++	+	++	++	+
Trifluoperazine hydrochloride	+++	+	++	++	+
Atypical					
Clozapine	0	+++	+++	+++	+++
Olanzapine	+	+	++	++	+++
Quetiapine fumarate	+/0	0	++	++	+
Risperidone	+	0	+	++	+
Ziprasidone hydrochloride	+	0	+	++	+

Note: 0 = minimal to none; + = low; ++ = moderate; +++ = high.

*Clozapine and olanzapine can cause diabetes mellitus independent of weight gain.

Most of the typical antipsychotics block alpha$_1$-adrenergic, muscarinic, and histaminergic receptors in addition to the dopaminergic receptors, which are primarily responsible for the side-effect profile of these drugs (Table 19-13). The low-potency drugs (eg, thioridazine, chlorpromazine) tend to be more sedating, be more anticholinergic, and cause more postural hypotension than the high-potency drugs (eg, haloperidol, fluphenazine hydrochloride). The high-potency drugs tend to cause more EPS. Weight gain can be seen with all of the typical antipsychotics, particularly with low-potency agents. Sexual dysfunction, including decreased libido, delayed (or retrograde) ejaculation, and erectile difficulties, are side effects common to all typical antipsychotics.

The side effects produced by a given drug can sometimes help in deciding whether or not to use that drug in a certain patient population. For example, suicidal patients should not receive thioridazine, mesoridazine besylate, or pimozide because of the cardiotoxicity associated with their overdose. The low-potency antipsychotics (thioridazine) should not be administered to patients with glaucoma, prostatism, or other contraindications to anticholinergic drugs or to patients taking other anticholinergic compounds such as tricyclic antidepressants. Description of neurologic side effects from antipsychotics (dystonia, akathisia, pseudoparkinsonism, tardive dyskinesia) and their management can be found in Chapter 9. The higher risk of tardive dyskinesia with the conventional neuroleptics is the single most important reason why the new-generation antipsychotics (like risperidone, aripiprazole, quetiapine fumarate, ziprasidone hydrochloride, and olanzapine) should be first-line treatment when use of antipsychotics is contemplated.

Plasma levels of antipsychotics may be increased by many other drugs, including some TCAs, SSRIs, beta-blockers, and cimetidine. Barbiturates and carbamazepine may decrease plasma levels of antipsychotics. Antacids can decrease the absorption of an antipsychotic. The antipsychotic drugs generally bind readily to proteins (85% to 90%) and should be administered with caution in combination with other highly protein-bound drugs like warfarin sodium and digoxin. Displacement and competition for binding sites could alter effective concentrations of both the antipsychotic and the other drugs. Antipsychotics antagonize the effects of dopamine agonists or L-dopa when these drugs are used to treat parkinsonism. Chlorpromazine, haloperidol, and thiothixene hydrochloride can block the antihypertensive effects of guanethidine sulfate. Antipsychotics may enhance the effects of CNS depressants such as analgesics, anxiolytics, and hypnotics.

New Generation Antipsychotics

Clozapine is structurally related to the typical antipsychotic loxapine succinate with a higher affinity for the D_4 than for the D_2 receptor. Clozapine has two principal metabolites, both with low pharmacologic activity. Risperidone is a benzisoxazole derivative with combined D_2 and $5HT_2$ receptor-blocking properties. It has no effect on muscarinic receptors but has some alpha-adrenergic antagonism. Olanzapine is a thienobenzodiazepine with particular affinity for both serotonin ($5HT_2$) and D_2 dopamine receptors and to a lesser degree D_4 and D_1 dopamine, muscarinic, alpha$_1$-adrenergic, and histaminergic H_1 receptors. Olanzapine has no alpha$_2$-adrenergic antagonism.

Clozapine has a 10-fold higher affinity for the D_4 than for the D_2 dopamine receptor and also binds preferentially to the mesolimbic and mesocortical dopaminergic tracts rather than the nigrostriatal tracts. The newer antipsychotics also preferentially block $5HT_2$ serotonergic receptors rather than D_2 receptors, which might account for their atypicality.

Clozapine may be particularly effective in treating patients with schizophrenia who do not respond to treatment with typical antipsychotics. It has also been used in some patients with severe EPS who cannot tolerate typical antipsychotics. Studies have shown that clozapine may be effective in the treatment of refractory schizoaffective disorder, other atypical psychoses, and bipolar disorder. New-generation antipsychotics may ameliorate negative symptoms, which in fact the conventional neuroleptics can sometimes cause (secondary negative symptoms), and they may have less propensity to cause EPS, including tardive dyskinesia. Olanzapine and quetiapine fumarate are more sedating than risperidone, ziprasidone hydrochloride, and aripiprazole.

Anticholinergic side effects, including blurring of vision, dry mouth, constipation, urinary hesitancy, tachycardia, and prolongation of cardiac conduction sedation and increased falls, can be seen with clozapine and olanzapine, particularly in high-risk patients (eg, those with dementia or delirium or those on other anticholinergic drugs). Risperidone, quetiapine fumarate, and ziprasidone hydrochloride have no significant anticholinergic effects.

Clozapine should only be administered to patients who will submit to weekly blood monitoring. It can lead to agranulocytosis in less than 1% of patients, with the risk being greatest in the first 6 months of treatment. Patients taking clozapine should be monitored for tachycardia and postural hypotension during the first month of treatment. The risk of seizures increases to 3% to 5% at doses of 600 mg/day and above. Patients should be treated for at least 2 months to see the maximum effect. Slow tapering of the clozapine dosage is recommended to prevent withdrawal symptoms, which may include marked agitation and rebound psychotic symptoms.

There has been no evidence of withdrawal symptoms following discontinuation of olanzapine. Olanzapine may increase transaminase values in up to 2% of patients. No blood monitoring is required because the elevations are transient and not clinically significant in most patients.

Plasma concentrations of clozapine may be increased by drugs that inhibit the P450-1A2 and 3A4 liver enzymes, such as cimetidine, nefazodone hydrochloride, and the SSRIs, particularly fluvoxamine maleate. Olanzapine is not associated with any significant hepatic isoenzyme P450 inhibition that might predict an adverse drug–drug interaction. Plasma concentrations of olanzapine can be decreased by smoking and carbamazepine and is increased in females. There is considerable evidence to indicate that clozapine and olanzapine cause significant weight gain and diabetes mellitus (independent of weight gain). All patients started on these drugs should be informed of these side effects, and weight, blood glucose, and lipids should be monitored regularly after starting the drug. Patients developing these side effects should be switched off the drug because there is evidence that weight gain and diabetes may improve after discontinuing the drug.

Off-Label Uses of Antipsychotic Agents

Antipsychotic agents, both the first and second generation, have been used for off-label indications in psychiatry (Table 19-14). Clearly for avoidance or minimization of tardive dyskinesia, second generation agents are preferred, such as low doses of risperidone, aripiprazole, quetiapine fumarate, ziprasidone hydrochloride, or olanzapine.

Using Antiparkinsonian Agents to Treat Extrapyramidal Symptoms

This group of drugs, which includes the anticholinergics and dopamine agonists, are used to treat some of the EPS caused by antipsychotics. Anticholinergic drugs, like biperiden hydrochloride, procyclidine, trihexyphenidyl, and benztropine mesylate, block M_1 muscarinic receptors predominantly located in the striatum. The dopaminergic agonists like amantadine hydrochloride increase dopamine release from the presynaptic terminals in the basal ganglia, restoring the dopamine-acetylcholine balance.

TABLE 19-14 Psychiatric and Nonpsychiatric Indications for Antipsychotic Agents

Psychiatric Indications	Nonpsychiatric Indications
• Psychoses associated with schizophrenia, schizoaffective disorder,* bipolar disorder,* depression,* dementias, other psychoses	• Treatment-resistant pain syndromes[†]
• Treatment-resistant depression	• Recurrent daily headaches[†]
• Treatment-resistant obsessive compulsive disorders*	• Refractory migraine[†]
• Treatment-resistant eating disorders, such as anorexia nervosa or bulimia*	• Intractable hiccup or severe vomiting[‡]
• Difficult-to-treat personality disorders*	• Pre-anesthetic drug regimens
• Posttraumatic stress disorder*	
• Body dysmorphic disorder	
• Behavioral aggression or agitation with dementia or other syndromes	

* In most of these indications, antipsychotic agents are mostly combined for short or long periods of time with the primary drug, which may be lithium, an anticonvulsant, an antidepressant, an anti-anxiety agent, etc.

† In these conditions, antipsychotics have been added in low doses to the primary therapeutic agent. Because tardive dyskinesia is a real possibility with the older drugs, lower doses of the new drugs are preferred.

‡ It is not fully known whether newer antipsychotic agents will be of help in these situations.

All the antiparkinsonian agents are equally efficacious in treating EPS, although there is some evidence to suggest that dopamine agonists, like amantadine, might benefit akinesia preferentially over tremor, rigidity, dystonia, and akathisia. It also appears that the antiparkinsonian agents, in general, are less effective in treating akathisia vs other EPS: beta-blockers or BZPs may be more effective (see Chapter 9). The different antiparkinsonian agents, their half-lives, and their dosages are listed in Table 19-15.

Anticholinergic side effects are most notably dry mouth, constipation, blurred vision, tachycardia, urinary hesitancy, and, in more serious cases, memory impairment, confusion, disorientation, and delirium. Amantadine hydrochloride may sometimes cause

TABLE 19-15 Antiparkinsonian Agents

Drug	Half-Life	Usual Daily Dose
Anticholinergics		
Benztropine mesylate (Cogentin)	>24 hours	1–2 mg tid
Biperiden hydrochloride (Akineton)	18–24 hours	2 mg bid
Procyclidine hydrochloride (Kemadrin)	12 hours	2.5 mg tid
Trihexyphenidyl hydrochloride (Artane)	5–10 hours	5 mg bid to tid
Dopamine Agonists		
Amantadine hydrochloride (Symmetrel)	14 hours	100 mg bid to tid

GI upset, anxiety, tremors, lethargy, ataxia, and, very rarely, an exacerbation of psychosis. There have been a few reports of tolerance to and abuse of antiparkinsonian agents in some patients with psychotic disorders. There are no absolute contraindications to the use of antiparkinsonian agents. Elderly patients and patients with prostatic hypertrophy, narrow angle glaucoma, or cardiac conduction abnormalities, or those taking other drugs with anticholinergic effects need to be monitored carefully.

PSYCHOSTIMULANTS

Amphetamine, first synthesized in 1887, was introduced into clinical use as Benzedrine in the United States in 1932. Its overuse, misuse, and abuse in the 1960s gave amphetamines a bad reputation, but interest in stimulant use has been recently renewed, most notably in depressed medically ill patients and patients with refractory primary depression. Psychostimulants (dextroamphetamine and methylphenidate) offer an attractive alternative to antidepressants like SSRIs for the treatment of depression among the medically ill because they lack many of the adverse effects of conventional antidepressants as well as possess a shorter latency in the onset of their therapeutic efficacy.

Amphetamine releases newly synthesized dopamine, thereby increasing the concentration of catecholamines in the synaptic cleft. Methylphenidate increases the release of intraneuronal dopamine from the granular pools into the synaptic cleft. The action of pemoline is not well understood. The half-lives of dextroamphetamine, methylphenidate, and pemoline are 12 to 20 hours, 2 to 7 hours, and 9 to 14 hours, respectively.

Indications

Stimulants have demonstrated efficacy in the treatment of depression in patients with general medical illnesses, including cancer, stroke, HIV infections, heart disease, dementia, head injury, and chronic pain syndromes. They are also helpful as an augmentation strategy in patients who have demonstrated a partial response to the SSRIs, the SNRIs, or the TCAs, or for the treatment of sexual dysfunction due to the SSRIs. They can also play a role in the symptomatic treatment of narcolepsy, ADHD, as adjuvants in pain management, and in combating the apathy seen in dementia, traumatic brain injury, or other organic brain syndromes.

Side Effects

The psychostimulants are capable of producing a range of CNS, cardiovascular, and GI disturbances that are generally dose related and reversible (Table 19-16). Their use in the medically ill, however, has been associated with relatively few side effects, even in the presence of underlying cardiovascular and CNS disease. All psychostimulants have abuse potential. However, clinical experience with the short-term use of psychostimulants in medical populations suggests little, if any, tendency toward tolerance or abuse. It is believed that the brief duration of exposure in the medically ill population and the low doses that are generally required to achieve a therapeutic effect are reasons why tolerance, abuse, and addiction are uncommon in this patient population.

There are no absolute contraindications to the short-term use of stimulants in the medically ill. Relative contraindications include a history of hypersensitivity to stimulants; history of psychosis or tics; pregnancy; uncontrolled hypertension or arrhythmias; history of abusing stimulants; or the concurrent use of MAOIs.

TABLE 19-16 Common Side Effects of Psychostimulant Use

Central Nervous System	Cardiovascular System	Gastrointestinal System
• restlessness	• palpitations	• nausea
• tremor	• tachycardia	• diarrhea
• irritability		
• insomnia		
• agitation		
• paranoia		
• tics		

Dosing

The recommended starting dose, peak doses, and dosage schedules are listed in Table 19-17. An initial dose of 5 mg of methylphenidate at 8 AM should be used, followed by observation of how the patient does 1 hour after the first dose. Pulse and blood pressure should be checked prior to and 1 hour after the first dose to determine if the patient shows evidence of sinus tachycardia or hypertension (pulse >100 beats/minute, systolic blood pressure >160 mm Hg, and/or diastolic blood pressure >90 mm Hg). The dose can then be increased by 5 mg every 2 to 3 days until the patient responds or has side effects. Typically, patients do not require more than 20 mg/day, often given in two divided doses: 10 mg at 8 AM and 10 mg at noon. Based on the authors' experience, doses greater than 40 to 60 mg of methylphenidate are rarely required.

A number of longer-acting preparations of stimulants have been marketed in the past few years for treatment of ADHD. These may allow once- or twice-daily dosing of children or adults. See Chapter 5 for additional information.

Typically, an initial dose of dextroamphetamine 2.5 mg is given at 8 AM and increased by 2.5 to 5 mg every 2 days until the patient responds or has side effects. In the authors' experience, doses greater than 20 mg are rarely required. Most patients need a single morning dose; however, some patients will need an additional dose in the afternoon. One should avoid doses late in the day to minimize the risk of insomnia.

Psychostimulants are usually continued for 6 weeks after remission of symptoms and then tapered and discontinued over a period of 1 to 2 weeks. Some patients, roughly one third, are discharged from the hospital on psychostimulants and are tapered from them as

TABLE 19-17 Dosages and Schedules of Psychostimulants in the Depressed Medically Ill

Drug	Starting Dose	Peak Daily Dose	Schedule
Dextroamphetamine	2.5–5.0 mg	15 mg	1 to 2 times daily
Methylphenidate	5.0–10.0 mg	30 mg	2 to 3 times daily
Pemoline	18.75 mg	75 mg	1 to 2 times daily

outpatients. Some patients will need long-term treatment with psychostimulants, which have been found to be safe and well tolerated.

OTHER PHARMACOLOGIC AGENTS

Calcium channel blockers, such as verapamil hydrochloride and nimodipine, have been used in anecdotal case reports or small controlled trials with evidence of some benefit in treating mania, although not all studies are supportive. However, large-scale studies are required for demonstration of efficacy and safety.

Studies have suggested that the dietary sugar myo-inositol (8 to 12 gm/day) is of benefit for unipolar and bipolar depression, although large-scale studies are needed for demonstrating efficacy. Interestingly, inositol has been used for lithium-induced side effects in short-term trials with some evidence of benefit.

L-tryptophan is now off the market in the United States, having caused eosinophilia-myalgia syndrome, probably as a result of contaminants in the production process rather than from the drug itself. It has been used in large doses as a hypnotic and in severe mania. Long-term benefits, side effects, and efficacy are yet to be determined. It is used along with lithium and other drugs.

Buprenorphine hydrochloride is an opioid with partial agonist activity at the μ receptor, which can be used sublingually and intranasally and may be useful for refractory depression and possibly bipolar depression.

L-thyroxine has been used in euthyroid or hypothyroid bipolar patients with a rapid-cycling course (four or more episodes in a year). Doses higher than thyroid replacement doses (0.1 to 0.5 mg/day) are used. Titration is done very slowly, with attention to osteoporosis and cardiac problems in long-term use. This treatment is best coordinated with a psychopharmacologist and an endocrinologist. This strategy helps some rapid-cycling or depressed bipolar patients achieve a measure of stability. Both L-thyroxine and liothyronine (T_3) (at doses of 25 to 50 μg/day) have been used to potentiate the effects of antidepressants in depression, although there is some evidence that T_3 is preferable.

Beta-blockers have been shown to have some use in treating performance anxiety symptoms (eg, stage fright) or to diminish the somatic symptoms in generalized anxiety disorder. Pindolol has been used at doses of 20 mg daily to speed the onset of action of SSRIs.

Much speculation has arisen around the role that omega-3-fatty acids (OM3FA), specifically docosahexanol acid, plays with psychiatric conditions and in particular depression. Previous clinical and epidemiologic studies regarding differences in rates of depression associated with dietary trends have suggested that communities with diets high in fish oil tended to have lower overall rates of depression. An association shown between lower serum cholesterol concentrations and increased suicide risk sparked additional interest. Evidence has suggested that an imbalance in the ratio of essential fatty acids (EFA), namely the N-6 and N-3 fatty acids, may be responsible for increased depressive symptoms associated with low plasma cholesterol. Examination of DHA and OM3FA in cases of depression have shown that serum total OM3FA were decreased in depressives compared with levels in healthy controls and in individuals with minor depression. DHA has been suggested to also play a role in postpartum depression. It has been found that a single pregnancy may deplete DHA levels and that multiple pregnancies may lead to a chronic and progressive depletion. Alcoholism has also been shown to decrease long-chain OM3FA from neuronal membranes, and alcoholism has clearly been demonstrated to have an increased association with depression.

A few preliminary trials have attempted to answer the question of a clinical role for these compounds in the treatment of psychiatric disorders, particularly bipolar disorders. However, until large-scale placebo-controlled trials demonstrate the effectiveness of DHA and associated OM3FA, the use of DHA as mono or supplemental therapy for use in depression or bipolar disorder cannot be recommended.

OTHER SOMATIC TREATMENTS

Somatic treatments other than medications have a long history in the treatment of psychiatric illnesses. Electroconvulsive therapy, transcranal magnetic stimulation, vagal nerve stimulation, hypnotherapy, biofeedback, light treatment, and psychosurgery are amongst the several treatments that have a place in the treatment of patients with a wide variety of psychiatric illnesses.

Electroconvulsive Therapy

Meduna used chemical (camphor) induction of seizures in 1934 in the first successful treatment of psychotic symptoms in schizophrenia. Cerletti and Beni introduced electroconvulsive therapy (ECT) in 1938, and it soon became used throughout much of the world. Improvements in anesthetic technique and monitoring further increased the safety of ECT. Its use declined in the 1970s and 1980s because of the availability of pharmacotherapy and adverse publicity. In recent years, there has been a resurgence of interest in ECT, with a more objective portrayal of this very effective treatment in the media. It is the only antidepressant with rapid onset of action.

ECT enhances noradrenergic transmission partly by increasing alpha$_1$-adrenergic receptors and decreasing alpha$_2$-adrenergic receptors (partly autoreceptors). It also desensitizes and down-regulates the cortical beta adrenergic receptors, up-regulates the 5HT$_2$ receptors, enhances dopaminergic function, and up-regulates gamma-aminobutyric acid (GABA) type B receptors. ECT also reduces cholinergic transmission, which may account for its amnestic effects.

Typically, most patients with major depression need about 6 to 12 treatments administered two to three times per week. The treatments are continued until maximum response is attained or adverse effects supervene. The cognitive deficits tend to increase cumulatively with an increasing number of treatments. Most psychotropic medications (except at times antipsychotics) should be discontinued on the day of treatment.

Indications and contraindications. ECT has demonstrated efficacy in major depression (with or without psychotic features), manic or depressed episodes of bipolar disorder, catatonic schizophrenia, and schizoaffective disorder bipolar type. It has possible efficacy in schizophreniform disorder, atypical psychosis, catatonia due to general medical conditions, Parkinson disease, delirium, and neuroleptic malignant syndrome.

Usually ECT is reserved for patients who have failed, refused, or are intolerant of pharmacotherapy. However, it is sometimes used as first-line treatment in patients who are acutely suicidal or homicidal, manifest extreme catatonic excitement or stupor, are markedly emaciated, in whom psychotropics are contraindicated (eg, during pregnancy), or who have had a good prior response to ECT. Of patients with major depression, 80% to 90% respond well to ECT, compared to only 50% of depressed patients who have failed adequate trials of pharmacotherapy. The presence of psychosis and melancholia in depressed patients is a possible predictor of good response to ECT.

Increased intracranial pressure (ICP) is an absolute contraindication to ECT because of the risk of cerebral herniation. Relative contraindications include space-occupying brain lesions (without increased ICP); recent myocardial infarction (within 1 month); aortic, ventricular, or cerebrovascular aneurysms; uncontrolled epilepsy; pheochromocytoma; retinal detachment; or high anesthesia risk (level 4 or 5 ASA rating).

Adverse effects. Common side effects include headache, tiredness, nausea, muscle aches, post-ECT confusion and sleepiness, and cognitive deficits. The latter includes amnesia (anterograde and retrograde), disturbances in language, perceptual learning, verbal fluency, naming abilities, and reaction time. Typically, the cognitive deficits resolve in a few weeks but can occasionally persist for a few months, particularly if the patient has undergone several bilateral ECTs or has an underlying dementia, obsessive personality style, secondary gain, or a strong expectation that such deficits will occur. The use of unilateral, nondominant electrode placement, brief pulse (vs sine wave), and suprathreshold stimulus are associated with a decreased likelihood of cognitive deficits. Because a course of ECT interferes with the long-term storage of new memories, patients invariably have poor recall of the period during which they were treated and for a period of several weeks prior to beginning treatment.

Serious side effects of ECT including death, complications due to anesthesia, myocardial infarction, arrhythmia, stroke, status epilepticus, fractures, or severe, persistent cognitive deficits are all extremely rare.

Transcranial Magnetic Stimulation

Transcranial magnetic stimulation (rTMS) is a new somatic treatment in psychiatric practice that has been adapted from neurology. Since the early to mid-1990s, reports (both open and controlled trials using sham rTMS) have indicated benefits for treatment-resistant depression (unipolar and bipolar), although some reports were equivocal or negative. The procedure remains in the realm of academic psychiatric research centers, which are working out the details of use including placement (left prefrontal for depression, right prefrontal for mania, etc), stimulus parameters (1 Hz vs 20 Hz, etc), frequency (daily vs less frequently), side effects, etc. Further, whether it can be used instead of or in conjunction with ECT has not been fully addressed. Preliminary studies have shown benefits in mania. Mixed results have been noted in OCD, and negative results were reported for one controlled study in schizophrenia. Once its eventual place in the somatic treatment of psychiatry is determined, the lack of anesthesia and an office-based procedural approach may offer many advantages for patients and clinicians.

Vagal Nerve Stimulation

Vagal nerve stimulation (VNS) is another treatment modality borrowed from neurology, where it has been approved for treatment of refractory epilepsy. At the present time, open data suggest benefits in refractory depression. A recent large multicenter placebo-controlled trial failed to demonstrate superiority to placebo in treatment-resistant depression. Larger trials in academic research centers will determine the place of VNS in psychiatric practice. The invasive procedure may limit its acceptance in patients who have failed previous antidepressant trials, including ECT.

Hypnotherapy

The term *hypnotherapy* encompasses a variety of conditions, assumptions, and techniques. There seems to be agreement that the hypnotic state requires a temporarily altered state of consciousness associated with deep relaxation and focused concentration. The specific methodologies for hypnosis are many, but the major points are to establish rapport with the patient, turn the patient's focus inward, move the patient away from preconceived ways of thinking, and encourage an unconscious analysis of the problem. Despite many years of controversy, hypnosis is now recognized as a useful adjuvant therapy, particularly for pain control.

Perhaps 90% of people can be hypnotized, with 20% to 30% being highly receptive to this modality. Caution should be used in patients with psychosis, organic psychiatric conditions, and antisocial personality disorders. The mechanism of action of hypnosis at present is unknown, with studies presently being done using PET imaging techniques. Earlier studies have suggested some changes in body chemistry when measuring catecholamines and serum cortisol, but the benefits may simply be due to improved skills of relaxation.

Controlled trials in asthma, *hyperemesis gravidarum,* and in anticipatory vomiting associated with chemotherapy found hypnosis to be of value in reducing symptoms and need for medication. In cases of irritable bowel syndrome unresponsive to conventional therapies, up to 60% of patients received some benefit from hypnotherapy, although the long-term effect was not studied. Hypnosis and imagery have long been recognized as helpful in reducing acute pain and have been used successfully in individual cases for anesthesia, particularly in oral surgery. Treatment of phobias and disorders of memory may also include hypnotherapy; combined with relaxation techniques, hypnotherapy is often included in behavioral treatment approaches.

Biofeedback

Biofeedback is a treatment modality that attempts to teach methods of self-regulation of bodily processes. It requires some form of physiologic information-gathering and a display that will allow the patient to achieve better control of the values fed back by the display. Commonly used information is that of skin temperature, galvanic skin responses, muscle tension measured by electromyography (EMG), and brain wave patterns displayed on an electroencephalogram (EEG). An example easily generalized to other uses is that of using thermal feedback of skin temperature to teach patients control of peripheral vasoconstriction or vasodilation. A monitor is placed on the patient's finger, a readout temperature is displayed, and imagery or relaxation techniques are used with feedback information to raise the temperature in the digit. This methodology has been very successful in some cases of Raynaud syndrome, vascular headache, and diabetic small vessel disease.

There is adequate scientific evidence to consider biofeedback as mainstream medicine and not simply relegate it to the alternative medicine sphere. EMG biofeedback has been shown to treat headaches caused by muscular contraction, even in chronic cases.

Migraine headaches have also been shown to respond to biofeedback. Circulatory disorders and delayed wound healing have benefited from thermal feedback. Controlled studies have shown biofeedback significantly more effective than relaxation methods alone. Biofeedback is the treatment of choice for fecal incontinence in patients who have impaired ability to feel rectal distention.

There are inconsistent results in the use of these techniques in irritable bowel syndrome and asthma. Although patients are able to lower their blood pressure using biofeedback, the effects are small and may not be consistently long lasting. A single study of patients with PTSD showed decreased medication requirements and a decreased relapse rate in those trained to increase their alpha and theta brain wave activity. There are no documented adverse effects from biofeedback.

Light Treatment (Phototherapy)

Bright light in the morning (2500 to 10,000 lux) using special lamps may be useful in seasonal affective disorder syndrome (SADS) for patients who experience winter depression. Exposure to the eye is better than to the skin. The duration is 2 hours for the lower intensity and 30 minutes for the higher intensity. Adverse effects are generally mild and respond to dose (duration) reduction. They include eye irritation, psychomotor activation, and insomnia. Long-term skin and eye complications have not been reported.

It is felt that this treatment may also be useful in jet lag and delayed sleep syndrome. Light therapy has also been applied to treatment-resistant depression and in some bipolar patients in conjunction with other treatments. Although preliminary data appear promising for some patients, large-scale studies are lacking for more definitive conclusions.

Psychosurgery

It has long been postulated that emotional behavior is regulated by specific brain circuits. Despite a long and controversial history, the use of neurosurgical interventions, commonly referred to as psychosurgery, remain an option for some severe, intractable psychiatric disorders. Four neurosurgical approaches, subcaudate, tractotomy, limbic leucotomy, anterior cingulotomy and anterior capsulotomy, for OCD remain procedures that are still actively used.

All of these techniques have traditionally involved making bilateral lesions in stereotactically defined brain regions. In subcaudate tractotomy, lesions are made under the head of the caudate nucleus in the substantia innominata. Anterior circulotomy involves placement of lesions in the cingulum bundle. Limbic leukotomy essentially combines the lesions made in the two previous procedures, while in the anterior capsulotomy the lesions are placed in the anterior limb of the internal capsule. From multiple studies, it has been estimated that 40% to 60% of patients with intractable OCD are considerably improved after surgery, but the conclusion that neurosurgery benefits patients with intractable disease must remain tentative until controlled clinical trials demonstrate efficacy and safety.

SUMMARY

Somatic treatments play a critical role in the treatment of most psychiatric disorders and may be quite helpful in many more. Developments in the understanding of some of these disorders as well as in basic neuropharmacology have led to improved antidepressant, anxiolytic, antipsychotic, and thymoleptic agents with greater specificity and fewer adverse effects. Nonpharmacologic somatic interventions such as electroconvulsive therapy, biofeedback, and light therapy also are most valuable for selected indications.

ADDITIONAL READINGS

Abrams R. *Electroconvulsive Therapy*. New York, NY: Oxford University Press; 1988.

American Psychiatric Association. *Practice Guidelines for Treatment of Patients with Bipolar Disorder.* Washington, DC: American Psychiatric Press; 1995.

Baldessarini R. Drugs and the treatment of psychiatric disorders—psychosis and anxiety. In: Hardman JG, Limbird LE, eds. *Goodman and Gilman's The Pharmacological Basis of Therapeutics*. 9th ed. New York, NY: McGraw-Hill; 1996:421-430.

Crowe RR. Electroconvulsive therapy: a current perspective. *N Engl J Med*. 1984;314:163-167.

Elkin I, Shea T, Watkins JT, et al. National Institute of Mental Health treatment of depression. *Arch Gen Psychiatry*. 1989;46:971-982.

Fugh-Berman A. *Alternative Medicine: What Works*. Tucson, Ariz: Odonian Press; 1996.

Gelenberg AJ. The use of benzodiazepine hypnotics: a scientific examination of a clinical controversy. *J Clin Psychiatry*. 1992;53(12 suppl):1-87.

Goodwin FK, Jamison KR, eds. *Manic-Depressive Illness*. New York, NY: Oxford University Press; 1990.

Hobbs WR, Rall TW, Verdoorn TA. Hypnotics and sedatives; ethanol. In: Hardman JG, Limbird LE, eds. *Goodman and Gilman's The Pharmacological Basis of Therapeutics*. 9th ed. New York, NY: McGraw-Hill; 1996:361-395.

Hollander E, Cohen LJ. The assessment and treatment of refractory anxiety. *J Clin Psychiatry*. 1994;55(2 suppl):27-31.

Hollister L. Clinical uses of benzodiazepines. *J Clin Psychopharmacol*. 1993;13(6 Suppl 1):64S-72S.

Kupfer DF. Long-term treatment of depression. *J Clin Psychiatry*. 1991;52(suppl 5):28-34.

Lin E, Van Korff M, Katon W, et al. Primary care physician role in adherence to antidepressant therapy. *Med Care*. 1995;36:519-526.

Masand PS. Weight gain associated with psychotropics. *Expert Opinion Pharmacother*. 2000;1:377-389.

Masand PS, Gupta S. Long-term adverse effects of novel antipsychotics. *J Psychiatr Pract*. 2000;6:299-309.

Masand PS, Gupta S, Dewan MJ. Selective serotonin reuptake inhibitors (SSRIs). In: Ananth J, ed. *Psychopharmacology: Treatment of Psychiatric Disorders*. Mumbai, India: Jaypee Brothers; 1999.

Masand PS, Gupta S, Dewan MJ. Selective serotonin-reuptake inhibitors: an update. *Harvard Rev Psychiatry*. 1999;7(2):69-84.

Masand PS, Tesar GE. Use of psychostimulants in the medically ill. *Psychiatric Clin N Amer*. 1996;19(3):515-547.

McElroy SL, Keck PE Jr, Friedman LM. Minimizing and managing antidepressant side effects. *J Clin Psychiatry*. 1995;56(suppl 2):49-55.

Pollack MH, Rosenbaum JF. Management of antidepressant-induced side effects: a practical guide for the clinician. *J Clin Psychiatry*. 1987;48:3-8.

Public Health Service Agency for Health Care Policy and Research. *Depression in Primary Care, Vol 2, Treatment of Major Depression*. Rockville, Md: US Department of Health and Human Services; 1993. AHCPR Publication, No. 93-051.

Schou MD. *Lithium Treatment of Manic Depressive Illness a Practical Guide*. 5th rev ed. New York, NY: Karger Publishing; 1993.

Chapter **20**

Psychotherapeutic and Behavioral Treatments

Stuart J. Eisendrath, MD
Mitchell D. Feldman, MD, M Phil

Although there have been tremendous advances in the pharmacologic treatment of psychiatric disorders, the primary care physician may represent the most potent treatment for persons with psychiatric problems. Several factors enhance the primary care physician's ability to carry out psychotherapeutic interventions. First, patients trust their primary care physicians and believe them capable of helping with emotional difficulties. Many patients feel more comfortable talking to their primary care physician than to an unfamiliar psychiatrist or counselor. Some patients may perceive a referral to a mental health specialist as a rejection by the primary care physician and will fear the stigma associated with seeing this specialist. As a consequence, many patients will fail to follow through with mental health referrals made by their primary care physician. Overall, only about half of outpatients referred for a mental health consultation complete the process.

A second factor that puts the primary care physician in an advantageous position to provide psychotherapeutic interventions is that patients typically come to their primary care physician with early signs of emotional distress. In fact, several studies have concluded that it is the emotional distress that activates the visit to the primary care physician in up to 60% of cases, even when a medical illness is present. The primary care physician is in an ideal position to intervene early in the course of psychiatric disorders to prevent more significant morbidity. The primary care physician can actually carry out primary or secondary prevention in some adjustments to different life stressors, such as menopause. For example, educating patients in advance about the emotional aspects of the disorder ("this often occurs in menopause") may help the patient cope with the stressor and prevent the onset of more serious or pathological reactions. Moreover, because much of the patient's distress is often focused on his or her health, the primary care physician is in a favorable position to address these concerns.

The third and possibly most significant factor is that the primary care physician has an ongoing relationship with his or her primary care patients. Continuity of care allows familiarity, trust, and confidence to exist, which can serve as a solid foundation for any form of psychotherapy. It also allows the patient to receive more integrated care that incorporates the biopsychosocial approach advocated by Engel (1995). Seeing the patient for brief visits may enable the primary care physician to deal with one aspect of the patient's difficulty and not overload the patient with too many psychological issues. Similarly, the primary care physician's goal is to achieve a modest change in the patient's emotional state; reconstructive personality therapy is inappropriate for primary care psychotherapeutic efforts.

This chapter reviews the patient-physician relationship and its impact on the diagnosis and management of psychiatric disorders. Different psychotherapeutic approaches relevant in the primary care setting are also discussed, and some limitations of psychotherapy conducted by the primary care physician are highlighted. Other behavioral strategies that the primary care physician can use to manage some conditions commonly seen in primary care settings are included.

PSYCHOTHERAPEUTIC AND BEHAVIORAL TREATMENTS AND THE PATIENT-PHYSICIAN RELATIONSHIP

The effectiveness of psychotherapeutic and behavioral treatments and the extent to which they are accepted by patients depend directly on the quality of the patient-physician relationship. Primary care physicians must focus on and build their relationship with patients. They can then use this connection to enhance the quality of historical data and promote patient adherence with these therapies.

The primary care physician has many opportunities to build the patient-physician relationship during the medical interview. Cohen-Cole (see Chapter 3) developed a model of the medical interview that divides the tasks that must be accomplished into three functions: (1) collecting information, (2) building rapport and responding to the patient's emotions, and (3) educating the patient and maximizing adherence. This model is reviewed here. Also provided is an explanation of how data-gathering strengthens the primary care physician's relationship with the patient and why it is necessary to carry out psychotherapeutic and behavioral treatments. This model also lays the groundwork for educating patients regarding mental health issues.

Data-Gathering

The first function of the medical interview is to gather data. To make a diagnosis of a psychiatric or behavioral disorder and initiate treatment, the primary care physician must gather complete and accurate information from the patient. To do this, the primary care physician must first optimize the environment in which she or he conducts interviews. The physical setting allows the primary care physician to express nonverbally what she or he regards as important. It is helpful to maximize privacy and minimize distractions such as the telephone and other potential interruptions that may disrupt the flow of the interview.

Next, the primary care physician must elicit accurate historical data from the patient. The goal is to establish a narrative thread so that the patient will tell the "story of the illness." Start the interview by surveying for all possible complaints the patient may have. By asking the patient if there is anything else to bring up after he or she has stated the chief complaint, the physician is able to increase the likelihood that more difficult psychosocial issues are brought to light. Many psychosocial issues are never uncovered in the primary care setting because the primary care physician prematurely closes off further inquiry. Research has shown that the patient's first stated complaint is rarely the most important one.

Data-gathering skills continue to be important after a diagnosis has been made and treatment initiated. This is especially true when treatment depends on efficient and accurate communication between physician and patient, as is true with all psychotherapeutic and behavioral therapies. These skills allow the primary care physician to efficiently monitor for any change in symptoms and to adjust the treatment accordingly.

Relationship-Building

The second function of the medical interview is to build the relationship with the patient. The success or failure of all psychotherapeutic and behavioral treatments depends on the

TABLE 20-1 Tasks to Develop and Maintain a Therapeutic Relationship
• Define the nature of the relationship
• Communicate professional expertise
• Communicate interest, respect, support, and empathy
• Recognize and resolve relational barriers to communication
• Elicit the patient's perspective

primary care physician's success in developing and maintaining a solid therapeutic relationship with the patient.

Lazare et al (1995) described five tasks (Table 20-1) that are necessary for the primary care physician to successfully develop and maintain a therapeutic relationship with the patient. First, the primary care physician must clearly define the nature of the relationship with the patient. For example, if the primary care physician intends to work with the patient in a long-term capacity using psychotherapeutic and behavioral treatments, this should be clearly explained beforehand. This is necessary because the patient-physician relationship will be different from the relationship the patient is likely to have had with a previous primary care physician. If the primary care physician intends to refer the patient for a mental health consultation under some circumstances, this should also be discussed. The primary care physician can educate the patient about what to expect when seeing a mental health specialist. For example, by giving an idea of how many sessions are typical, what types of problems can be focused on, and the confidentiality of the relationship, the primary care physician may increase the patient's likelihood of following through with the referral.

Assuming the primary care physician continues to work with the patient, the second task necessary to building a therapeutic relationship is for the primary care physician to communicate professional expertise. This can be accomplished by presenting a professional and competent demeanor and by communicating knowledge about the patient's medical history and treatment. If treatment is offered to the patient, the physician should be prepared to explain why that treatment was selected and what the patient is likely to experience. For example, anticipating the usual time course of response to psychotherapy or medications is often essential to promoting adequate adherence.

The third task is to communicate interest, respect, support, and empathy. The primary care physician must join the patient by communicating interest and warmth. If the patient feels that the primary care physician is truly interested in him or her and will be available to provide support as they work together on difficult emotional issues, they are much more likely to engage in and maintain the challenging work that many psychotherapeutic and behavioral treatments require. Asking open-ended questions such as "What have you thought may be causing your symptoms?" or "What worries you the most about your condition?" helps to build rapport and understanding.

A central way for primary care physicians to build the relationship with their patients and help them to feel understood is by using empathy appropriately. Empathy indicates a person's appreciation, understanding, and acceptance of another person's emotional situation. Note that the primary care physician does not have to feel what the patient feels or to have gone through it in order to use empathy effectively. In fact, empathy can be thought of as a powerful therapeutic tool or technique. Nonverbal behaviors such as nodding, smiling, and touch can also communicate empathy.

Empathy can effectively strengthen the patient-physician bond so that other, more structured nonsomatic therapies are much more likely to be accepted by the patient. Empathic statements can be easily recalled by using a simple mnemonic, **R-S-V-P-R.** Statements and examples of each follow:

- **R**eflection: You seem a bit sad right now.
- **S**upport: I'd like to help you work on that.
- **V**alidation: I can understand why that might make you feel sad.
- **P**artnership: We can work together to improve your depression.
- **R**espect: I admire how well you have dealt with this despite all of the sad things that have happened to you.

The fourth task in building and maintaining a relationship with the patient is to recognize and resolve various relational barriers to communication. These barriers may be physical (eg, when possible, lower the bed rails when interviewing a hospitalized patient) or they may be psychological, social, or cultural.

Working with patients from different cultures can be particularly challenging. Many of the concepts central to psychiatric treatment are alien to persons who have not grown up in a Western culture. Physicians must recognize when these cultural barriers exist and attempt to modify their communication style and treatment recommendations accordingly. Patients from many other cultures may find it inappropriate if the primary care physician asks too many personal questions or attempts to explore their emotional issues. The primary care physician must clearly explain why he or she is interested in that information and that it is a routine component of medical care in the United States.

The fifth and final task is to elicit the patient's perspective. Not only will this help patients to feel understood and respected by their primary care physician, but it is an essential step in formulating and carrying out a treatment plan. For example, a patient with clear signs and symptoms consistent with a major depression may believe that their fatigue and sleep disruption are actually due to environmental allergies. This patient is unlikely to comply with their primary care physician's request that they attempt to schedule more active time outdoors. Any nonsomatic treatments suggested for patients must take the patient's explanation of their illness into account.

PSYCHOTHERAPY

Although there are a variety of definitions of psychotherapy, perhaps the broadest is this: Psychotherapy is an effort to treat psychiatric disorders using verbal communications. There are many schools of psychotherapy (Table 20-2); however, they all share some common features:

- *Establishing a trusting relationship* between the psychotherapist and the patient. Although often tenuous initially, the patient's sense of trust increases in working with the therapist.

TABLE 20-2 Approaches to Psychotherapy
• Cognitive
• Behavioral
• Interpersonal
• Psychoanalytic/psychodynamic

- *Providing a conceptual framework for understanding the psychiatric disorder.* The patient learns there is some basis for the unpleasant feelings she or he is experiencing; eg, depression is related to feeling helpless in a work or love situation.
- *Offering the patient hope* that a resolution or improvement of the patient's condition is possible. The patient learns that change is possible.
- *Allowing the patient to feel accepted* by the therapist despite real or imagined flaws. Patients learn they are not so flawed as the therapist investigates their distress with them.
- *Restoring the patient's sense of control.* Whether it is by connection with the therapist or by learning new ways of coping, the patient feels more in control of his or her life.

Some of the principles underlying these therapies are discussed more fully in Chapter 1.

Cognitive Therapy

Cognitive therapy techniques have been developed by a number of clinicians, particularly Albert Ellis and Aaron Beck. These approaches are based on the theory that an individual's thoughts strongly influence his or her emotional states. These thoughts may be based on inaccurate and distorted perceptions that are learned over many years. For example, jumping to a negative conclusion or catastrophizing leads an individual to constricted behavior and depressed mood. If an individual forecasts a disaster occurring on a routine basis, it may deepen or cause depression. By changing and challenging these underlying thoughts, individuals can gain more control over their emotional states. Therapy using these approaches is often more time-limited (eg, 5 to 10 sessions over several months). It is an extremely useful approach with considerable evidence of success for conditions such as depression, panic, and posttraumatic stress disorders. Cognitive therapy is often combined with behavioral therapy and called cognitive-behavioral therapy.

Another variation of cognitive therapy is termed *problem-solving therapy (PST)*. In this therapy, the patient and therapist collaborate to enumerate the problems the patient is facing and then rank them to decide which to focus on first. Then the collaborators develop a list of possible solutions and rank these in order to be tried. Problem-solving therapy can be a very practical and effective approach that a patient can learn and use on his or her own as a specific skill.

Behavioral Therapy

Behavioral approaches to psychotherapy are based on the theory that the patient has "learned" to react in certain pathological ways to life stressors and that teaching new ways to react may be more adaptive for the individual. For example, phobias consisting of inappropriate reactions to a nonthreatening stimulus may be unlearned by teaching patients to relax with hypnosis as they approach the phobic stimuli in their imaginations. For obsessive-compulsive disorder, a behavioral technique called exposure-response prevention is often used. In this approach, objects or situations that produce anxiety are organized into a hierarchy ranked by the discomfort produced. Then the individual begins to expose himself, usually starting with the least discomfort. The patient then moves up the scale. When anxiety occurs, the person avoids performing their typical obsessive-compulsive ritual. Patients gradually learn that the disaster they are magically trying to avoid does not take place. This approach is often effective in time-limited situations. Other behavioral approaches include interventions such as biofeedback, relaxation, imagery, hypnosis, assertiveness training, and conditioning techniques. These approaches aim at enhancing the individual's sense of control in various situations and can often be taught effectively in the primary care setting. This is shown in the following relaxation script:

> Close your eyes and focus on your breathing. Listen to my voice, but if your mind wanders you can just go on by focusing on my voice again. Begin to breathe using your diaphragm. You can feel this by placing one hand on your abdomen and noticing that your abdomen moves out as you breathe in. This is a very peaceful way of breathing. As you breathe out, let the air escape from your nose effortlessly and then continue breathing in the air using your diaphragm. Then begin to focus on your muscle tension. You can start with your feet. Tighten all the muscles in your feet for 10 seconds and then let the muscles relax. Then you can move up to your legs. Tighten the muscles in both your upper and lower legs for 10 seconds and let the muscles relax. As your muscles relax they become loose and limp. Next tighten the muscles of your abdomen and trunk for 10 seconds, then let them relax and go limp. Next focus on tightening the muscles of your hands and arms for 10 seconds. Then let the tension go and let the muscles go limp and relax. Next focus on the muscles of your head and neck for 10 seconds and then let them relax. Then focus on all the small, fine muscles of your face and tense them for 10 seconds and then let them relax. Now go back to your breathing and continue your diaphragmatic breathing and notice how relaxed you've become. When you feel ready, you can open your eyes and enjoy the relaxation you've created.

Other behavioral strategies are used with other psychiatric problems. For example, a primary care physician can often motivate a psychomotorically retarded depressed patient to begin some movement or exercise, such as getting out of bed, walking a short distance, or gradually increasing levels of activity. This type of behavioral activation can be quite useful. In depression, it is also helpful to make another behavioral prescription: encourage the patient to do some pleasurable activity each day. Lewinsohn et al (1986) have found that performing pleasurable activities each day can be as effective as cognitive therapy in some patients. It appears that pleasant activities, particularly when they include an element of mastery (eg, a hobby, gardening), are the most effective.

Interpersonal Therapy

Interpersonal therapy focuses on how interpersonal relationships and interactions affect mood. This type of therapy, though used for a variety of conditions, is most studied in the treatment of depression. Therapy focuses on four interpersonal situations leading to depression: (1) unresolved grief; (2) role conflicts (eg, arguments with a boss); (3) role transitions (eg, retirement, divorce); (4) inadequate social supports. Interpersonal therapy has specific strategies to deal with each of the four situations. For example, someone with unresolved grief may be encouraged to write a letter or carry on a conversation with the deceased. Reviewing the relationship with the lost person, including both positive and negative aspects, and ventilating feelings about the lost person are also encouraged. This approach is usually carried out in a time-limited manner, ranging from 3 to 16 sessions.

Psychodynamic Therapy

One of the earliest schools of modern psychotherapy, originally referred to as psychoanalytic and later called psychodynamic, developed in the first half of the 20th century. This school explains behavior as being motivated by unconscious factors, which are things such as traumatic incidents and disappointing relationships in childhood. These factors then stimulate current behavior without the individual being aware of it. So-called transference reactions occur where the person acts toward people in his or her current life as if they were someone from their past, without being aware that they are doing so. Psychodynamic approaches are aimed at helping the person to gain insight into the motivations for their behavior with the idea that this will diminish psychiatric symptoms. Although highly effective for some individuals with certain types of problems, others do not appear to benefit greatly from this technique even when substantial insight has been achieved. This approach usually requires frequent sessions (generally at least weekly) and lengthy periods of treatment (generally several or more years).

Selecting the Appropriate Therapy

Although there is little data to confirm which psychotherapy is best overall, there is evidence that specific conditions respond well to specific psychotherapies. For example, obsessive-compulsive disorder responds robustly to behavioral strategies that include exposure-response prevention. Anxiety disorders, such as generalized anxiety and panic disorder, respond well to cognitive-behavioral approaches. Interpersonal and cognitive therapies have been demonstrated to be effective for depression. Many recent studies have been randomized controlled trials that indicate that cognitive-behavioral and interpersonal psychotherapies are effective tools for the clinician. The success of these treatments is often equal to that of pharmacologic interventions with none of the potential adverse side effects. For example, in an intriguing study of individuals with obsessive-compulsive disorder, behavioral therapy produced successful results equivalent to fluoxetine. The success was evident on positron emission tomography, which showed a similar restoration of normal brain metabolism patterns in both the fluoxetine and the comparison behavioral therapy study subjects.

Overall, there is ample evidence to suggest that for many psychiatric disorders, psychotherapy is equivalent to pharmacotherapy in producing remission of symptoms, although generally it works more slowly. The choice of treatment should be based on factors other than efficacy, such as patient preference, cost, and availability of competent mental and behavioral health care. The decision of whether to try a particular patient on psychotherapy, medication, or combination treatment has not been clearly established in evidence-based studies for many conditions.

In addition, several recent studies suggest that combining pharmacotherapy with psychotherapy may be the best approach for some patients. For example, a recent randomized controlled trial of patients with panic disorder found that patients in the drug (imipramine) plus cognitive-behavioral therapy arm of the study had a significantly faster and more durable response than patients randomized to imipramine or cognitive-behavioral therapy alone. Similarly, studies of patients with major depression suggest that a combination of pharmacologic and nonpharmacologic treatment leads to superior response rates and lower rates of relapse in vulnerable patients.

SPECIFIC PSYCHOTHERAPEUTIC STRATEGIES

Unlike psychotherapy conducted by a mental health specialist, the following interventions, which can be carried out by a primary care physician, have more modest but still important goals:

- Restore baseline psychological functioning.
- Prevent serious decline in functioning.
- Increase self-esteem by expanding coping strategies.

It is not necessary for the primary care physician to obtain in-depth information from patients, such as childhood psychological development, for these strategies to work. Instead, these interventions focus on the here and now and are aimed at the patient's strengths and encourage the patient to continue to make progress on his or her own.

One of the most useful approaches to primary care psychotherapy, the BATHE technique, is described in Stuart and Lieberman's *The Fifteen Minute Hour*. The authors advocate a *BATHE* approach for every patient visit. For example:

- Explore the *Background* of what psychosocial events are going on in the patient's current life after getting an overview of the patient's signs and symptoms and performing whatever physical examination is necessary.
- Note the patient's *Affect* as the background is described.
- Inquire about what is *Troubling* the patient the most; asking "What worries you the most?" may help sharpen this question.
- Ask *How* he or she is handling the problem.
- *Empathize* with the patient with statements such as, "That must have been hard—I can see that you are really suffering."

This technique may be extremely helpful even when nothing else can be done for the patient: it builds trust in the patient-physician relationship and helps the patient feel understood.

Elements of the different forms of psychotherapy that were discussed earlier can be woven into the BATHE approach. The connection between one's emotional life and somatic symptoms can be explored so that the patient becomes aware of these linkages. For example, explaining that divorce frequently leads to depressive feelings and somatic complaints may help individuals understand their experiences. Educating patients that there may be a connection between their anger over a situation and their migraine headaches may help them begin to see the need to make changes in their life situation. Even reminding the patient that there is a choice may be highly therapeutic to an

TABLE 20-3 Specific Psychotherapeutic Techniques
• Reframing
• Clarifying the meaning of the illness
• Projection of the problem
• Role reversal

individual who has gotten so bogged down in a situation that he or she feels hopeless and without options.

Specific techniques that the primary care physician can use to assist a patient during a brief session are listed in Table 20-3. These interventions do not require a complex assessment of the patient's psychodynamic motivations. They are based on a current assessment of the patient's existing emotional state. In many instances they may provide an excellent opportunity for the primary care physician to help the patient cope with difficult situations.

Reframing is a powerful psychotherapeutic technique that the primary care physician can use. Reframing occurs when the primary care physician offers patients another way of viewing their life situations, problems, or themselves. Reframing is so successful because it does not require the problem or situation to change. As Epictetus said centuries ago, "It is not things themselves that bother us, but rather our attitude about those things." Helping an individual to see a situation differently depends, of course, on the primary care physician's understanding of how the patient sees the situation and then being able to provide an alternative view.

Milton Erickson, a well-known psychiatrist and hypnotherapist, used reframing with great success. A patient once came to see Erickson with feelings of depression, doubting his ability to become a success in sales because he had a mild stuttering problem that became worse with anxiety. Erickson suggested to the patient that his stuttering could actually be an asset. Most customers would not find a stuttering salesman to be slick or sleazy and would be more likely to trust him. With this different viewpoint, the patient became less anxious about his stuttering and became highly successful in his sales career.

Reframing is a particularly useful technique for the primary care physician to consider when a patient is having a difficult time adjusting to a medical problem. It may allow a patient to see the situation from a different perspective.

Case Vignette

Mr Brown is a 42-year-old man admitted to the coronary care unit (CCU) with a myocardial infarction. After his physician gives him his diagnosis, Mr Brown becomes anxious and poorly compliant with his medical care. He gets out of his hospital bed and does pushups in his CCU room. The physician speaks with the patient and his family and learns that Mr Brown was very physically active before entering the hospital and prided himself on his strength. It becomes clear that the patient sees the myocardial infarction as a lessening of his power and masculinity. Mr Brown's physician tells him that it takes a strong man to go along with all of what the physicians and nurses were asking of him. In some ways the hospitalization could be a positive opportunity for him to show his real strength. The patient appears to accept this alternative viewpoint and becomes more compliant during the rest of his hospitalization.

Clarifying the meaning of illness is another useful technique the primary care physician can use with medically ill patients. It is critical that the primary care physician gain some understanding of what the illness means to the patient if the primary care physician hopes to treat the patient with a biopsychosocial perspective. The BATHE technique is an excellent way to gain an understanding of the specific meaning an illness has for a patient. In particular, questions like "What troubles you most about the illness?" or "What is the illness interfering with most in your life?" or "Who is it affecting most besides yourself?" are highly useful.

Case Vignette

Mr Allen is a 75-year-old man who underwent a below-the-knee amputation because of peripheral vascular disease. Even though he was having an excellent physical recovery, he is in a depressed state when seen several weeks after discharge from the hospital. Mr Allen's primary care physician presumes that his depression is related to his altered self-image and worries about mobility. When asked what most troubles him about his surgery and whom he thinks it will affect in addition to himself, Mr Allen responds with a much different answer than the physician expects, which clarifies the illness' meaning. Mr Allen states he is very worried about whether he will be able to perform sexually and that his wife will have a hard time coping with this situation. This elucidation of his concerns leads to some joint sessions with Alan's wife to discuss his worries. With her input, Alan's concerns are greatly lessened and his depression lifts.

Another intervention that is useful with a variety of patients is *projection of the problem*. When faced with a difficult situation, some patients become so stuck in feeling guilty or ashamed that it is difficult for them to feel any self-esteem. One way to help such individuals is to ask them to project the problem onto someone else they know and ask how they would feel about the other person feeling or reacting as they are doing. This degree of distance and objectivity often allows the patient to feel more comfortable with their view of him- or herself.

Case Vignette

Mrs Martin is a 40-year-old woman who became severely depressed after her husband was fired from his job, causing major family financial distress. Mrs Martin has responded well to a trial with antidepressants but is critical of herself for needing them and for having gotten depressed in the first place. Her primary care physician asks her what she would think if one of her friends had gone through the stressor, depression, and response to treatment that she had. Mrs Martin responds that she would tell her friend she admires her for showing courage and getting help for her problems. After this psychotherapeutic exploration, she becomes more accepting of her own responses to stress.

Projection of the problem is particularly useful for medical situations in which a patient may feel guilty about an illness. In these instances a specific form of projection of the problem, role reversal, is often very effective.

Case Vignette

Mrs Nance, a 51-year-old woman, underwent a mastectomy for a carcinoma. Several weeks after the surgery she begins to feel depressed. Her primary care physician identifies this depression on a postoperative follow-up visit and asks her what is troubling her most about the surgery. She responds that she is concerned her husband will no longer feel she is an attractive woman and that he might prefer someone else. Her primary care physician inquires if she would feel less love for her husband if he had undergone a similar disfiguring surgery. She responds that of course she would continue to feel love for him and that he is more to her than a perfect body. This perspective helps Mrs Nance gain another attitude about her husband's reactions. The primary care physician also suggests that she talk with her husband about how he actually feels about her surgery. With this encouragement, she does so and feels relieved at his supportive response.

Most of these therapies involve the physician working one-on-one with the patient. At times it may become apparent that the patient's problem is not so much within himself or herself but part of an interpersonal problem within an intimate relationship or within a poorly functioning family system. The patient may benefit simply from having the broader interactional problems pointed out by the physician. At other times psychotherapeutic work between the dyad or with the entire family may be necessary. Although many of the general principles and conceptual frameworks described here may be used with relational units, there are also specialized approaches for working with couples and families.

PSYCHOTHERAPEUTIC APPROACHES TO COMMON PROBLEMS IN PRIMARY CARE SETTINGS

Depression

Some specific psychotherapeutic interventions have been developed for treating depression. Many are derived from Aaron Beck's cognitive theory of depression (Beck et al, 1979). Beck describes a number of cognitive distortions—errors in thinking—that are "depressogenic." One of Beck's followers, David Burns (2001), describes these errors for the lay public in his outstanding book, *Feeling Good*. Some of the most common errors are described below:

- *All-or-nothing thinking.* An individual sees things as black or white, such as performance that is either perfect or a complete failure.
- *Overgeneralization.* The individual sees a single negative event as a never-ending pattern of defeat.
- *Jumping to conclusions.* An individual jumps to a negative conclusion such as forecasting a negative outcome or believing that someone is reacting negatively without collecting definite facts.
- *Catastrophizing.* An individual exaggerates the importance of a mistake or problem.
- *Emotional reasoning.* An individual assumes that his or her negative emotions actually reflect the way things really are without realizing distortion could be taking place.

Burns outlines a number of techniques that can be used to help a patient recognize and change these distortions. Homework, such as keeping track of depressive moods during a week and noting cognitive distortions that occur with the onset of the depression, may be quite useful. If the primary care physician uses the BATHE technique described earlier, it is often apparent what type of cognitive distortion the patient (without realizing it is a distortion) is using. The primary care physician is then in an excellent position to clarify the depressogenic viewpoint that the patient is using and suggest alternatives.

Case Vignette

Mr Mikel is a 63-year-old salesman who is complaining of vague abdominal pain. After medical evaluation fails to reveal any etiology, his primary care physician notes that Mr Mikel has a depressed affect; the primary care physician explores what is going on in Mr Mikel's life and learns that his company was acquired by a larger corporation and that he is anxious about his future there, expecting he will be laid off. The primary care physician suggests that Mr Mikel may be jumping to a conclusion about the situation (negative forecasting) and asks if there are any other possibilities he might envision. Mr Mikel suggests that the corporation might want him to stay with the company because of his excellent performance and experience. In discussing the situation further, the primary care physician learns that Mr Mikel appears to be seeing the situation as a negative one because he feels depressed (emotional reasoning) and tells Mr Mikel that this may be occurring. Mr Mikel responds by giving further information: he qualifies for an exceptional severance package if he decides to leave the corporation and has a solid retirement program in place. During numerous visits that extend over the course of a 2-month period, Mr Mikel's depressive mood clears and he feels more in control of his work situation. He decides to leave his corporation and start a part-time consulting business that will give him and his wife more leisure time to travel. He adapts to this lifestyle extremely well.

Anxiety

Anxiety, in either generalized form or panic attacks, is a common symptom that precipitates a patient's visit to the physician's office. Cognitive psychotherapy can be highly effective in reducing anxiety. Beck and Emery (1985) have extended cognitive theory to the anxiety disorders and suggest that anxiety is often a consequence of negative cognitive distortions. For example, a patient experiencing a panic attack who tells herself that she is going to die is likely to amplify distress. The primary care physician can explain to the patient that she has a heightened sensitivity to bodily sensations and that it only *feels like* she is going to die (emotional reasoning). In other words, the patient can remind herself of this distortion when a panic disorder occurs and, by doing so, lessen the distress she feels.

Beck and Emery have suggested the **AWARE** technique for anxiety disorders:

- **A**ccept the anxiety.
- **W**atch your anxiety level and rate it.
- **A**ct despite your anxiety.
- **R**epeat the steps until the anxiety diminishes.
- **E**xpect the best.

This approach advocates that the patient monitor his or her anxiety levels and look for a correlation between stressors and cognitive distortions. If anxiety does occur, it should not be regarded as catastrophic but rather as an unpleasant feeling that will pass. The primary care physician should encourage the patient to act by confronting the anxiety. For example, if an individual with panic disorder and agoraphobia feels anxious about going out to a shopping mall, he or she should be encouraged to approach and eventually go to the mall for progressively longer periods. It is important to educate the patient that continual confrontation of the anxiety will tend to lessen it, while trying to avoid it may increase it. Primary care physician support and reassurance about confronting their anxiety helps patients who are prone to jumping to negative conclusions about their ability to improve.

Teaching self-control strategies to patients with anxiety disorders can be quite useful. For example, teaching a Jacobson approach with progressive muscular relaxation can help a patient who is feeling acute anxiety to gain control. Similarly, teaching a patient controlled diaphragmatic breathing can help reduce hyperventilation in panic attacks.

Adapting to Chronic Disease

The primary care physician plays a central role in helping patients cope with chronic disease. Providing empathic support can lessen the suffering that patients experience. Educating patients about their disease and reducing unwarranted concerns is extremely useful. By becoming a partner in managing a chronic disease, the physician may help decrease the patient's sense of isolation in facing the disease. In some instances the primary care physician and patient may find it difficult to deal with chronic disease because they both use an acute illness model to conceptualize it. For example, the primary care physician may try to cure a patient of a chronic pain syndrome rather than care for the patient over the longer term. When this occurs, the physician's high level of expectation is typically not met and the primary care physician may end up feeling frustrated, resentful of the patient, or doubtful of his or her own skills and competence. To be successful, the primary care physician must diminish his or her expectations to what is realistically achievable. The following equation is often helpful in understanding how primary care physician expectations are central to primary care physician self-esteem:

$$\text{Self-esteem} = \text{Realistic achievement} - \text{Expectation}$$

In theory, there is a broad range of what can be achieved; however, in practice, there is a fairly narrow range of what physicians can realistically accomplish for most patients. What is more easily modified is the expectation that the primary care physician brings to his or her work. When it is excessive, the primary care physician will not feel a sense of accomplishment no matter what is achieved. When it is reduced to reasonable levels, the primary care physician can feel satisfied even when the outcome is not perfect. Helping patients to identify and modify their unrealistic expectations can also be extremely helpful.

Case Vignette

Dr Wagner, who has recently completed her residency, is feeling frustrated by the lack of progress she is making with her large caseload of patients with many chronic illnesses. She has come to work at a public clinic after her residency and sees primarily indigent patients who appear to make little progress despite her vigorous efforts. She discusses her feelings with a more senior primary care physician, who comments that perhaps she might try realigning her expectations. Instead of expecting her patients to dramatically improve, she might consider that she is providing a real service by helping the more disadvantaged patients maintain themselves without deteriorating. Viewed from this perspective, Dr Wagner feels more satisfied with her clinic work.

Patients also may have difficulty understanding their own role in chronic illness. In acute illness, the patient commonly plays a fairly passive role. The acute disease process usually requires a biological intervention, and it is appropriate for the patient to delegate control for the treatment of the illness to the primary care physician. In chronic disease, however, the patient who continues to delegate primary responsibility to the primary care physician is at risk. To successfully cope with the disease, the patient must accept significant responsibility for dealing with it. From the patient's perspective, he or she must relinquish the idea that the primary care physician will provide a cure and realize he or she must be responsible for his or her care to be successful. This reconceptualization of roles occurs in successful management programs such as many pain control programs in which the patient is taught to assume more responsibility for self-care.

PHYSICIANS' EMOTIONAL REACTIONS TO PATIENTS

One of the best tools that a primary care physician can use to psychotherapeutically care for his or her patients is the set of feelings that the patients stimulate in the primary care physician. These are sometimes referred to as counter-transferences (see Chapter 15). A variety of reactions are often produced in primary care physicians: anger, frustration, tenderness, warmth, sexual excitement, jealousy, irritation, sadness, sympathy, depression. Inexperienced primary care physicians may not recognize or may try to suppress such feelings, rationalizing they are "unprofessional." More experienced primary care physicians know it is important to pay attention and perhaps even discuss their feelings with a colleague. By being aware of such feelings, the primary care physician can use them to help the patient. For example, the feelings that are present in the primary care physician often reflect feelings the patient is also experiencing.

Case Vignette

Dr Fitzgerald begins to feel rather frustrated and helpless in making suggestions for possible medical interventions to deal with Mr Dale's ulcer disease. Although his primary care physician regards the condition as eminently treatable, Mr Dale rejects any suggested treatment, saying he had already tried something similar. Dr Fitzgerald recalls that Mr Dale lost his wife 1 year earlier, yet she found that she had little sympathy for him. In fact she felt eager to end the appointment. Recognizing this reaction (feeling frustrated, helpless, and irritable) as a possible sign that Mr Dale might be depressed, she screens for and is able to make the diagnosis of major depression and begins treatment. Dr Fitzgerald establishes that this episode of major depression is Mr Dale's only occurrence of a psychiatric disorder and is related to his pathological grief reaction.

When the primary care physician begins to feel irritable, frustrated, depressed, and rejected, it may be a valuable clue that the patient suffers from depression. Rather than acting immediately on his or her feelings—and limiting his contact with the patient—the primary care physician in the example above used her feelings in the process and helped establish an accurate diagnosis that would have been easy to miss. Similarly, other feelings in the primary care physician can help identify other problems in patients. For example, when the patient stimulates anger in the primary care physician, there is a high likelihood that the patient is angry about something. When the primary care physician feels confused in obtaining a clear history, it is possible that the patient has cognitive dysfunction. Even when the physician's reaction to a patient is not negative, he or she may use the information therapeutically, as the following example suggests.

Case Vignette

Ms Gwenn is a 30-year-old teacher who relishes telling her physician, Dr Blair, the details about some of her sexual affairs when she comes in to complain of her various somatic complaints. On occasion, Dr Blair becomes sexually interested in her. By discussing her case with a colleague, Dr Blair realizes that there is a pattern in her behavior. Whenever Ms Gwenn has been rejected in a relationship, she comes in with a somatic complaint and sexually stimulating story. She appears to use the stories as a way of capturing his attention. With this understanding, Dr Blair is able to tell her that he will see her on a regular, time-contingent basis to follow her medical problems, whether or not her symptoms improved. With this reassurance, Ms Gwenn markedly decreases her sexually seductive behavior. She eventually accepts a referral for psychotherapy to learn more of why her relationships keep failing.

LIMITATIONS OF PSYCHOTHERAPEUTIC AND BEHAVIORAL INTERVENTIONS

Psychotherapeutic and behavioral interventions clearly have their limitations. For example, when a patient manifests persistent vegetative symptoms of depression such as sleep disturbance, appetite change, or anergia, most clinicians consider treatment with pharmacotherapy. It would take a highly skilled primary care physician to treat major depression with psychotherapy alone. As noted earlier, there is evidence that antidepressants and psychotherapy may be most effective together. This type of synergy is seen in a variety of conditions. Obsessive-compulsive disorder is an example of where serotoninergic medications can be combined with behavioral techniques to great advantage.

Psychotherapy provided by a primary care physician may be limited by the population being treated. For example, individuals with significant personality disorders may be quite refractory to psychotherapeutic efforts. These patients often may see problems as external to themselves and feel little motivation to change their contribution to the situation. In other cases, these individuals obtain gratification from defeating the psychotherapeutic efforts and do not realize that it is a Pyrrhic victory. When treating individuals with personality disorders, the primary care physician should keep the goal of small gains in mind. Indeed, the most common limitation in treating patients psychotherapeutically is likely to involve the patients' readiness for change. If patients have not reached the point where they want to make a change, it is extremely difficult for the psychotherapist to impose change externally.

Perhaps the most important limitation to psychotherapeutic efforts occurs when safety issues are prominent. For example, highly suicidal or homicidal patients require hospitalization until their impulses are under control. It is hard to proceed with psychotherapy when lives are at stake.

Similarly, it is hard for the primary care physician to implement psychotherapy when he or she feels uncomfortable with the patient. Some patients may activate such strong feelings in the primary care physician, such as anger or resentment, that it is difficult for the primary care physician to remain in a psychotherapeutic stance. Either referral to or consultation with a psychiatrist is then indicated.

SUMMARY

Primary care physicians have many tools to use when treating psychiatric problems that occur in everyday practice. Although medications have much to offer, psychotherapeutic and behavioral interventions by the primary care physician may also be highly effective. This chapter has provided a brief overview of some psychotherapeutic techniques the primary care physician can readily employ. Behavioral strategies may also be useful for managing some common problems in practice. With experience, the application of these techniques and strategies may be a source of considerable satisfaction for the primary care physician.

ADDITIONAL READINGS

Barsky AJ. Hidden reasons some patients visit doctors. *Ann Int Med.* 1981;94(part 1):492-498.

Barsky AJ, Wyshak G, Latham KS, et al. Hypochondriacal patients, their PCPs, and their medical care. *J Gen Intl Med.* 1991;6:413.

Beck AT, Emery G. *Anxiety Disorders and Phobias: A Cognitive Perspective.* New York, NY: Basic Books; 1985.

Beck AT, Rush AJ, Shaw BF, et al. *Cognitive Therapy of Depression.* New York, NY: Guilford Press; 1979.

Burns DD. *Feeling Good.* 2nd ed. New York, NY: Avon Books; 2001.

Cole S, Bird J. *The Medical Interview: The Three Function Approach.* St Louis, Mo: Mosby Year Book; 2000.

Eisendrath SJ. Brief psychotherapy in medical practice—keys to success. *Western J Med.* 1993; 158:376-378.

Elkin I, Gibbons RD, Shea MT, et al. Initial severity and differential treatment outcome in the National Institute of Mental Health Treatment of Depression Collaborative Research Program. *J Consult Clin Psychol.* 1995;63(5):841-847.

Engel GL. The clinical application of the biopsychosocial model. *Am J Psychiatry.* 1980;137:535-540.

Feldman MD, Christensen JF. *Behavioral Medicine in Primary Care: A Practical Guide.* New York, NY: McGraw-Hill; 1997.

Jarrett RB, Rush AJ. Short-term psychotherapy of depressive disorders: current status and future directions. *Psychiatry.* 1994;57(2):115-132.

Lazare A. The interview as a clinical negotiation. In: Lazare A, Putnam S, Lipkin Jr M, eds. *The Medical Interview: Clinical Care, Education, and Research.* New York, NY: Springer-Verlag; 1995:50-62.

Lazare A, Putnam S, Lipkin Jr M. Three functions of the medical interview. In: Lazare A, Putnam S, Lipkin Jr M, eds. *The Medical Interview: Clinical Care, Education, and Research.* New York, NY: Springer-Verlag; 1995:3-19.

Lewinsohn PM, Munoz RF, Youngren MA, et al. *Control Your Depression.* New York, NY: Fireside Publishers; 1986:73-107.

Matthews DA, Suchman AL, Branch WT. Making "connexions": enhancing the therapeutic potential of patient-clinician relationships. *Ann Int Med.* 1993;118:973-977.

McMullin RE. *The New Handbook of Cognitive Therapy Techniques.* New York, NY: WW Norton & Co, Inc; 2000.

Smith Jr GR, Rost K, Kashner TM. A trial of the effect of a standardized psychiatric consultation on health outcomes and costs in somatizing patients. *Arch Gen Psychiatry.* 1995;52(3):238-243.

Stuart MR, Lieberman JA. *The Fifteen Minute Hour: Applied Psychotherapy For The Primary Care Physician.* 2nd ed. Westport, Conn: Praeger Publishers; 1993.

White CA. *Cognitive Behaviour Therapy for Chronic Medical Problems: A Guide to Assessment and Treatment in Practice.* Chichester, NY: John Wiley & Sons; 2001.

Chapter 21

Restructuring Primary Care Practices to Improve Recognition and Management of Mental Disorders

David S. Brody, MD

Recognizing and managing mental health disorders in primary care is a challenging task. It requires time to do the following:

- Identify patients who might have a mental health problem.
- Fully evaluate patients identified.
- Educate and motivate mentally ill patients to accept a mental health diagnosis and adhere to treatment recommendations.
- Provide long-term monitoring of adherence and outcomes.

It also requires knowledge of specific diagnostic criteria and management guidelines. It is not surprising therefore that the recognition, management, and outcomes of mental health disorders in the primary care setting have been shown to be far from optimal. For example, the literature indicates that the underdiagnosis of depression, inadequate dosage and duration of treatment with antidepressant medications, infrequent follow-up, lack of adjustment of therapy according to patient response, and poor patient adherence to antidepressant medications and referrals contribute to less favorable outcomes than are possible. Recently, concern has been expressed that primary care physicians are prescribing selective serotonin reuptake inhibitors (SSRIs) to patients who either do not need them or who are likely to benefit more from other forms of treatment.

A number of barriers contribute to these difficulties. Patients usually present with somatic symptoms rather than mood or emotional symptoms. They may be reluctant to accept a mental health diagnosis because of their concerns about the meaning of the diagnosis (eg, "I must be crazy"), its cause (eg, "I'm weak or a failure"), its treatment (eg, "It will be embarrassing or ineffective"), or its impact (eg, "I will lose my job"). Physicians may lack the time and training necessary to adequately address these problems. Also, they may believe that such problems are outside their scope of responsibility or that the patients are not likely to improve, even if they put time and effort into managing them. The health care system may also create barriers if there is difficulty accessing and communicating with mental health specialists.

Some exceptionally well-trained and committed physicians may be able to overcome these barriers on their own. Most physicians, however, need selected tools and organizational changes in their practice in order to overcome these barriers. Tools can help physicians save time by expediting the collection of information from patients for the purposes of screening, diagnosis, further assessment, and outcomes monitoring. Tools can also help to expedite the provision of information to patients about their mental health problem and its management. Tools such as management guidelines, algorithms, and information tables that profile commonly used psychotropic medications can increase physicians' knowledge of mental health disorders and promote greater adherence to standards. Tools can also be used to decrease patients' resistance to accepting a mental health diagnosis and treatment by educating patients about their mental health problem and its management and enabling them to play a more active role in their care. Tools have also been used to increase recognition of mental health disorders, improve documentation, and help organize care so that nothing is missed or forgotten.

Redefining the functions of the office support staff, such as nurses and secretaries, may be necessary to ensure that there is consistent availability and use of these tools. The staff may also perform important functions, such as patient education and follow-up of outcomes and treatment adherence, tasks that don't necessarily need to be done by a physician. Other organizational changes can be made to increase the availability of input from mental health specialists.

This chapter includes a discussion of the use of tools and organizational changes to facilitate the recognition and management of mental disorders in primary care. This discussion focuses on depression because the role of tools and organizational changes has been most thoroughly evaluated for this problem.

TOOLS FOR THE PRIMARY CARE PHYSICIAN

Tools for the primary care physician are available as individual entities, as well as part of a comprehensive and coordinated series of tools or a tool kit. Two tool kits for treating depression in primary care have been developed. The MacArthur Initiative Depression Tool Kit can be accessed at www.depression-primarycare.org. The Depression in Primary Care Tool Kit can be obtained through the *International Journal of Psychiatry in Medicine* at http://psychiatry.mc.duke.edu/ijpm/index.html. After connecting to this Web site, click "Abstracts and Editorials," then "Volume 30, Number 2," then click "The Depression in Primary Care Tool Kit." Both tool kits can be easily downloaded for use in a primary care practice. Tools have been developed for the following four categories: (1) assessment, (2) patient education, (3) management guides, and (4) outcomes monitoring. Although a vast array of tools are available, physicians should feel free to select only those tools that will be most helpful.

Assessment Tools

Numerous tools have been developed for depression screening, none of which is clearly superior to the others for screening purposes (see Table 21-1, which lists the Web sites for some of these instruments). Most of these instruments serve primarily as screening measures rather than diagnostic measures. Higher scores on these questionnaires increase the likelihood of a depressive diagnosis. However, additional questions that are not in the instrument must be asked of patients with high scores in order to ascertain the presence or absence of a *Diagnostic and Statistical Manual of Mental Disorders,* fourth edition (DSM-IV), diagnosis, such as major depression or dysthymia.

The use of screening instruments in primary care has been shown to increase the recognition of depression by a factor of 2 to 3, but it has not been consistently shown to improve treatment or outcomes when used as the sole intervention. Only a few instruments designed for use in primary care serve as both screening and diagnostic measures, of which PRIME-MD® has been the best validated and most widely used. PRIME-MD®, developed for Pfizer Pharmaceuticals in New York, was originally designed as a clinician-administered instrument. PRIME-MD® is now available in an entirely self-administered version called the Patient Health Questionnaire (PHQ-9), which has been recently validated in 3000 primary care patients and has comparable operating characteristics as the original PRIME-MD®.

TABLE 21-1 Web Sites for Screening Instruments

- Beck Depression Inventory (BDI): www.uea.ac.uk/~wp316depression.pdf

- Center for Epidemiologic Studies Depression (CES-D):
  http://chipts.ucla.edu/Assessment_Instruments/asmt_dp2html

- Duke Anxiety-Depression Scale (DADS): http://healthmeasures.mc.duke.edu/

- Geriatric Depression Scale (GDS)—Long Version:
  www.stanford.edu/~yesavage/GDS.english.long.html

- GDS-short version: www.stanford.edu/~yesavage/GDS.english.short.score.html

- Primary Care Evaluation of Mental Disorders (PRIME-MD®)*: pdf file available from
  Robert Spitzer, MD, e-mail address: RLS@columbia.edu

- PRIME-MD® Patient Health Questionnaire (PHQ-9):
  www.cmecenter.com/primedmtoday/

- The Zung Self-Rating Depression Scale (SDS):
  www.wellbutrin-sr.com/hcp/depression/zung.html

*This is largely a physician-administered instrument. The other instruments listed in this table are self-administered.

PRIME-MD® contains a two-item screening tool and a nine-item diagnostic instrument. The screening tools ask whether or not the patient has often been bothered by depressed mood or anhedonia during the past month. The two-question screen is:

During the *past month* have you *often* been bothered by:

1. Little interest or pleasure in doing things ☐ Yes ☐ No
2. Feeling down, depressed, or hopeless ☐ Yes ☐ No

This two-item screening instrument has been found to be as good as longer screening questionnaires. It can identify 96% of patients with major depression; however, like other screening instruments, more than half of the patients who screen positive will not have this disorder.

Patients who respond positively to either or both of these questions are instructed to complete the nine-item diagnostic evaluation instrument, the PHQ-9 (see Appendixes 1 and 2 in Chapter 3). The criteria for diagnosing a major depressive disorder or other depressive disorder are listed at the bottom of the questionnaire. This nine-item instrument also measures severity of depression symptoms. Response scores for each DSM-IV symptom of depression range from 0 for "not at all" to 3 for "nearly every day." A total score is calculated by adding the scores for each of the nine symptoms. Higher scores indicate greater depression symptom severity.

Screening tests are available for other mental health problems commonly seen in primary care, including bipolar disorder, panic disorder, social phobia, substance abuse, and domestic violence (see Additional Readings for references).

The PRIME-MD® screening and diagnostic questionnaire can be administered to all patients or only those whom you have some reason to suspect might be depressed. Valenstein et al (2001) found that the most effective screening strategy for this type of questionnaire in a busy primary care practice was to give nurses the responsibility for distributing, collecting, and placing completed questionnaires in the chart. This strategy resulted in both increased recognition and treatment of depression.

After diagnosing a mood disorder, additional information should be collected to aid in developing a management plan. This information includes an assessment of suicide risk, past history and treatment of mental health problems, psychiatric comorbidity, and recent losses and other sources of stress. Tools, available on the Web sites noted earlier, can be used to collect virtually all of this data through self-administered questionnaires. For physicians who are interested in providing counseling, the Depression in Primary Care Tool Kit contains a self-administered education and counseling needs assessment. Depressed primary care patients most frequently request education and counseling as part of their treatment. This questionnaire assesses patients' attitudes about depression and identifies barriers to patient acceptance of a diagnosis of depression and adherence to treatment recommendations. It also identifies maladaptive beliefs or cognitions that may be contributing to their emotional distress.

Patient Education Tools

A key component of depression management is helping patients accept a diagnosis and activating them to seek help, adhere to management recommendations, and practice lifestyle changes that can promote recovery. This process can be time-consuming and sometimes adversarial. Patient education materials have been developed to save physicians time in this process and to reinforce and supplement the issues they have discussed with their patients. A variety of patient education materials are available on the MacArthur Foundation Web site noted earlier, as well as on a number of other Web sites (see Table 21-2). These materials can be used to educate patients about what depression is and how it is treated, as well as to provide more specific information on antidepressant medications and various types of psychotherapies.

In addition, self-help manuals and books can help patients learn strategies to reduce and/or prevent emotional distress. Cognitively and behaviorally oriented self-help books have been shown to significantly improve symptoms of depression for up to 2 years. Some of the more popular self-help books are listed in Table 21-3.

TABLE 21-2 Selected Web Sites for Patient Education Materials

- Aetna Intelihealth: www.intelihealth.com/depression

- Agency for Healthcare Research and Quality: http://text.nlm.nih.gov (select "AHCPR Supported Guidelines" and then "Depression in Primary Care")

- American Medical Association: www.ama.assn.org/consumer/specond.htm

- Depression Awareness Recognition and Treatment Program of the National Institute of Mental Health: www.nimh.nih.gov/publicat/index.cfm

- National Alliance for the Mentally Ill: www.nami.org/

- National Depression and Manic-Depressive Association: www.ndmda.org

- National Foundation for Depressive Illness: www.depression.org

- National Mental Health Association: www.nmha.org.ccd

- Psychology Information Online: www.psychologyinfo.com/depression

Treatment Guides

It is often difficult to keep up with the literature; to remember when to start antidepressant medications; to determine whether the dose needs to be increased, the medication changed, or a second medication added; and to determine how long to continue a medication after symptoms have resolved. The Agency for Health Care Policy and Research

---

TABLE 21-3 Self-Help Materials

Depression Books

Burns DD. *The Feeling Good Handbook.* New York, NY: Penguin Books; 1989.

> This book is based on cognitive therapy. It contains chapters on depression, anxiety, fears, and phobias, as well as a chapter on medications. It contains homework assignments and work.

DePaulo Jr RJ, Horvitz LA, Jamison KR. *Understanding Depression: What We Know and What We Can Do About It.* New York, NY: John Wiley & Sons; 2002.

> This is one of the best books available for patients and families.

Emery G. *Getting Un-Depressed.* New York, NY: Simon & Schuster, Inc; 1981.

> This book focuses on common concerns and issues faced by women who are depressed. Self-management recommendations are based on cognitive therapy.

Fassler DG, Dumas LS. *"Help Me, I'm Sad:" Recognizing, Treating, and Preventing Childhood and Adolescent Depression.* New York, NY: Penquin Books; 1998.

> This book explains what depression is and how it is treated in a way that is helpful for older children, adolescents, and their parents. It is informational rather than self-help.

Gold MS. *The Good News About Depression.* New York, NY: Villard Books; 1986.

> This book is not really a self-management guide. Rather, it describes what depression is, who treats it, and how it should be managed. There is an emphasis on the biological aspect of the disorder and its treatment.

Lewinsohn PM, Munoz RF, Youngren MA, Zeiss AM. *Control Your Depression.* New York, NY: Prentice Hall Press; 1978.

> This book is based on social learning theory. It provides instruction on self-control strategies, relaxation techniques, social skills training, and modification of maladaptive beliefs. It includes homework assignments and worksheets.

Styron W. *Darkness Visible.* New York, NY: Vintage Books/Random House; 1992.

> This book, by the Pulitzer Prize–winning author of *Sophie's Choice,* describes his personal experiences in having a major depressive disorder, his treatment failures, and then a successful treatment. Any individual who is having or has had a depressive disorder will be able to identify with aspects of this beautifully written and emotionally moving account.

Solomon A. *The Noonday Demon: An Atlas of Depression.* New York, NY: Simon & Schuster; 2001.

> This book examines depression in personal, cultural, and scientific terms. The author describes the vast range of available medications and the efficacy of alternative treatments.

TABLE 21-3 (continued)

Stress Management Books

Davis M, Eshelman ER, McKay M. *The Relaxation and Stress Reduction Workbook.* 3rd rev ed. Richmond, Calif: New Harbinger Publications; 1988.

> This is a very basic instructional manual. It covers topics such as relaxation techniques and time management.

McKay M, Davis M, Fanning P. *Thoughts & Feelings: The Art of Cognitive Stress Intervention.* Richmond, Calif: New Harbinger Publications; 1981.

> This workbook is based on the principles of cognitive therapy. It presents chapters on topics such as problem-solving, systematic desensitization, and values clarification. Homework assignments and worksheets are included.

Depression Pamphlets

Depression: What You Need to Know [pamphlet]. Distributed by the National Institute of Mental Health. Ordering information: D/ART/Public Inquiries, National Institute of Mental Health, Room 15–C-05, 5600 Fishers Lane, Rockville, MD, 20857.

> This pamphlet reviews the diagnosis, causes, and treatment of depression. It contains a brief discussion of the types of activities that patients as well as their families and friends can do to reduce depressive symptoms.

has developed guidelines for managing major depression in primary care. These guidelines have been updated and are summarized in the MacArthur Initiative Depression Tool Kit. More detailed algorithms on managing depression are provided in Chapter 8. Both tool kits contain tables on the use of antidepressants. The tables include information on dosing side effects and mechanisms of action, as well as counseling guidelines. These tools can be placed in the charts of patients who are being treated for depression.

Outcomes Monitoring Tools

An important component of depression management is regular systematic assessment of outcomes. Simply asking patients if they feel better or less sad may miss significant improvement in areas such as sleep, appetite, or, most important, functioning. At the other extreme, it is important to accurately determine that the depression has fully resolved and not merely improved. The PHQ-9 can be used to monitor changes in depression symptoms. Functional status questionnaires, such as the SF-36 or SF-20, can be used to assess changes in various domains of functioning. See www.rand.org/health/surveys for copies of these instruments. Flowcharts are included in both tool kits to facilitate charting and review of this information.

IMPLEMENTING OFFICE-BASED SYSTEMS TO FACILITATE CARE

The effectiveness of the tools you use will depend on the organizational strategies that are developed for their implementation. Questions to be addressed include some or all of the following: Where will the tools be stored? For which patients will they be used? Who will be responsible for their implementation? How will they get to the chart or the physician? The selected tools must be easily accessible. To the extent possible, responsibility for

TABLE 21-4 Depression Disease Management Responsibilities That May Be Delegated to Office Staff

- Distributing and collecting assessment questionnaires
- Placing guidelines and other relevant materials in the medical chart
- Providing and reviewing patient education materials
- Providing basic education about depression and its treatment
- Helping patients schedule appointments with mental health specialists
- Monitoring outcomes and patient adherence to medications and referrals by phone or at follow-up visits, using structured questionnaires
- Providing general support and encouragement

their implementation should be delegated to the office staff. Responsibilities that may be delegated are listed in Table 21-4.

Research to date indicates that simply using a screening questionnaire to identify patients who may be depressed does little to improve the treatment or outcomes of depression. However, use of a depression-screening questionnaire can lead to improved outcomes if other systems are also in place to improve patient care, monitor outcomes and patient adherence, and educate patients about depression and its management. For this reason, the US Preventive Task Force recommends screening adults for depression only in practices where there are systems in place to ensure accurate diagnosis and effective treatment and follow-up.

Relatively simple, low-cost system changes can make a big difference. For example, having a nurse periodically contact by phone patients being treated for depression to systematically evaluate outcomes and adherence has been repeatedly shown to improve outcomes. Calling patients several weeks after a referral to a mental health specialist is likely to decrease the nonadherence rate for these referrals by 50%. Providing feedback to physicians in the office on their rates of recognition of depression and outcomes of treatment, compared to benchmarks, can improve quality of care and outcomes. Having a nurse review selected patient education materials on depression with the patient can improve patient satisfaction.

Increasing access to input from mental health specialists may also improve care. This increased access can be accomplished by developing relationships with psychiatrists who are willing to see your patients for one or two visits, establish a diagnosis, develop a treatment plan, and then educate you and your patient about how to implement that plan. Patients are likely to accept a mental health referral if you are able to refer them to a specific mental health specialist and if the patient understands that the purpose of that referral is to help you provide the best possible care.

Integration of mental health specialists into primary care settings can improve communication, reduce patient resistance to seeing these specialists, and enhance continuity of care. Over time, this integration has the potential to improve primary care physicians' skills in detecting and managing depression. A program in Hamilton, Ontario, brings psychiatrists and therapists into the offices of 88 family physicians in 36 practices. These mental health specialists work in the primary care practices at specified intervals, which may vary from several times per week to once every 3 weeks, depending on the size of the practice and the number of referrals generated. Investigators found that the primary care physicians, therapists, and psychiatrists all expressed great satisfaction with this shared mental health care program, which is based in primary care. The primary care physicians indicated that the program increased their skills, helped them feel more comfortable handling mental health problems, and led to greater satisfaction with the mental health care provided to their patients. Identified problems included finding space for the mental health specialist to see patients in the primary care office and scheduling difficulties.

THE FUTURE—AUTOMATED MENTAL HEALTH DISEASE MANAGEMENT SYSTEMS

Many key components of an effective depression disease management program can be automated. Through the use of interactive voice response systems, the Internet, or personal digital assistants, primary care physicians can collect assessment data from their patients, receive reports that contain severity and diagnostic information and treatment recommendations, and monitor their patients' progress and medication adherence at specified intervals. This type of information should reduce both the overuse and underuse of psychotropic medications and may even enable primary care physicians or their staff to provide brief structured psychological treatments efficiently and effectively. Further, these systems can enable patients who suspect that they might be depressed to assess themselves and monitor their progress. They can inform patients about their diagnosis and its management; address common concerns about the meaning, cause, and treatment of depression; encourage them to follow recommended treatments; and educate them about what else they can do to expedite their recovery. These systems can also identify patients who are not improving as expected and determine whether this is due to adherence problems or inadequate treatment. Appropriate additional interventions, such as telephone care management or psychiatric consultation, can then be provided. Finally, these systems can provide a variety of performance reports to both providers and health care plans. Information from these reports can be used to continuously improve treatment and outcomes and to appropriately compensate primary care physicians who provide high-quality care for depression.

These types of systems have been developed but have not been formally evaluated. Information about one such system can be obtained from the following Web site: www.oqsystems.com. It is hoped that these systems will improve the outcomes of depression in the primary care setting; reduce unnecessary costs, such as those related to the overprescription of SSRIs; and be embraced by primary care physicians, patients, behavioral health care systems, and health care plans.

SUMMARY

There are many barriers to effectively managing psychiatric disorders in primary care settings. However, a variety of readily available tools that are not part of the usual medical practice setting can be used to overcome these barriers with only modest effort and expense. These tools can help increase both patient and physician satisfaction by improving the care provided and also improving patient outcomes. These tools include physician and patient education and outcome tracking and monitoring tools. Systems-based approaches can also be implemented in certain practice settings. Disease management approaches to specific disorders such as depression are being developed similar to approaches used for other chronic illnesses.

ADDITIONAL READINGS

Brody DS, Dietrich AJ, DeGruy F, Kroenke, K. The Depression in Primary Care Tool Kit. *Int J Psychiatry Med.* 2000;30:1-12.

Gray GV, Brody DS. Automating psychiatric tasks: taking quality to the next level. *Dis Manage Managed Care Interface.* October 2001:65-69.

Hirschfield RM, Williams JB, Spitzer RL, et al. Development and validation of a screening instrument for bipolar spectrum disorder: the Mood Disorder Questionnaire. *Am J Psychiatry.* 2000;157(11):1873-1875.

Hunkeler EM, Meresman JF, Hargreaves WA, Fireman B, et al. Efficacy of nurse telehealth care and peer support in augmenting treatment of depression in primary care. *Arch Fam Med.* 2000;16:143-149.

Katon W, Robinson P, Von Korff M, et al. A multifaceted intervention to improve treatment of depression in primary care. *Arch Gen Psychiatry.* 1996;53:924-932.

Katon W, Von Korff M, Lin E, et al. Collaborative management to achieve treatment guidelines, Impact on depression in primary care. *JAMA.* 1995;273:1026-1031.

Katzelnick DJ, Simon GE, Pearson SD, et al. Randomized trial of a depression management program in high utilizers of medical care. *Arch Fam Med.* 2000;9:345-351.

Kroenke K, Spitzer RL, Williams JB. The PHQ-9: validity of a brief depression severity measure. *J Gen Intern Med.* 2001;16:606-613.

McFarlane J, Parker B, Socken K, et al. Assessing for abuse during pregnancy. Severity and frequency of injuries associated entry into prenatal care. *JAMA.* 1992;267:3176-3178.

Physician Consortium for Performance Improvement. *Clinical Performance Measures: Major Depressive Disorder: Tools Developed by Physicians for Physicians* [pamphlet]. Chicago, Ill: American Medical Association; 2003.

Pignone MP, Gaynes BN, Rushton JL, et al. Screening for depression in adults: a summary of the evidence for the U.S. preventive services task force. *Ann Intern Med.* 2002;136:765-776.

Rost K, Nutting P, Smith J, et al. Improving depression outcomes in community primary care practice: a randomized trial of the Quest intervention. *J Gen Intern Med.* 2001;16:143-149.

Simon GE, Von Korff M, Rutter C, et al. Randomized trial of monitoring, feedback, and management of care by telephone to improve treatment of depression in primary care. *Br Med J.* 2000;320:550-554.

Spitzer RL, Kroenke K, Williams JBW, et al. Validation and utility of a self-report version of PRIME-MD, the PHQ primary care study. *JAMA.* 1999;282:1737-1744.

Stein MB, McQuaid JR, Laffaye C, et al. Social phobia in the primary care medical setting. *J Fam Pract.* 1999;49:514-519.

Stein MB, Roy-Byrne PP, McQuaid JR. Development of a brief diagnostic screen for panic disorder in primary care. *Psychosom Med.* 1999;61(3):359-364.

Valenstein M, Vijan S, Zeber J, et al. The cost-utility of screening for depression in primary care. *Arch Intern Med.* 2001;134(5):345-360.

Weaver MF, Jarvis MAE, Schnoll SH. Role of the primary care physician in problems of substance abuse. *Arch Intern Med.* 1999;159:913-924.

Wells K, Sherbourne C, Schoenbaum M. Impact of disseminating quality improvement programs in managed primary care: a randomized controlled trial. *JAMA*. 2000;283:212-220.

Whooley M, Avins A, Miranda J, Browner W. Case-finding instruments for depression: two questions are as good as many. *J Gen Intern Med*. 1997;12:439-445.

Williams JW, Hitchcock NP, Cordes JA, et al. Is this patient clinically depressed? *JAMA*. 2002;287:1160-1170.

INDEX

C

Organophosphates, anxiety-producing
    substances, 158
Orgasm, 260–262
OSAS, see Obstructive sleep apnea syndrome
Osteoporosis, caused by psychotropics, 302
Outcomes monitoring, 451
Ovarian disease, polycystic, caused by
    psychotropics, 302
Overgeneralization (cognitive error), 14, 438
Oxazepam, see also Benzodiazepines;
    profile of anxiolytics, [table], 404
OXC, see Oxcarbazepine
Oxcarbazepine, see also Mood stabilizers;
    profile of mood stabilizers, 411–412, [table],
        409–410

P

P450 enzymes, 391
Pacing, delirium symptoms, 199
Pain
    abdominal, in irritable bowel syndrome, 293
    behavior, 331
    chronic, 329
    clinics, 331
    hypnotherapy for, 423
    management, opioid addiction, 118–119
    medical conditions and, 329
    neuropathic, antidepressant treatment for, 389
    psychogenic, 329
Pain disorder, 329–331
    "disorder of the Ds" (disability, drugs,
        depression, doctor-shopping,
        dependency), 329, 330
    management, 330
    posttraumatic stress disorders and, 334
    somatization disorder, 148–149, 323, 324
    somatoform, 329
    treatment-resistant, antipsychotics for, 417
Paint, anxiety-producing substances, 158
Pandora's box, 33, 34
Panic attacks
    chest pain and, 285
    hyperventilation, 440
    psychiatric emergencies, 64, [table], 65
Panic disorder, 160–163
    cognitive-behavioral therapy, 434
    criteria, [table], 162
    interpersonal presentations (difficult patient
        situations), 344
    psychotherapeutic approaches in primary
        care, 440
Paranoia
    drug-induced, 184

hostile, angry patients, 350
    interpersonal presentations (difficult patient
        situations), 344
Paranoid delusions, 180
Paranoid personality disorder, 186–187,
    [table], 186
Paraphilias, 263–264
    antidepressant treatment for, 389
Parasitosis (delusion), 315, 328
Parasomnias, 228, 239
    management, 243
Parental figures, unhappiness and, 5
Parents
    bonding with child, 22
    child's romantic, erotic feelings and jealousy,
        5, 24–25
    power struggles with children, 23, 24
    preparation for child's birth, 21–22
    schoolchildren's peers and, 27
    traits, and child temperament, 21
    values, superego and, 4, 5
Paresthesias, antidepressant side-effect
    management, 397
Parkinson disease, 312
    antiparkinsonian agents, 416–418,
        [table], 417
    dementia, 215
    depression and, 138
    sleep disorders and, 242
    subcortical dementias, 207
Paroxetine hydrochloride, see also Selective
    serotonin reuptake inhibitors;
    cancer patients, 310
    depression treatment, 143–144
    dose and plasma level data, 387
    half-lives and active metabolites, 395
    panic disorder treatment, 162
    side-effect profile, 388
    2D6 isoenzyme inhibition, 391
Parsons, Talcott, 340
Passivity, oral stage of development and, 5
Patient confidentiality, see Confidentiality
Patient education
    depression, 140–141
    self-help materials, [table] 450–451
    tools, Web sites, 449
Patient health questionnaire (PHQ–9), 42,
    51–54, 136–137, 447–448
    outcomes monitoring, 451
    Web site, 448
Patient history, see History-taking
Patient interview, see Interview, medical
Patient privacy, see Privacy
Patient restraints, 61